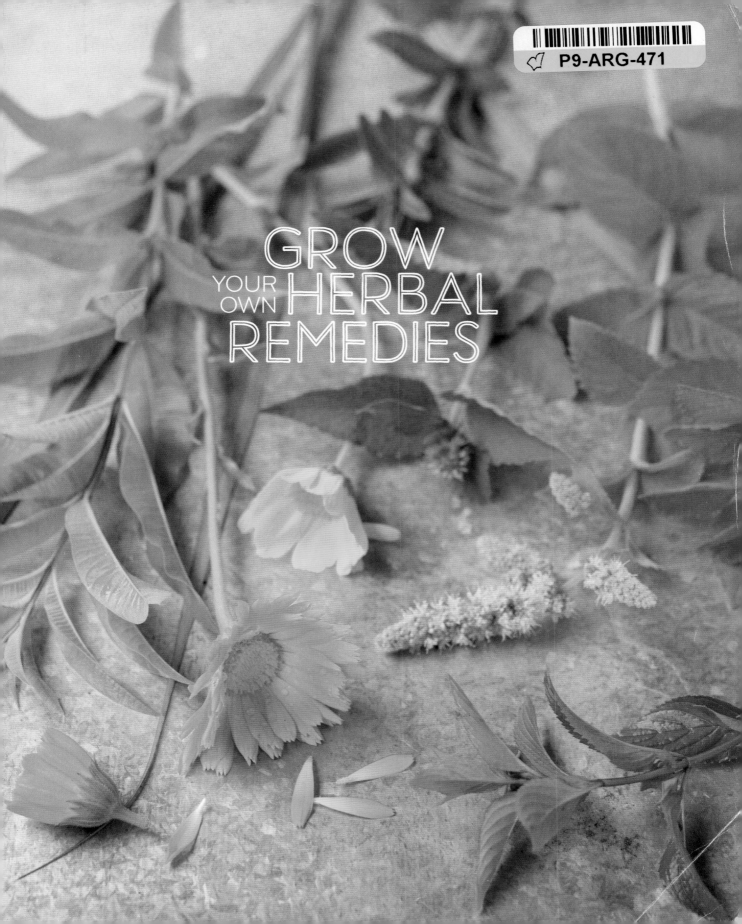

GROW
YOUR
OWN HERBAL
REMEDIES

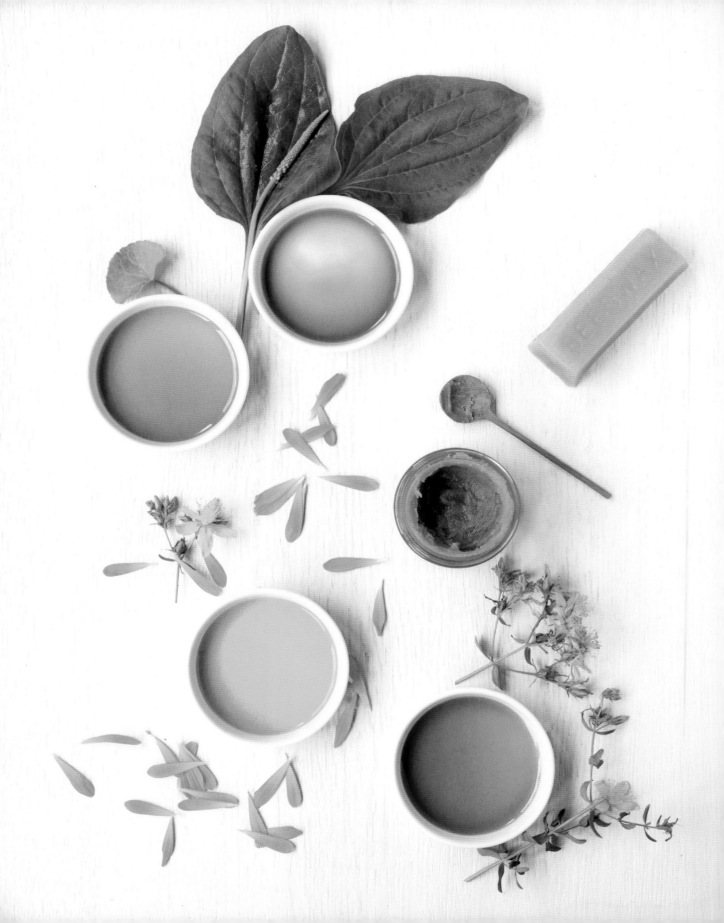

GROW YOUR OWN HERBAL REMEDIES

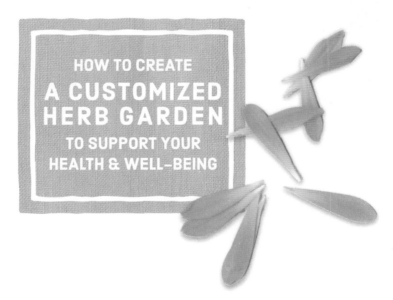

HOW TO CREATE A CUSTOMIZED HERB GARDEN TO SUPPORT YOUR HEALTH & WELL–BEING

MARIA NOËL GROVES

Photography by Stacey Cramp

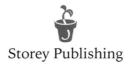

Storey Publishing

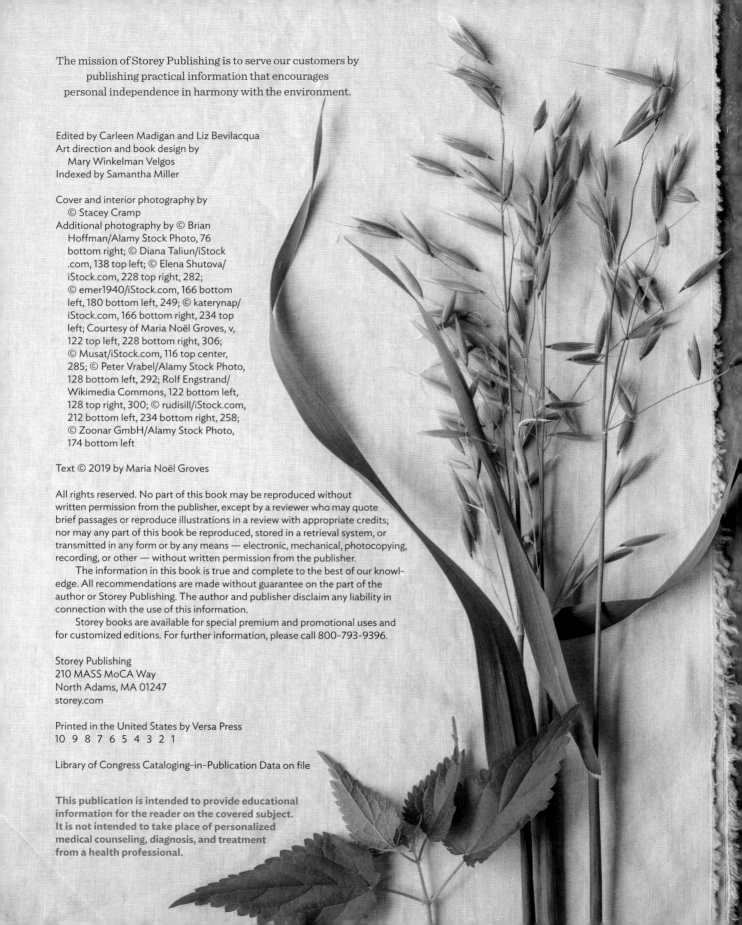

The mission of Storey Publishing is to serve our customers by publishing practical information that encourages personal independence in harmony with the environment.

Edited by Carleen Madigan and Liz Bevilacqua
Art direction and book design by
Mary Winkelman Velgos
Indexed by Samantha Miller

Cover and interior photography by
© Stacey Cramp
Additional photography by © Brian Hoffman/Alamy Stock Photo, 76 bottom right; © Diana Taliun/iStock .com, 138 top left; © Elena Shutova/ iStock.com, 228 top right, 282; © emer1940/iStock.com, 166 bottom left, 180 bottom left, 249; © katerynap/ iStock.com, 166 bottom right, 234 top left; Courtesy of Maria Noël Groves, v, 122 top left, 228 bottom right, 306; © Musat/iStock.com, 116 top center, 285; © Peter Vrabel/Alamy Stock Photo, 128 bottom left, 292; Rolf Engstrand/ Wikimedia Commons, 122 bottom left, 128 top right, 300; © rudisill/iStock.com, 212 bottom left, 234 bottom right, 258; © Zoonar GmbH/Alamy Stock Photo, 174 bottom left

Text © 2019 by Maria Noël Groves

Storey books are available for special premium and promotional uses and for customized editions. For further information, please call 800-793-9396.

Storey Publishing
210 MASS MoCA Way
North Adams, MA 01247
storey.com

Printed in the United States by Versa Press
10 9 8 7 6 5 4 3 2 1

Library of Congress Cataloging-in-Publication Data on file

Dedicated to . . .

Mimi Mandile, my mother and number one fan, who introduced me to herbal gardening and still lets me raid her garden periodically, as well as to my ever-supportive father, Jim Mandile.

Harriet Bean, who lovingly planted many of the herbs on this property during the 30 years she lived here before us and still keeps in touch.

Shannon Groves, my awesome husband, who always believes in me, joins me on adventures, and shares this wonderful land with me, helping to make it even more beautiful each season.

My teachers: Nancy Phillips and Rosemary Gladstar, who inspired me to cultivate herbs in the garden; Michael Moore, for fostering a love for wild-crafting and medicine making; and Christine Tolf, for opening my heart to flower essences.

Reishi, my sweet rescue mutt, who keeps me company, reminds me to take breaks, and never misses the opportunity to stop and sniff the flowers.

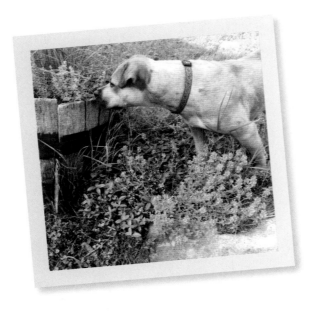

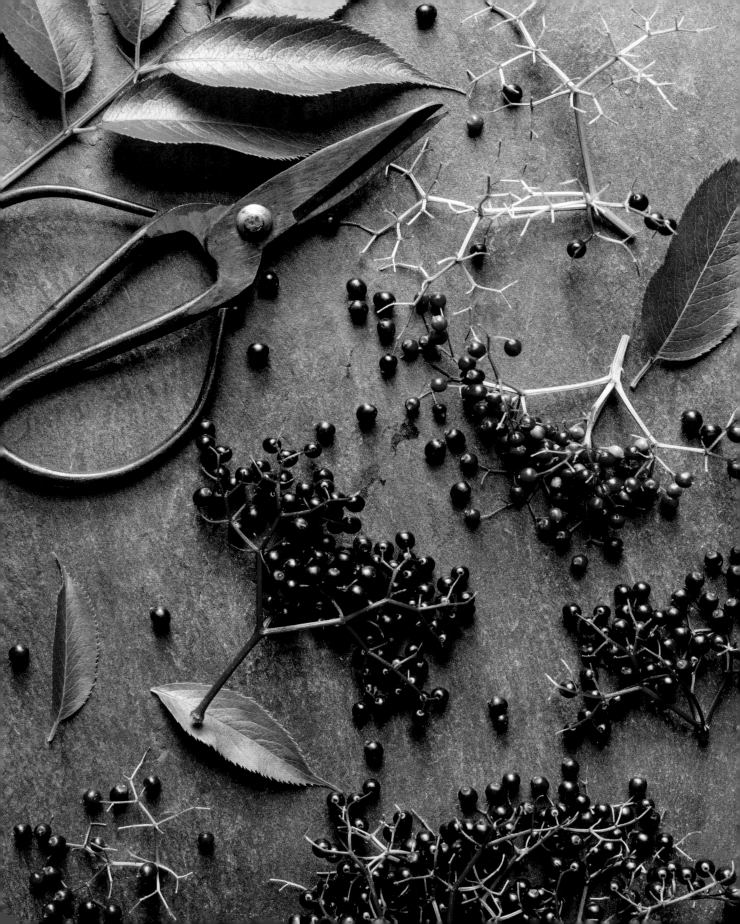

Contents

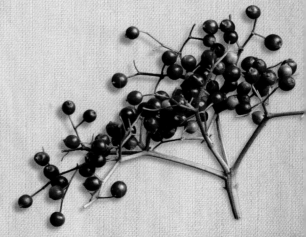

PART THREE

HEALING GARDEN HERBS

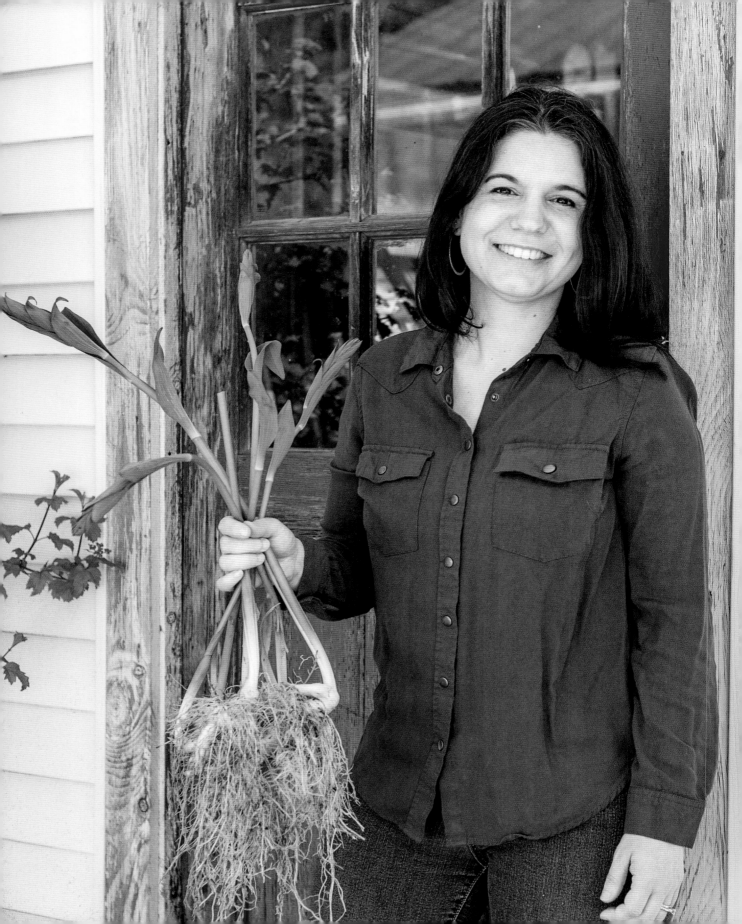

At the Garden Gate

MEDICINAL HERB GARDENING usually begins with one of two questions: "What should I grow?" Or "How can I use the plants I already have?" Everyone loves a good "top five" list of herbs you *must* plant to serve your health needs. But if every herbalist created a top five list, you can bet those lists would differ *vastly* from one person to the next. The truth is that the best herbs for *you* to grow will depend on your health needs, your growing conditions, and which plants resonate most with you. When you connect with the plants in this way, you'll get so much more out of your very own remedy garden.

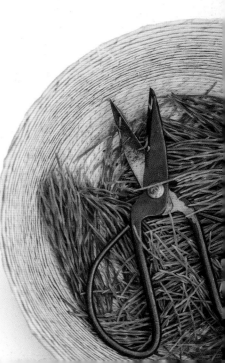

WHY GROW MEDICINAL HERBS?

So many excellent companies already make and sell fabulous herbal products, why on earth go through the trouble to grow your own plants and make your own herbal remedies? This question never crossed my mind when I first began to explore herbalism. First, I worked the supplement aisles of a popular local natural foods store, then I put my shiny new journalism degree to work covering the "herb beat" for *Natural Health* magazine. I quickly learned which herbs you could use for what and realized I wanted to become an herbalist to understand the plants on a deeper level. But making *my own* medicine seemed unnecessary.

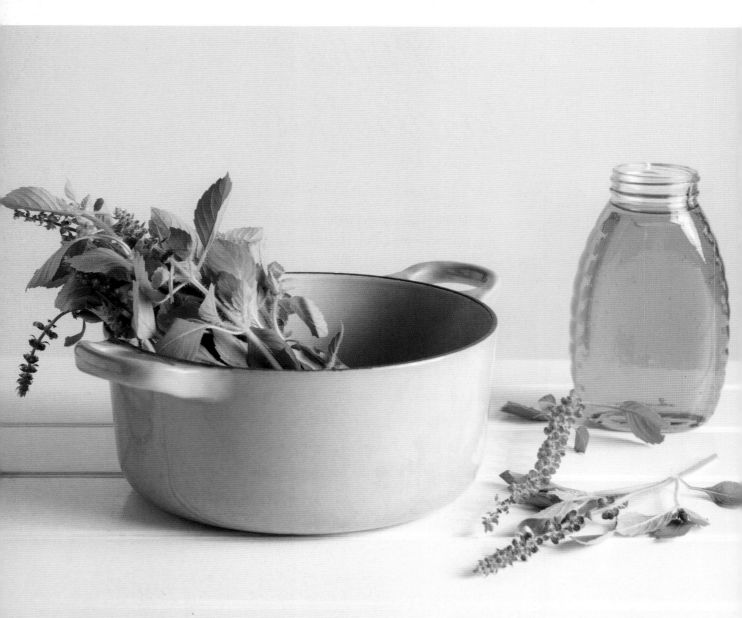

Growing your own herbs allows you to create custom remedies and capture the healing qualities of plants at their peak.

Lucky for me, I landed on study programs with herbalists who believed in getting your hands dirty: first with Nancy Phillips and Rosemary Gladstar (herbal farming and gardening advocates and gurus), then with my primary teacher, Michael Moore (a devout wildcrafter). I came home from herb school and realized: I need plants. I need to be connected with them. I need to be able to custom formulate remedies. Working with the plants directly and making my own remedies — including those for my clients — makes me a better herbalist, a healthier person, a more effective practitioner, and a more whole human being.

Believe it or not, the remedies you make from the plants in your backyard can be just as good as — and often superior to — products you buy. But that's not the only reason why you should grow your own herbal remedies.

TOP SIX REASONS TO GROW YOUR OWN HERBAL REMEDIES

- **Freshness.** Freshness matters, as does the ability to make things *exactly* the way you want them. This, on a chemical level, is what makes *your* remedies stronger than what you buy.
- **Less expensive.** You can make potent remedies for a fraction of the retail cost. That 1-ounce bottle of tincture that cost you $15? You can make *16 ounces* for less. Teas are practically free.
- **Customization.** Don't simply stuff your pantry with as many remedies as you possibly can. Think critically about the best plants for you (which is what this book is about). Start with small quantities, gradually building an herbal medicine cabinet tailored exactly to you and your family. You can also craft your own blends, which are often more effective than

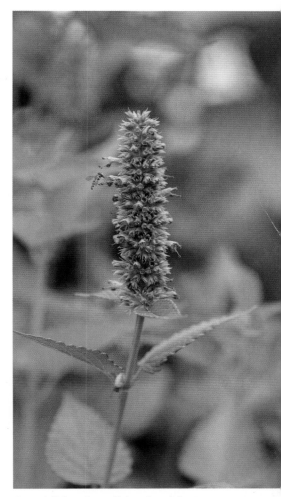

Grow delicious, beautiful, and useful herbs like Korean mint, which is almost impossible to find.

What Is an "Herb"?

Herbalists define "herb" broadly to include *any* plant or plant part used to promote health. Even mushrooms (*completely* different creatures entirely) become honorary "herbs." But if you're talking to a botanist, an "herb" refers *only* to leafy plants that die back in winter and lack woody stems (as opposed to shrubs and trees). Horticulturists and garden centers may also use this definition and/or limit "herbs" to culinary plants, often with subdued leafy mounds of growth. For a chef, "herb" refers to the *leaves* of culinary herbs, as opposed to seeds, roots, and barks, which are spices. Herbalists are generalists. If it grows from the earth and helps us feel better, it's an herb.

prefab store-bought formulas, and they're fun to create. The recipes in this book serve as a starting point.

- **Self-sufficiency and empowerment.** Being able to step into your backyard or open your medicine cabinet when you aren't feeling well, take a plant, and feel better — that's what it's all about. You don't need to run out to the store. It's right there for you and your family. The more you learn the plants and gain confidence in your skills as a home herbalist, the stronger you will feel in your ability to make yourself, your family, your community, your landscape, and the planet healthier.

- **Sustainability, stewardship, and confidence.** When you grow your own herbs, you not only ensure you have access to amazing quality plants whenever you need them. You develop a connection with the plants themselves and gain confidence in the quality and identity of the herbs you use. You promote sustainability for plants that might be grown and harvested unethically in commerce, and you become a steward of your land and the plant kingdom, a reciprocal relationship where you help the plants and they help you. In doing so, you also provide food, habitat, and diversity for a deeper ecology on your property that includes birds, bees, butterflies, mycelia, and earthworms.

- **Connection.** Plants are much more than a source of medicine; they have personalities. When you grow, harvest, and make medicine with a plant, you get to know your medicine on a deeper level. It means more than white or green powder in a pill. You commune with the individual plants and your

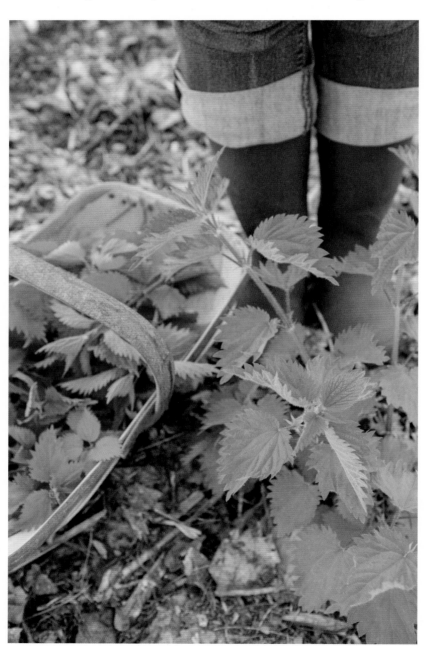

Only herbalists plant stinging nettles in their gardens! In spite of its weedy nature and painful sting, nettle is rich with valuable nutrition. Find an out-of-the-way spot for it to thrive.

local ecosystem at large. Nature heals, whether you're nibbling on some Korean mint or simply looking out the window at its beautiful purple blooms and the bees pollinating it.

What's in a Name? Latin Names and Plant Families

I've included the genus and species for every herb in the plant profiles that begin on page 246. These two names together identify the exact plant in question. If you're purchasing starts or seeds, use the Latin name to ensure you're getting the plant you want. Common names can be misleading. (And labeling mistakes happen, so you'll still want to confirm the plant's identity before you harvest it.)

Often, multiple species can be used interchangeably, which is indicated by "spp." as in "*Monarda* spp." for bee balm. In the description, I'll suggest specific favored species (such as *M. fistulosa*) to seek out. Plants with an " × " between the genus and species (such as peppermint: *Mentha* × *piperita*) are hybrids that won't grow true to seed, but you can propagate them by other methods like root division and cuttings. Plants with a long history in horticulture — like calendula, elder, rose, and echinacea — may have many *varieties* developed for ornamental purposes. Unless I've specified

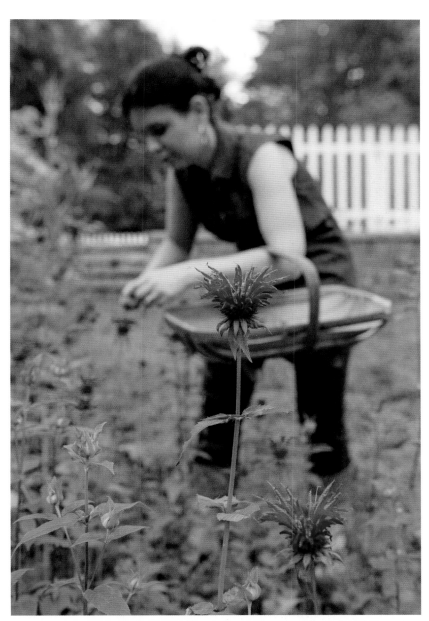

There are many species and varieties of bee balm you can grow. The bright red *Monarda didyma* attracts hummingbirds and can be used for medicine, but *M. fistulosa* is stronger medicinally.

certain varieties in the profile, stick with the original plants for optimal medicinal potency.

I've included the plant family because I want you to gradually learn and recognize plant patterns and family resemblances.

You'll often find similar physical features, growing conditions, and/ or medicinal properties among various plants in the same family. Popular plant families in the medicinal garden include mint, rose, daisy, and parsley.

YOU DON'T NEED A GREEN THUMB — OR EVEN A GARDEN

You definitely do not need to be an amazing gardener or have perfect growing conditions to add herbs to your landscape. Herbs are far more forgiving than vegetables and flowers, and less tasty to the local fauna. In fact, if you've got soil in your yard, you probably already have medicinal herbs whether you've planted them or not. The plant world is generous that way. If your home doesn't include a patch of soil to tend, you can bring it in with containers inside, on the steps, and along the driveway. Or you can ask friends, neighbors, and local organic farmers if you can harvest some of their herbs or weeds.

I chose the herbs in this book specifically because they're easy to grow (or thrive abundantly, wild, in backyard environments), incredibly useful medicinally, safe, and easy to harvest and use to make remedies. I have a close, personal relationship with these plants, having cultivated or wildcrafted all of them numerous times in my 25 years working as an herbalist, particularly the 13 years that I've tended them on my property.

I didn't come to this land with gardening know-how, and even though many herbs already grew on the property, I've had my challenges: poor, acidic, sandy soil; early frosts; legions of hungry critters; and shade from enormous pines around and throughout the yard. I don't have a lot of time to tend to my plants or spend hours harvesting and processing them. I'm eternally grateful for mulch, timed drip irrigation, and low-fuss plants that produce plenty of medicine without much effort.

Most of the herbs in this book will thrive in a pampered garden bed with full sun, rich soil, and regular doses of water. But many herbs adapt to a wide range of conditions and neglect yet still produce year after year. You won't find any divas (sorry, ginseng) or plants that require colossal time or effort for a puny harvest (goodbye, astragalus and nigella) in this book. You'll learn basic gardening know-how in chapter 1. For the land-challenged, check out your container options on page 22.

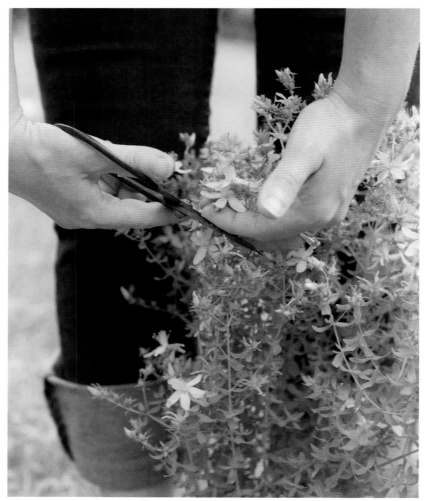

No garden? No problem! Grow plants in containers or forage common "weeds," like this St. John's wort, from clean, wild spaces.

WHAT SHOULD YOU GROW?

Here are the things you'll want to consider when choosing your herbs.

Herbs that address your health needs. What types of health benefits would you like in your life? Do you want herbs that taste good and look beautiful? Weeds that nourish your body better than store-bought vegetables? Something to help you sleep? First aid remedies for your little ones' boo-boos? Think about daily tonics as well as the ailments you and your family face most often and start there.

Plants for your growing conditions. Whether you garden in New Mexico or New Hampshire, you could grow almost all of the herbs in this book with soil amendments, irrigation, and careful placement. But start with what you've got versus what you can create. If you've got a shady yard, opt for plants that thrive in dappled sunlight. A hot climate? Go for tropicals. Dry? Low-water plants. Soggy? Find some herbs that like wet feet. You'll have more success with these plants and can always expand as your garden and skills grow.

Herbs that resonate with you. This may be the least tangible thing to learn because it's solely dependent on your individual relationship with individual plants. Use your intuition to see which

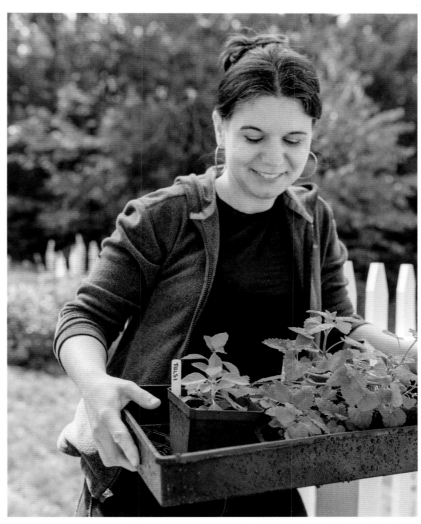

Holy basil (tulsi) and lemon balm are among some of my favorite incredibly useful and easy-go-grow herbs for the garden.

plants call to you. When you try them, see if they resonate — even if you don't notice a major "effect" right away, you'll usually sense that you generally like or don't like how you feel when you take them. Which herbs actually have the desired outcome? Does valerian lull you to sleep or make you feel agitated? Does nettle make your body sing with nourishment or feel drained from peeing all day?

You want to know this before you plant a huge patch of it and put up a half gallon of tincture or tea. Play with the plants, start with small quantities, and tune in to what your body tells you it likes best.

Also bear in mind that your herb garden does not need to begin with a hundred plants. Start with one to five that really call to you, get to know them really well, then expand from there.

HOW TO USE THIS BOOK AND CHOOSE YOUR PLANTS

I don't know your growing conditions or which plants resonate with you, but I do know which easy-to-grow plants tend to work best for specific body systems and everyday health concerns. Whether you're a newbie or already have some gardening and herbal skills up your sleeve, it helps to start with a body system approach. This is the same approach I took in my first book, *Body into Balance: An Herbal Guide to Holistic Self-Care,* as well as my Home Herbalist Series study program. Rather than choosing from a laundry list of plants, target a particular purpose, and then look at each plant's nuances. What are each plant's specific indications? What side benefits does each plant offer? What are the cautions? Where does it like to grow?

Even though this book is organized into "gardens" for each health topic, I don't necessarily expect (or want) you to plant every single one of the featured plants in one plot in your yard. Feel free to pick the ones that seem best suited for your health needs and the growing conditions on your property. It may make sense to plant the herbs you choose in different places in your yard. Nettle stings and spreads while calendula needs a full-sun pampered garden bed. Just because different herbs blend well in a tea doesn't mean they play nice next to each other in the garden. You'll be better off foraging for nettle if it grows wild nearby or planting it in a damp, part-shade, out-of-the-way spot where it won't sting you every time you pop into the garden for some culinary herbs.

Most of the herbs in this book will grow well in temperate gardens from USDA Hardiness Zones 4 to 9 with moderate moisture, decent soil, and partial shade to full sun. Within one yard you'll often have microclimates of shade, soil, and moisture where you can tuck plants into their niches. But if your yard has *very* specific site specs — really cold, hot, dry, wet, relentlessly sunny, or shady — check out the site suggestions on page 312 to hone your plant selection and read the profiles in part 3 for more tips.

PLANT ID AND SAFETY

Medicinal herbs, particularly those covered in this book, *generally* have a solid safety record with rare and minor side effects. That said, I encourage my students and readers to empower themselves by sticking with some basic safety rules.

- **Do your research.** Check a plant out in at least three different sources to get a sense of what it can be used for and any potential safety issues. Incorporate a mix of mostly herbalist/clinician perspectives with some evidence-based/scientific ones. You can safely use only this book, but you'll gain even greater insight into herbal medicine by gathering a variety of perspectives.

- **Listen to your body and intuition.** Ultimately, your own experience with the plant will determine which herbs work best for you. Intuition can guide you to which plants to try (assuming you've also done research, especially for safety), then tune in to your body to determine whether or not the plant resonates and if it has the desired effect.

- **Correctly identify your plant.** Mistakes happen. *All the time.* Garden centers mislabel plants, something unexpected may grow where you planted seeds, friends share improperly identified plants from their garden, and so forth. It's most important to key out and identify plants you wildcraft, but always double-check new plants in the garden that you haven't used before. Get yourself a good field guide. One of the most common, lethal mix-ups is to mistake foxglove leaves for mullein, comfrey, or other plants. Identification is unfortunately beyond the scope of this book, but you'll find information

about how to identify plants on my website (see Resources, page 316).

- **Check for herb-drug reactions.** If you're on any medications, check for any potential interactions with herbs. You can ask your pharmacist to check it in the pharmacy's database. If you're on several medications or ones like blood thinners that interact with many herbs, seek an herbalist or naturopathic doctor's guidance on what herbs you can safely take, and keep your doctor in the loop.

- **Start low, work up.** Using the dosages in this book as a general guide, start low and work up. Start below the recommended dose, especially if you're a "sensitive person" — just a few drops of tincture or sips of tea. This way you can gauge your response and ensure the plant agrees with you. Work your dose up to the recommended range. If it doesn't seem to work, increase your dose (within the range). If it still doesn't work, try another plant or seek professional guidance.

- **Know your limits.** Self-empowerment doesn't mean you need to know and do it all. Get regular checkups and develop a good health care team that you trust to refer to, especially in potentially dangerous, life-threatening conditions (e.g., copious bleeding, anaphylactic shock, difficulty breathing, serious acute infections, severe dehydration, heart attack) as well as conditions that don't respond promptly to natural therapies. These are times to turn to modern medicine, not your garden.

HOW HERBAL MEDICINE WORKS

In herbal medicine, we aim to get to the root of the problem and choose herbs that help bring the body back into balance, alongside diet and lifestyle changes. While this book will introduce you to safe, effective herbs for common health concerns, I delve much more deeply into healing in my first book, *Body into Balance: An Herbal Guide to Holistic Self-Care.* There, I discuss each body system in depth, with protocol points for various conditions. While both books can be used independently, the two work particularly well as a companion set. In one, you'll understand each body system and see the big picture. Here, you learn how to grow, harvest, and use the plants, and you get many more recipes to inspire you in your healing journey.

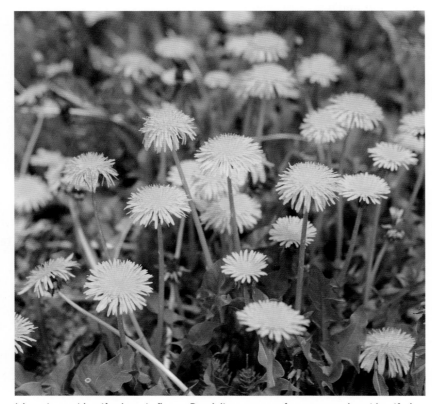

It's easiest to identify plants in flower. Dandelions are easy for most people to identify, but many different plants have similar flowers and leaves and could be confused if you don't take the time to correctly identify them.

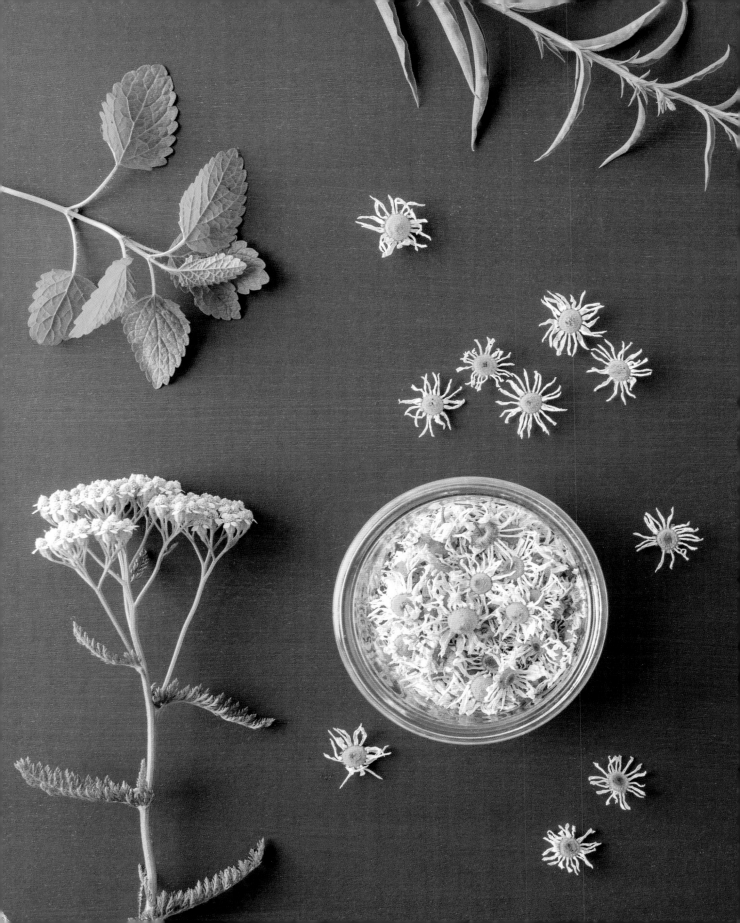

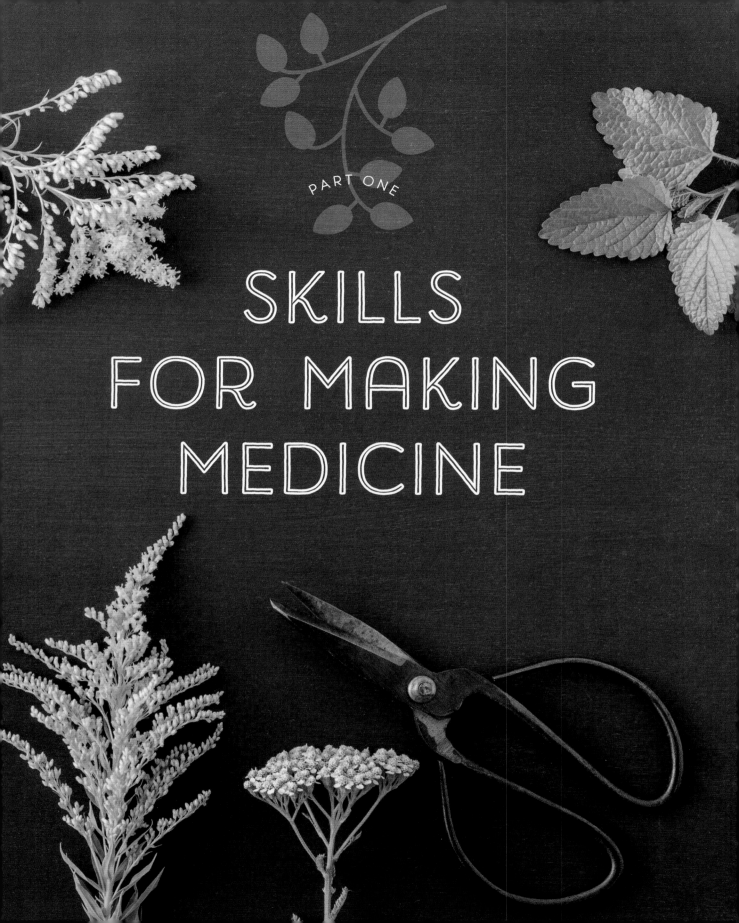

SKILLS FOR MAKING MEDICINE

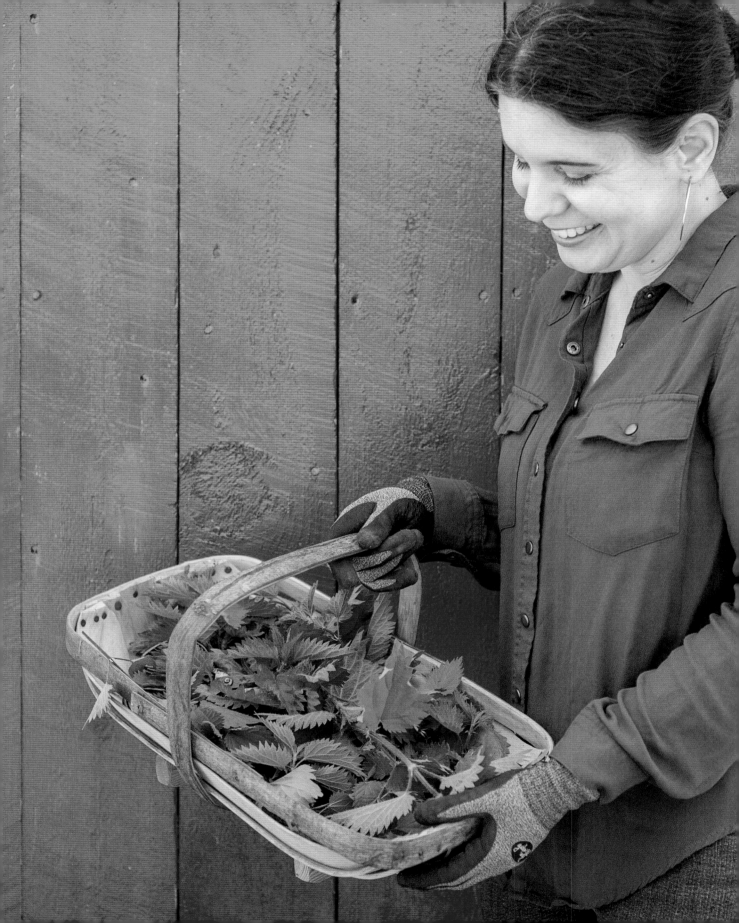

Growing, Harvesting, and Preserving

HERBAL GARDENING may seem daunting, but these plants are generally easier to grow than food crops, flowers, and ornamentals. Cultivating your own herbs helps you connect with your medicine and ensures you have easy access to high-quality plants that suit *you* best. With very little effort, you can grow and make medicine with benefits that exceed those of what you buy in the store. Here are a few pointers on getting your green thumb going.

PLANTING, CARE, AND MAINTENANCE

Of all the plants you could grow, herbs tend to be the least fussy. Most of the plants in this book thrive in a plush, vegetable-worthy garden bed with rich, well-drained soil, regular watering, and full sun. Yet they'll often tolerate drier and poorer soils, partial shade, and other less favorable conditions. Herbs will meet you where you're at, but you can make them even happier by understanding each plant's favored habitat and tending to your soil ecology. This approach takes time, but it's not that difficult or expensive.

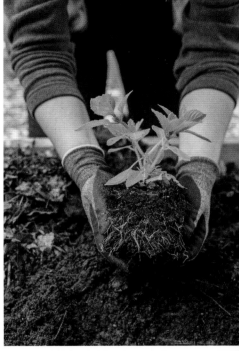

Planting day! If possible, choose a dreary spring day with rain in the forecast, or water regularly after planting. Hot, sunny weather quickly dries out and kills young plants.

Thirteen years ago, my husband and I purchased a home nestled within a state park. The previous owner cultivated medicinal herbs for personal use here for decades. It sounds like a dream, but we also have had our challenges: weeds galore (the sheep sorrel! the crabgrass!), acidic and sandy soil, hungry wildlife, a short season, and limited sun thanks to the enormous pine trees that encircle the property. Through mulching, laying manure (friends' horses and my chickens), and gradually expanding the property with new beds each year, it's been a joy to watch the soil structure — and the plants — become more vital. During those first few years, we never saw earthworms. Now our garden beds are rich with good dirt and slithering friends, and the herbs are ecstatic.

Finding the Best Site for Your Plants

The first step to a successful garden is to observe. Watch your property throughout the season. Watch which plants grow where. (Horsetail and jewelweed? That's a damp spot.) Where does the sun land hot on the soil, where are the pockets of shade? Where does snow accumulate in winter? Where is the first place it melts and disappears? If you have a hill, chances are the top will have drier, sandier, or rockier soil while the bottom will be moist and rich.

Different plants may prefer different soil types — slightly sandy, rich in humus — yet most plants will thrive in well-drained soil rich in organic matter. Consider running a soil test to get a baseline, especially if you want to add amendments like lime, greensand, and blood meal, otherwise you're flying blind and spending money on products you might not need. Check in with your local extension office or organic land care organization for tips and testing companies.

Look for microclimates. Buildings, fences, and stone walls create microclimates of cool shade or reflected sun and heat. They also offer protection from wind, light frosts, and animal traffic. Note your north-facing (very shady), south-facing (very sunny), and east/west-facing (part shade) spots. Consider planting the same type of plant in three locations, then see where it thrives.

Building Your Bed

Regardless of what your soil is like, you can take my approach: build beds using a lazy lasagna gardening method. Choose your garden bed location and size, and decide whether or not you're going to frame it with wood, brick, stones, or other material or simply edge it with a lawn edging tool. For a formal bed that you'll harvest

and tend to regularly — such as culinary herbs — don't make the bed too wide, as you'll want to be able to work the bed without stepping in it. Three to 4 feet in width usually works well. If you can, build your bed in the fall to plant in spring. This will give the soil a chance to settle and time for beneficial microbes to kick in. That said, you *can* build and plant your beds in the same day if that's the time frame you've got.

- **Loosen the soil (optional):** Using a broad fork, break up compact soil without overworking it. You can skip this step, but it makes better-quality soil that goes deeper into the ground.
- **Cardboard or newspaper base:** Lay flattened cardboard boxes (not technically organic due to glue but very effective and easily available) or several layers of wet black-and-white newspaper over the area. This smothers grass and most weeds and eventually breaks down into the soil once the bed is established.
- **Edge or frame it:** Use your edger tool to cut a perimeter around your bed, or place/build your bed frame. If you can't afford stone, untreated pine boards are easy and relatively affordable, lasting 5 to 10 years in our yard. Use boards 2 inches thick and 6 to 8 inches wide. Cedar costs more but lasts longer. (Pressure-treated wood

lasts longer but leaches toxic chemicals into your soil.)
- **Fill it:** Start with twigs and small branches (for drainage) and a thick layer of leaves or straw. Then add loam and compost. Continue layering this way if you have space and material

until the bed is full. Use compost covered with leaf mulch for the top layer. The soil will settle over time.
- **Plant it:** When you're ready to plant your seedlings, pull back the mulch and dig a hole a tad larger than the plant.

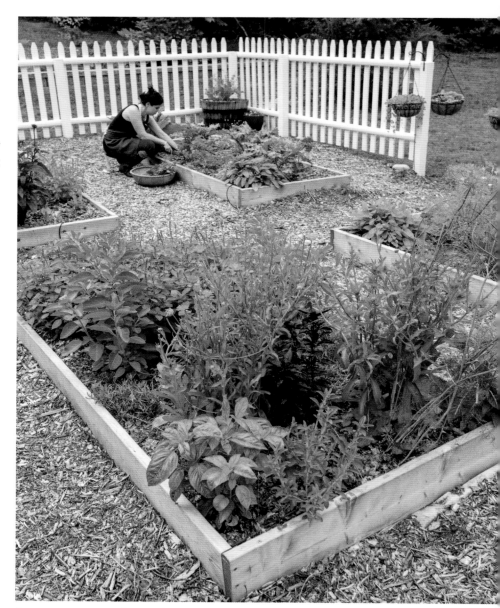

Space out your young plants so they won't get too crowded as they grow throughout the season. Tomato cages help keep floppy calendula upright.

Gently remove the plant from its pot and unravel the roots if they're bound. Place the plant flush with the soil line in the hole, fill in with soil, and gently tamp down the soil around it. If desired, make a small indentation in the soil to help catch water (or raise it up a bit in waterlogged areas). Water well, and surround with mulch. Keep an eye on newly planted seedlings, watering periodically until they get established. If possible, plant when the forecast predicts light rain (as opposed to hot sun). Wait to plant most annuals and tender perennials until the threat of frost has passed. Tender perennials are herbs that will live year-round only in warm climates and often perish if exposed to frost. If possible, "harden off" new seedlings by placing them outdoors for increasingly longer periods, or at least wait to plant until a week of mild weather is forecasted before planting.

Getting Supplies

Purchase organic compost and loam from landscape supply companies that deliver by the truckload or square yard, or scavenge loam from another area of your yard (like that spot where you've been dumping glass clippings and leaves for years). Get well-aged manure from your own livestock or local farms. Horse manure may contain more weed seeds, but it's often readily available. We brought a small flock of chickens to our property as part of our soil improvement project, and they've been tremendous. We apply coop shavings to the beds in fall and winter, then cover them with leaf mulch. (For safety, avoid harvesting crops in these beds until 90 to 120 days after application.) Compost grass clippings, garden waste, and kitchen waste to use, too.

MULCH

Mulch is your friend! It prevents weeds, holds moisture, builds organic matter, improves drainage, feeds earthworms, and improves the microbial and fungal diversity in your soil. Yes, it may encourage slugs and ticks and reduce the activity of self-seeding herbs, but the benefits outweigh the risks. Use what you've got: pine needles, wood chips, newspaper, straw, grass clippings, sawdust, wool, leaves — leaves are by far my favorite. If it's practical, run them through a shredder or drive over them with the mower. This keeps the leaves from smothering the soil, helps them break down faster to enrich the soil, and allows perennials to pop out. In the fall, our lawn mower collects leaves in the bag, and we dump them in a pile or directly on the garden beds. I collect extra bags from friends and students. Ensure

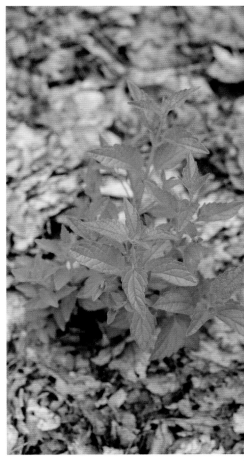

Chopped leaf mulch saved from the previous fall helps hold moisture, reduce weed pressure, and gradually enriches the soil ecology.

they come from unsprayed yards without invasive seeds like bittersweet berries. Avoid excessive amounts of oak, hemlock, or chestnut leaves. Wood chips work well for woodland plants and trees, but they take longer to break down and temporarily rob nitrogen from the soil (sprinkle some organic fertilizer or blood meal onto the area to offset the nitrogen loss). We get a truckload of free wood chips every few years

when the road crews trim around the power lines — perfect for my beds of shrubs and trees along the forest's edge as well as for garden walkway paths.

SOIL AMENDMENTS AND FERTILIZERS

Aged manure and compost make fantastic fertilizer, and you might not need any more than that. North Country Organics Pro-Gro works well as an all-purpose fertilizer to sprinkle in with new plants and in spring when the plants could use a boost. Neptune's Harvest fish and seaweed emulsion is also popular (unfortunately, it encourages our raccoon and skunk population to dig up everything looking for fish). Biochar improves nutrient and water retention. Depending on your soil's needs (as evidenced by the soil test), organic amendments could include blood meal, fish emulsion, seaweed, greensand, lime, wood ash, and other nutrient-rich materials. Check with your local nonprofit organic association to find out where to get a soil test and buy these items. They may offer bulk orders, and well-stocked feed and farm stores sometimes carry organic fertilizers. You might not need all these fancy amendments, though. Compost or manure and mulch usually do a fabulous job balancing and improving a variety of soil types over time.

Sun

Most herbs prefer partial to full sun with a few exceptions, which gives you quite a bit of flexibility. The "sun" icon refers to how much sunlight and exposure a plant likes or will tolerate.

 Full sun: Bright sunshine most of the day. Large fields, south-facing spots, and against walls and buildings. Six to 10 hours of sunlight/day.

 Partial shade: These locations have sun for part of the day and shade at other times, or dappled sun, near trees or in the shadow of a taller plant. East- and west-facing spots next to buildings, walls, and along forest edges. To create partial shade in a full-sun landscape, plant taller shade plants or use a shade cloth. Partial-shade-loving plants may need protection from bright sun at the height of day. Tolerates 3 to 6 hours of direct sunlight/day.

 Shade: Usually not 100 percent shade but mostly shady, north-facing sites next to buildings, in the forest, or under the shade of tall plants, trees, vines, or shade cloth. Less than 3 hours of direct sunlight/day.

Water

All plants need water, but how *much* they need varies. Water refers not only to how much water comes down on the plant in the form of watering, rain, and irrigation but also how much moisture occurs naturally in the soil due to conditions (near wetlands, a ditch, bottom of a hill), as well as the water retention capacity of the soil. For example, basil loves to be watered regularly, but it rots out if it gets waterlogged. Bacopa revels in sludgy soil, while cayenne peppers thrive in a minimal amount of moisture.

Many herbs do fine without regular watering as long as they're planted in decent soil, mulched, and kept moist enough with periodic rainwater. Some prefer regular irrigation. Water your plants deeply and thoroughly in the morning, focusing on the root zone, and keep them top-dressed with plenty of mulch. Watering cans and hoses with a watering attachment work in a pinch, but this method is time consuming and may not be the most effective approach. Drip irrigation systems on a timer are an investment for years to come, do an excellent job tending your plants, and can easily be expanded each year.

The moisture icons in the plant profiles (page 246) tell you how much (or if) you need to water a plant and what kinds of soils and sites it prefers. Keep in mind that shady sites hold moisture better than sunny spots. Most herbs fall into the one- or two-drop category.

Zero drops: Low-water, drought-resistant plants prefer sandy soil and often hail

from the American Southwest or Mediterranean regions. In damp environments, consider raised terra-cotta pots minimally watered on stone walls or against buildings. They usually like heat and full sun. Examples include California poppy, cayenne, horehound, and thyme.

One drop: Relatively low water, poor to good soil. May tolerate or enjoy regular irrigation but don't *need* it except during very dry spells. Examples include ashwagandha, black cohosh, catnip, and goldenrod.

Two drops: In sunny spots, water regularly. If the soil is rich, consistently moist, in part shade, and/or well mulched, these herbs may not need to be watered regularly. Examples include blue vervain, bee balm, elder, and lemon balm.

Three drops: Daily watering and/or wet feet. Good for swampy spots, damp soil, containers in a dish of water, and locations next to water features. Examples include gotu kola, bacopa, and horsetail.

Know Your Zone

Knowing your USDA Hardiness Zone (see Resources on page 316) and the zone that a plant prefers will help you choose the perennials most apt to survive in your location. The zone assesses the number of consecutive frost-free days, which also indicates how

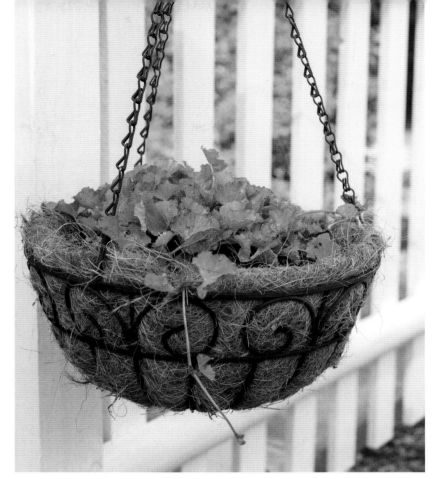

Growing frost-tender plants like gotu kola in hanging baskets or containers enables you to quickly move them indoors if frost threatens and during wintertime. It also keeps hungry woodchucks at bay.

much heat or cold a plant can handle. You may be able to push a plant's boundaries with extra TLC if you live on the edge of a plant's zone. For example, in hot climates, you may need to plant the herb in a shady spot or just grow it like an annual in cooler months. In cold climates, opt for a protected site and/or cover it in winter.

Weed and Pest Control

The bane of a happy gardener, weeds and pests are what make gardening hard work. My goal: cultivate the best garden with

the least amount of effort. I *love* feeding weeds and bugs to my chickens. It's so satisfying to watch them gobble up my garden enemies! But the fewer weeds and bugs I have to deal with at all, the better. Manage weeds from the get-go with mulch. Use several layers of newspaper or cardboard (covered with some wood chips and/or leaves) to smother existing weeds. Prevent weeds seeds from sprouting in open soil by applying a thick layer of leaves. Catch weed sprouts as early as possible, *especially* before they set seed. Make a habit of pulling a few weeds

every day as you walk through the garden. If hand-pulling isn't enough, a CobraHead or a Korean-style Ho-Mi hand plow helps dig out tough weeds (the Ho-Mi helps with planting, too). The first year I lived here, I didn't know what any of the plants sprouting in my garden were, so I let *everything* go to seed — big mistake! But it *does* get easier each year that you stay on top of those weeds.

Pests range from earwigs and other insects to munching rodents, deer, woodchucks, and porcupines. For insects and disease, your best defense will be good soil, vital plants, and careful monitoring. Fortunately, most herbs are resistant to most diseases and not terribly tasty to pests. Spraying plants with garlic, cayenne, or soapy water and erecting good fences all help deter pests. But rather than wage war on every critter that comes through your yard, stick to planting less disease- and pest-prone species and work to improve your garden ecology. Each year, you'll notice that your plants stay healthy and lush with minimal intervention. Many insects (Japanese beetles, caterpillars) and diseases (powdery mildew) take hold after the plant passes its prime, so make a point to harvest roses, marshmallow, nettle, and bee balm before they turn.

STARTING FROM PLANTS OR SEEDS

You've got a few options for getting plants into your garden: planting seeds or seedlings or propagating from existing plants. I highly recommend starting with seedlings and perennial starts rather than seeds, at least at first.

Seedlings: An Easy Way to Start

Compared to starting a plant from seed, starting with a seedling or potted plant will be *vastly* easier and more successful and will enable you to harvest your herbs much sooner. Plant your herb seedlings in spring. Trees and shrubs should go in as soon as the ground can be worked. Wait until after the threat of frost for annuals and tender perennials.

Starting from Seed

Seeds are more economical, but they are also more challenging to grow. A few plants grow easily from a packet of seeds sown right into the garden and are worth a shot: dill, calendula, California poppy, Korean mint. Check your seed packets for instructions, some (like the aforementioned) do better if you sprinkle the seed

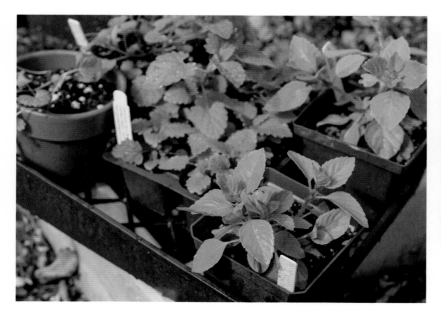

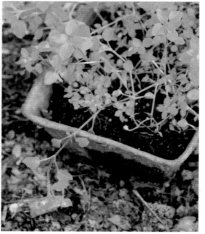

Beginning gardeners can ensure success by starting with seedlings rather than seeds.

Know Your Plant Lifespans

Some herbs need to be planted anew each year, a few live on a specific two-year cycle, and others will outlive you, all of which depends on your zone and freezing temps.

Annual: Dies after frost or setting seed. Replant or let self-seed. Examples include calendula and dill.

Perennial: Returns each year. Most herbs are perennial, including lemon and bee balm.

Biennial: Produces only herbaceous growth the first year, flowers and fruit/seed the second year, then dies. Examples include burdock, mullein, and the deadly foxglove.

Tender perennial: Survives winter only in warm climates, otherwise treated as an annual or brought indoors in cold climates. Examples include lemongrass, lemon verbena, gotu kola, bacopa, ashwagandha, and rosemary.

Short-lived perennial: Dies off easily or within about 3 years. Examples include artichoke (in warm climates), Korean mint, St. John's wort, and some mallows.

In It for the Long Haul

Most of the plants discussed in this book can be harvested the same season you plant them, but a few take longer to get established. This might be a deciding factor for whether or not you want to grow a particular plant, especially if you want to make medicine pronto or don't anticipate being in the same place for very long. In some cases — like wild cherry bark and birch — you can usually find established wild trees to prune instead. Generally speaking, while you could harvest the roots of most perennial plants within the first year or two of planting, some take longer to "ripen."

It can take several years for shrubs and trees to begin producing flowers and berries. This will depend on the age of the plant you planted as well as the species and growing conditions. (Pay more for an older tree, and it may produce more quickly than a spindly bare root sapling.) Most will grow faster and produce more flowers and fruit with full sun, good soil, and regular moisture.

Garlic: planted in fall, harvest the following summer

Biennial roots: fall of first year or spring of second (before it flowers)
Examples: mullein, burdock

Most perennial roots: 2–3+ years (but if you're weeding babies out, use 'em)
Examples: yellow dock, marshmallow, valerian, elecampane

Echinacea roots: 3–4 years

Black cohosh roots: 3+ years

Mimosa bark/flowers: 2+ years

Roses/hips: 3–5 years

Elderflowers/berries: 3–5 years

Hawthorn flowers/berries: 3–10 years

Linden flowers: 5–10 years

Most bark: 2–5 years (or as soon as they're big enough to prune)
Examples: cramp bark, wild cherry, mimosa, birch

in the garden in late fall. So why might you want to grow plants from seed at all? Some plants are more readily available as seeds than as seedlings. Also, if you need an abundance of one type of plant, seeds will be less expensive than seedlings.

To successfully grow herbs from seed, you'll need to pay attention to directions on your seed packet for when to plant and how deep to plant them. When starting seeds indoors, use a special seed starting mix, not regular garden soil. Water regularly and evenly without letting the soil get too soggy (which causes the spread of a fungal condition called "damping-off") or dry (death to those poor little seedlings). Consider using grow lights, a heated mat underneath, and a gentle oscillating fan — this will encourage better growth than growing them in a sunny windowsill does.

MAKING MORE PLANTS

You don't necessarily need to buy plants *or* seeds. You could propagate from established plants you already have — spreading more in different areas of your property — or swap plants with fellow gardeners.

Root division. Most perennials can be propagated by root division. Simply dig up and divide or shovel off a part of a preexisting plant. This works best with perennials that produce a crown of roots or grow by root runners. Good candidates include most plants in the mint family (bee balm, for example). For trees and shrubs such as elder, carefully remove root suckers with their attached roots to start new plants; they'll need good soil and plenty of TLC for that first year to ensure they survive. You may wish to sever a sucker from the mother plant *in* the ground several weeks before you dig it up to give it a chance to establish its independent root system. For both these methods, the best time to divide plants will be in early spring while they're relatively dormant.

Cuttings. Cuttings can be snipped from actively growing plant shoots. Cuttings of some plants (gotu kola, bacopa) only need to be placed in water for a few weeks or months to establish roots, which can then be planted in soil. Or dip the cutting in rooting hormone, then place it directly in containers of dirt. Attend to the cuttings as if they're young seedlings until they're established with a strong root system. Candidates for cuttings include plants in the mint family, stevia, passionflower, and lemon verbena.

Self-sown seedlings. Some plants self-sow, and you can dig up and move these babies to new spots in spring or late fall. Chamomile, Korean mint, calendula, blue vervain, fennel, and dill readily self-seed.

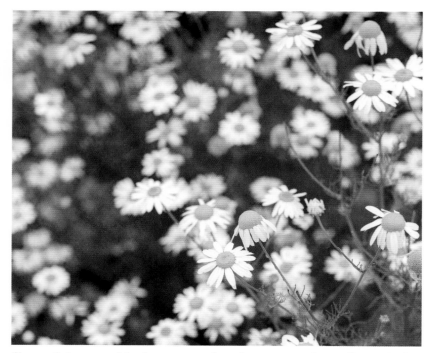

Chamomile is an annual that is easy to grow from direct-sown seed or seedlings and will often self-seed.

CONTAINER GARDENING

Containers add a pop of color and design to gardens, they allow you to create microclimates within a small space, and they can contain misbehaving plants. For people without access to land, container gardening transforms patios, porches, and rooftops into an herbal oasis.

Consider the Pros of Container Gardening

Attractive garden design: Pots cost more money than planting something in the ground but less than hardscaping (stone walls, picket fences, statues).

Expansion of your gardenable space: Place planters on steps, walls, patios, porches, rooftops, walkways, and other plant-friendly spots, whether you have an in-ground garden or not. Grow plants such as gotu kola, lemon balm, and culinary herbs indoors for winter or if you have no outdoor space.

Portability: The freedom to easily move from one location to another benefits tender perennials (lemongrass, gotu kola) that live outdoors in summer, and inside during winter, and plants like basil that you want to save from those first few frosts to extend their lifespan.

Containment: Potting up voracious root runners prevents plants like mint and bee balm from running amok in your garden or yard.

Decorative protection: Hanging planters add vertical space, eye-catching design, and keep tender leafy plants like gotu kola out of hungry animals' reach.

Container Cons

Containers cost money, especially if you opt for new large pots (which are generally preferred), ceramic pots, and artfully designed pots.

Soil dries out quickly, and plants require more water, fertilizer, and attention than when grown in the ground.

Not all plants like to be contained, particularly those that have big root systems or like to spread.

Container plants probably won't grow as big and lush as the same plant planted in a plush garden bed.

Outdoor potted plants are more susceptible to cold in winter. Plants that would've survived in the ground might freeze down to the roots and die in a pot. Surround your plastic pots with a mound of wood chips to the top of the pot to protect them for the winter. Terra-cotta and ceramic pots break during a hard freeze — they need to be brought indoors in winter or emptied of soil to store in a garden shed.

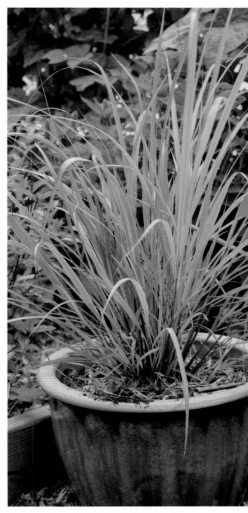

Growing lemongrass (a tropical, tender perennial) in a pot enables you to overwinter it indoors.

Create Microclimates

Use terra-cotta pots for plants that like dry soil (rosemary, cayenne).

Choose plastic and glossy ceramic to retain moisture (bacopa, gotu kola, basil).

Place container plants (cayenne, passionflower, lemongrass) on sunny steps, on walls, or near buildings to add heat and protection from elements.

Place containers in part shade, a moist corner, or a dish of water for plants that like it wet (bacopa, gotu kola).

Use different soil and watering schedules according to plants' needs.

Container Tips

Choose wisely. Containers generally work best for annuals that die at the end of the season and tender perennials that you want to bring indoors in winter. Most potted plants won't survive the outdoors in winter in cold climates unless you mulch them into a pile of wood chips.

Save money on pots by using terra cotta or plastic, scouting out thrift shops or discount stores, asking for hand-me-downs from gardeners, and repurposing buckets and other vessels (repaint if desired, and drill holes in the bottom for drainage).

Go big. Small pots — including the pots seedlings arrive in — will *not* sustain long-term growth, will require more attention (water, fertilizer), and will stunt your plant's growth.

Work your way up. Plants do better if you gradually upgrade the size of the pot by about 2 inches in diameter when the roots begin to fill the pot. (I admit, I don't always do this and just go right for the big pot.) You want adequate room for the roots to grow but not so much space that the soil stays waterlogged between watering, especially for plants like rosemary that hate excess moisture. Root-bound plants should be repotted.

Water correctly. Potted plants dry out quickly and will need more regular watering — often daily or twice daily. If your plant is wilting, it needs water, and next time don't let it go that long. Plastic and glazed ceramic work better for plants that need to retain water. Hanging planters pose the greatest challenge.

Watering tricks. Timed drip irrigation is not that expensive and can be a godsend for outdoor containers. For an attractive low-tech alternative that works well for indoor plants, too, consider Plant Nanny stakes (into which you place repurposed wine bottles filled with water) or an olla. Self-watering containers and window boxes are available in a variety of sizes, with plenty of DIY plans available online.

Fertilize. Plants can easily run out of nourishment when their roots are confined by a container because they can't reach through the ground to access nutrition elsewhere once they've depleted the limited nutrient supply in the immediately surrounding soil; overwatering can make matters worse by washing away nutrients when the excess water flows out of the container's drainage holes. Add fertilizer (e.g., seaweed emulsion, nettle-comfrey leaf tea) to the watering can or soil periodically or dress with compost. Plants that go dormant in winter should not be fertilized until spring.

Ensure good drainage to avoid plants getting waterlogged and rotten, except for the very few plants that like wet feet (bacopa, gotu kola). If your planting vessel doesn't have drainage holes already, drill several small ones at the bottom.

Catch drainage. Indoors in particular, you'll want to place your pots in a dish to catch any overflow of drainage water, as the overflow could ruin your floors and furniture with water and mold.

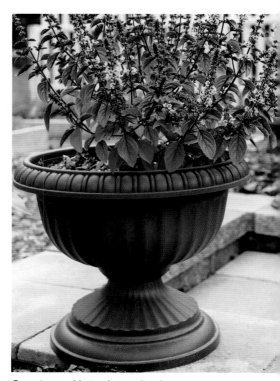

Containers add visual appeal and new garden space but require extra TLC.

Container-Friendly Herbs

Anise hyssop*	Chives	Mint*
Bacopa	Fennel*	Parsley
Basil	Gotu kola	Passionflower
Bay leaf	Korean mint*	Rosemary
Cayenne	Lemon balm*	Thyme
Chervil	Lemongrass	

*These plants fare better in large pots of 20 inches or more in diameter. Feel free to try other plants as well, especially if you've got a big pot like a whiskey barrel.

Avoid watering so much (or so infrequently) that water drains out — it pulls nutrients from your soil.

Find the happy place. Every plant has a happy place, and you may need to move a pot around at first, whether outdoors or (especially) indoors, to find the right mix of environmental factors such as sunlight and warmth. Browning tips, yellowing leaves, and long leggy stems are all signs that a plant is not happy. Lack of sun tends to be a problem indoors — consider a sun lamp.

Use good soil. You *might* be able to get by outdoors with a mix of compost, loam, and chopped leaves or perlite, but plants in containers do best with potting soil.

Watch for pests. Potted plants — especially indoor potted plants — are already at a disadvantage, so they're more susceptible to pests. Insects thrive indoors where the habitat is favorable for the pests (no predators, no rain, no cold). Wash leaves and use sticky traps, nontoxic sprays, pruning, and other methods to help control infestations. Extension services offer pest identification, prevention, and management tips.

Pop in flowers for extra color. Heartease pansy is a personal fave — it blooms all season long, doesn't need much water, and the flowers are pretty in infused water, in tea blends, and as a garnish.

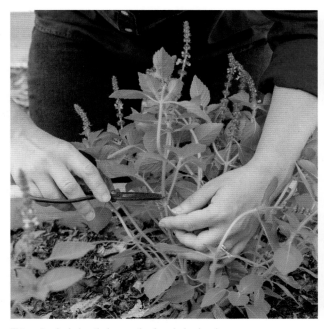

Trimming holy basil above a leaf node looks clean.

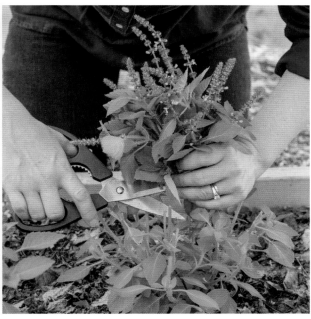

The "bad haircut" method speeds the harvest.

HARVESTING

Many new herbalists panic when it comes to harvesting time, not sure what to do and when best to do it. It's really easy! For specifics, refer to individual plant profiles (page 246). Generally speaking, though, harvest when that particular plant looks, smells, and tastes potent, flavorful, healthy, and vital. Basically, when it's "happy." Aromatic herbs possess more flavor harvested earlier in the day. If you're planning to dry herbs, harvest them after the dew has evaporated (and, if you're relying on warm, sunny weather for the dehydration process, check the forecast). Harvest flowers just as they open. Harvest roots and barks in spring or fall. That's the *ideal* scenario, but fit this process into your schedule. If that means you're out there late at night with a headlamp jumping at a frost warning or digging a root mid-June, so be it!

Leaves and Aerial Parts

"Aerial" refers to the aboveground parts of the plant, which may be in flower or not. Harvest in a way that encourages future growth while also giving you enough material for making remedies.

For herbs with leaves and stems that branch off from the main stem (most plants), harvest the top one-quarter to two-thirds of the plant, making sure to leave at least a few sets of leaves behind. The plant will look and recoup better if you trim *just* above a leaf node — this is where the new growth will take place. That said, if you're short on time, have a lot of plant material to harvest, or are working with a sprawling plant like thyme, you can give it a "bad haircut": bunch the material together in your hands and hack across the top portion in a straight line. The plant will look scraggly at first, but will grow back just fine.

For plants that do not branch or leaf out — like chives, parsley, and lemongrass stalks — you'll instead cut the plant right down to the ground, but leave one-third to two-thirds of the plant untouched. Chives and lemongrass's grassy tops (not the tightly rolled stalk part) can also be trimmed from the top.

Flowers and Buds

Pinch off the newly opened blossoms, including any green sepals or bracts at the base of the flower. Typically, the whole flower head is left intact (calendula, red clover, chamomile), but you may opt to remove only the petals (rose, dandelion). When drying flowers, lay them out in a single layer and consider using a dehydrator. You want to make sure the middles are *completely* dried or they will ferment and mold in storage.

Bark

Harvest bark in early spring when the sap is rising but the tree hasn't yet leafed out, or in fall once the leaves have begun to change color and drop. In a pinch, though, you *could* harvest bark at any time of the year; for example, when you're

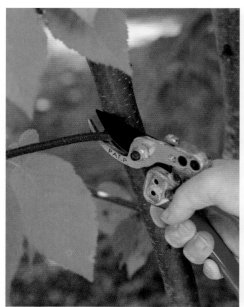 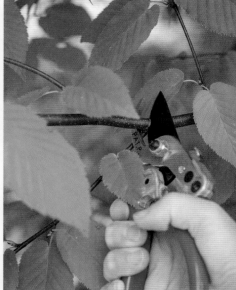

When harvesting bark, prune young branches with a thinning cut (left) or heading cut (right).

pruning the tree for vigor and shape. The medicinal part of bark is the inner bark — not the outer bark (which is more astringent and protective for the plant) nor the inner woody pith. The inner bark is often juicy, green, and aromatic.

Do not remove bark directly from a live tree. Prune the branches off first, aiming for twigs and branches up to approximately 1½ inches in diameter — you won't need to remove the outer bark from these young branches. How you prune will determine the tree or shrub's future growth. A "heading cut" is made above a strong node and will encourage the tree to bush out from that spot. A "thinning cut" removes the branch to the base of the trunk, junction, or the ground. You may

opt to take down a whole tree or take advantage of a blow-down after a storm; you'll need to remove the outer bark from wider branches and the trunk. I prefer harvesting bark from smaller branches and twigs — it's easier.

If there are any leaves on the pruned limbs, pull those off. Then use a knife or peeler to scrape off the bark and use clippers to trim up the twigs — this is what you'll use to make medicine. Sometimes the bark peels off easily, and you can just slice it down the length or mash it a bit between two rocks, then strip it by hand.

If you decide to tincture bark, consider adding 10 percent glycerine or honey. Bark's usually rich in astringent tannins, which precipitate out, making your tincture

gloppy and less potent over time. Glycerine helps stabilize and stall the process.

Roots

As with bark, roots are best harvested in spring or fall rather than when the plant is focused on putting out leafy growth and flowers, yet exceptions can be made if needed.

A garden fork loosens the soil around the plant and may suffice for digging up the roots. Depending on the plant and land, use a sharp spade or hori hori, particularly good for slicing a chunk off of a root crown. You can also work out the root with a digging stick, hori hori, or CobraHead. While this requires a little extra effort, it works well for roots that travel, like burdock and nettle, or those that are not hard to bring up, like mullein and valerian.

Once you've got your roots out of the ground, bang them against the ground or a rock to loosen and remove some dirt. Rinse them off with the power-wash setting of your garden hose sprayer and/ or dunk them in cold water and swish around vigorously. If dirt remains, remove with a potato scrubber and cold water. Roots should be processed fresh. Chop roots into smaller pieces with a hatchet, loppers, clippers, or wood chipper to dehydrate them or use fresh. Dry in a single layer in the oven at 100 to 120°F (38 to 49°C).

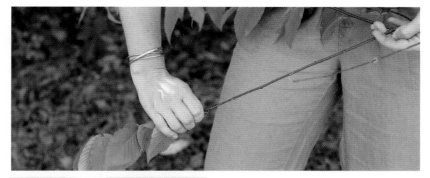

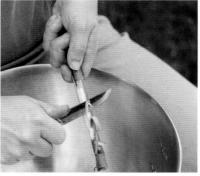

Harvest twigs and small branches for bark. Simply chop twigs, and peel bark from thicker branches.

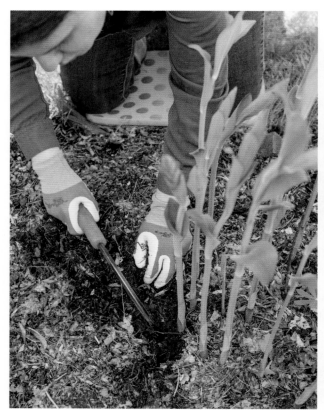 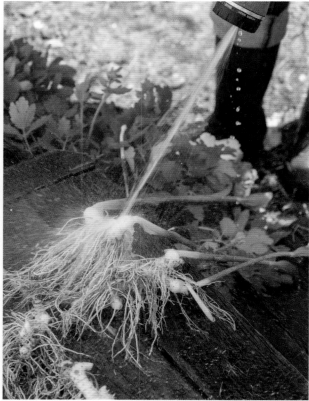

The CobraHead is one of several root-digging tools (left). The power-wash setting on a garden hose cleans roots quickly and easily (right).

PRESERVING HERBS

You've harvested your herbs, now it's time to *do* something with them! Those fresh plants might go straight into a remedy recipe (chapter 2) such as a tincture, or you may want to dry or freeze the plant for later use. First, if you haven't already, you'll want to pick through your plant material to remove anything that's buggy, dead, hitchhiking (live bugs, other plants), or otherwise undesirable, then move on to the next step.

Drying

Keep dried herbs on hand for making tea, cooking, and year-round remedy making. It's cheap and easy to dry herbs, particularly if you're not sure when or how you want to use them later. Most dried herbs, flowers, and fruits keep for at least 1 year in good storage conditions (page 30), longer for roots, bark, and mushrooms. They often keep well; most of what you buy online and in stores is already 1 to 3 years old. As long as your dried herbs still look, smell, and taste good, you can use them.

Dried herbs can take up a considerable amount of pantry and cabinet space, though. *Most* herbs can be used fresh or dried, with a few that are best fresh or best dried.

Milky oat seed, St. John's wort, and motherwort are nearly useless when dried and should *always* be used fresh. Dried skullcap, lemon balm, echinacea, California poppy, valerian, and rosemary can be used in recipes but will not be anywhere near as strong or effective as their fresh counterparts. Passionflower, calendula, lemon verbena, lemongrass, and linden make lovely dried herbs but lose potency more quickly than other dried herbs (in about 3 to 8 months). Take *extra*special care when drying these herbs

Should I Wash My Herbs?

Except for roots, we usually don't wash herbs. That's because introducing water will increase the risk of spoilage for drying herbs and several types of herbal preparations (glycerites, honeys). Simply ensure you're picking plants that are relatively clean (from dirt, pollen, animal manure, pollutants) and discard any questionable material.

If your plants are dirty, wash them off with a hose before you harvest them, let them air-dry, then harvest them. If you've harvested herbs that really do need to be cleaned, use cold water and a salad spinner, gently towel dry, then let them finish air-drying before proceeding with your processing. If you can dust off the dirt with a clean, dry brush or towel, do that instead. Roots should be washed in cold water as discussed on page 26.

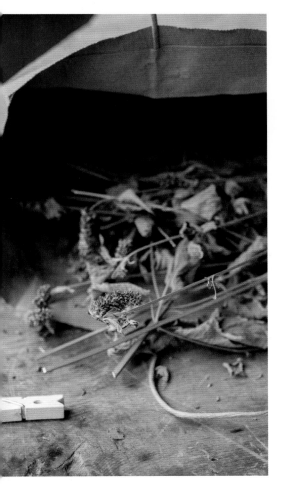

A brown paper bag, loosely packed, cinched shut, and placed on the car dashboard does an excellent job drying aerial parts of herbs.

to maintain maximum quality. In general, make tinctures with fresh plants if you have the option, dried if you don't.

Herbs best dried are wild cherry, elderberry and flower, horsetail, and alder due to potential toxicity or negative side effects in their fresh states. No matter what you're doing with them — even making a tincture — *these* plants should be dried first, with the exception of horsetail, which is fine tinctured fresh. (Fresh horsetail or elder can also be cooked instead.)

DRYING METHODS

Every herbalist will offer a different "best" way to dry herbs. The best method for *you* will depend on convenience, materials, space, climate, and the plant (and part) you're drying. Flowers, roots, and berries should be dried in a single layer. Leave aerial parts on the stem; use flowers whole;

fruit whole or cut into smaller pieces; mushrooms sliced; and roots chopped. Some mushrooms and roots are impossible to chop once dried.

Your goal is to have thoroughly crisp-dry plants. Any residual moisture could ferment or rot the plant in storage — this is a particular problem for flower heads and berries. Once your plant is dried, remove it promptly to process and store. Herbs get dusty and less potent if they sit around too long.

Air-Drying

In the iconic herbal kitchen, herbs hang by the rafters or over the woodstove, drying in bundles. Bring a few stems together with string or an elastic bland to hang them from pegs, or lay them flat on screens, preferably out of direct sunlight in a well-ventilated, dry area. Air-drying works best for leaves and flowers and (if the air is

dry enough) chopped roots and could take a few days to a week or longer. Use it for juicy herbs like basil and comfrey that turn black easily during the drying process. Air-drying works well if your air is dry. In high humidity, though, herbs won't get crisp-dry at room temperature. You could *start* your plants with air-drying to remove most of the moisture, then use a low-heat method to crisp them.

Low-Heat Drying

As humidity increases, bump up the heat and ventilation to dry your plants. Ideal maximum drying temperature for most herbs runs from 95 to 110°F (35 to 43°C) depending on the plant and outside humidity (higher for fruit, roots, mushrooms). Low-heat methods dry herbs quickly, which may actually result in *better* quality dried herbs versus those left to sit for

days or weeks air-drying. Check your plants every 6 to 24 hours and move them around if some areas are drying faster than others. Commercial herb growers construct drying sheds, hoop houses covered with shade cloth, or tobacco trailers to dry herbs this way.

Paper Bag in the Car

This is my favorite method for aerial parts and leaves! Loosely pack your bag with herbs, cinch it shut with a clothespin, and place it in the windshield of your car on a warm, sunny day. (If it's hot out, place the bags on the car seat or in a clean trunk.) Crack the window if it's really hot or your plants are particularly juicy. The bag protects the plant from direct sunlight and helps wick away moisture. A basket of herbs with another basket over it also works.

Dehydrator

Make sure your dehydrator is good quality and able to hit 95 to 110°F (35 to 43°C) for leaves and flowers, 125 to 135°F (52 to 57°C) for fruit, and somewhere in between for roots and mushrooms. Cheap dehydrators tend to

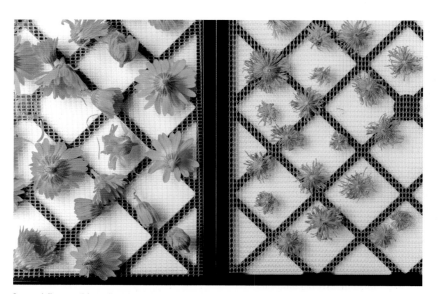

Spread flowers like calendula in a single layer in the dehydrator to ensure they dry completely through to the middle of the blossom.

get too hot, which is a particular problem for aromatic plants. If you notice a strong herb smell, it's too hot. Always get a bigger dehydrator than you think you'll need! Dry herbs in a single layer. Roots, fruit, and flowers dry *best* in a dehydrator. For herbs like basil and comfrey that turn black easily, make sure the dehydrator is not too hot and your plants are in a *single* layer. The Excalibur brand is good but pricey. Resourceful folks make their own. Make sure you can control the temperature.

OTHER METHODS

Some people use the stove and the microwave, but these are too hot for most herbs. Attics, sheds, and greenhouses work well. Hang herbs from a clothesline or suspended screens/racks or in brown paper bags. Make sure your drying space is clean, won't rust, is free of pests like mice and rats, and that you don't forget about your herbs.

Garbling

"Garbling" is the technical term (yes, really) for processing dried herbs to remove the leaves from the stem and break everything up into small "cut and sifted" pieces. The less broken down a plant is, the better it retains its quality in storage, but it's far easier to *use* your herbs if they're broken down a bit, and you can fit more material in a jar once they're cut and sifted.

Once your herbs are crisp-dry, hold them over a large bowl or bin and garble by hand, stripping the leaves off the stem and removing any additional large stems (for prickly nettle, raspberry, and comfrey leaves, wear clean gloves). Then crumble up the herbs with your hands.

Or, create a "rubbing screen." Cover a box or bin with galvanized hardware cloth, stainless steel mesh, or a plastic screen (something that won't rust) and rub the herbs back and forth so that the broken leaves fall through into the bin while stems remain on top for easy removal. You may want different sizes of mesh for different plants.

Store flowers, fruit, roots, and mushrooms exactly as they come out of the dehydrator — no garbling necessary. You may be able to more finely chop up roots and mushrooms with a compact or conventional blender, wood chipper, or meat grinder.

Storing Dried Herbs

Heat, light, oxygen, and moisture degrade the quality of your herbs. Store dried herbs and shelf-stable remedies in a cool, dark, dry spot like a pantry or cabinet. Glass jars with tight-fitting lids work best. If you don't plan to use an herb for several months, use a mason jar vacuum sealer to further enhance the shelf life. This option isn't practical if you plan to open the jar more often.

FREEZING

Freeze herbs — especially culinary herbs — that lose their oomph once dried, such as basil, chives, and lemongrass stalks. Depending on the herb and how you want to use it, you can do this in several ways. Always label your products so you know what they are and how long they've been in storage. Store them in thick, freezer-safe bags or containers with as little air

Once your herbs are crisp-dry, "garble" them: remove the leaves and flowers from the stem. If desired, crush lightly to make them "cut and sifted" for easy use.

as possible. These should be used up within a few months to a year to avoid freezer burn.

Ice Cubes

Freeze chopped or puréed herbs in ice cube trays to plunk into recipes. Simply place chopped herbs in the tray covered with water, broth, juice, or other suitable liquid, depending on how you want to use the herbs. Once frozen, pop the cubes into a labeled bag or container. Any herb works. Great for smoothies, soups, sauces, and floral ice cubes (page 96). You can also juice herbs or make a slurry in water and then freeze that. Concentrated tea and herb broths freeze well, too (pages 36 and 153).

Frozen Paste

Oil locks in flavor and protects herbs from deterioration in the freezer — a trick I learned from culinary herbalist Susan Belsinger. Purée fresh leaves with your oil of choice (olive oil, or something mild for baked goods). Fill a ziplock bag, flatten, and squeeze out as much air as possible. Freeze flat. Then you can easily pull off a chunk of frozen herb-oil to add to soups, stews, sauces, and baked goods. Good candidates include lemon balm (for cake), basil (for pesto), cilantro (for salsa), curry paste, and parsley.

Herb Butter

Fold finely chopped herbs into softened butter. Shape, freeze, and store to pull out for later use in cooking or on bread. Great for chives, parsley, chervil, lemon balm, and savory or sweet blends.

Vacuum Seal

A few rugged herbs stay fresh when simply frozen in a bag or container, particularly chives and lemongrass stalks. If you have a surplus, you can keep whole herbs fresher longer by vacuum sealing them, which works well for parsley and to some extent for cilantro and basil (use immediately upon opening the bag). The freezer breaks down the cell walls of these tender herbs, making them a bit mushy, so they're best used in cooked recipes.

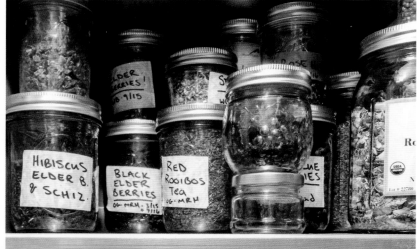
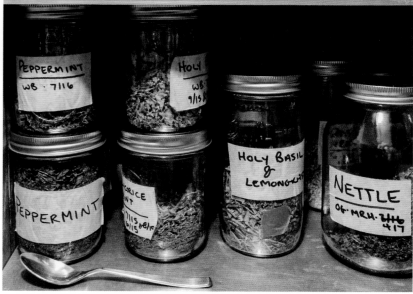

Store dried herbs and shelf-stable remedies in a cool, dark, dry cabinet or pantry. Masking tape makes great labels.

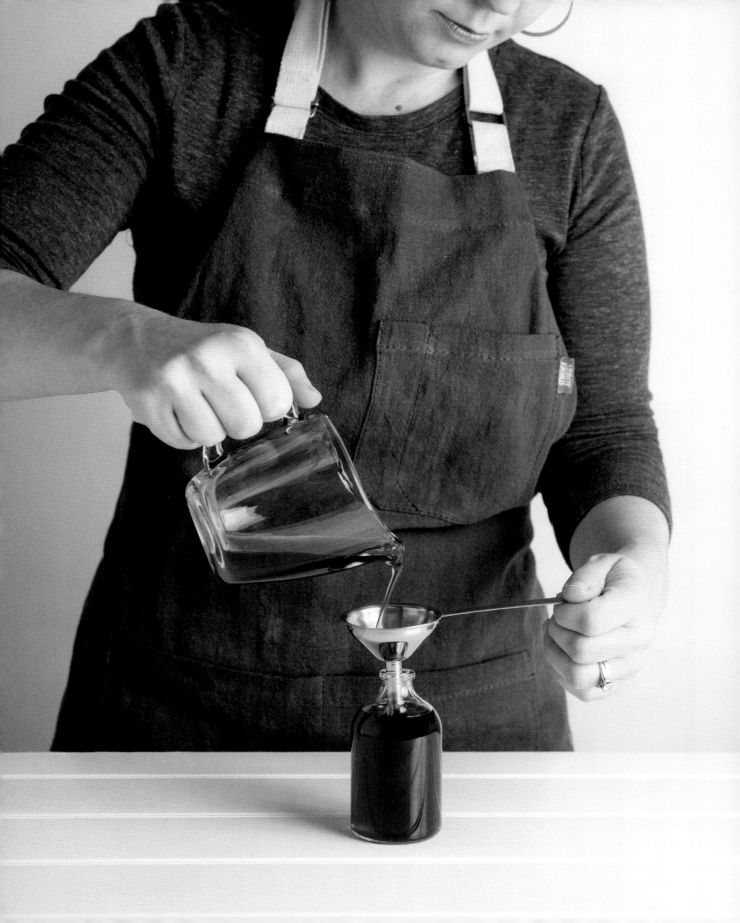

CHAPTER
TWO

Mastering
Basic Remedies

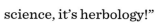

CRAFT STELLAR herbal remedies in your
kitchen that surpass anything you
can buy in stores. It's amazingly easy
and fun. The basic method for most
recipes: shove herbs in a jar, cover
them with something (e.g., alcohol,
vinegar, honey), then strain them
after a few weeks. Or simmer them
on the stove, then strain them.
As my teacher Michael Moore
would say, "This isn't lab
science, it's herbology!"

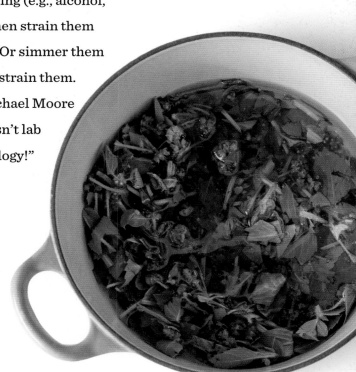

Aside from eating plants directly, extracting them in water is the purest, simple, affordable, and easy way to take medicinal herbs. Hot water extracts a wide range of constituents from a plant, including aromatics and minerals, delivering them in an easily digested form. Most herbal remedies involve extracting constituents with a solvent. In the case of water, it's hydrating, healthy, gentle, and safe for anyone.

Some tea connoisseurs believe that "tea" can *only* be made with the tea plant (i.e., *Camellia sinensis* — green tea, black tea, white tea). The rest are "herbal tisanes." Poppycock. Remember, herbalists are generalists. Any plant (or mushroom) extracted in water is a tea in my book. Even broth could be construed as tea.

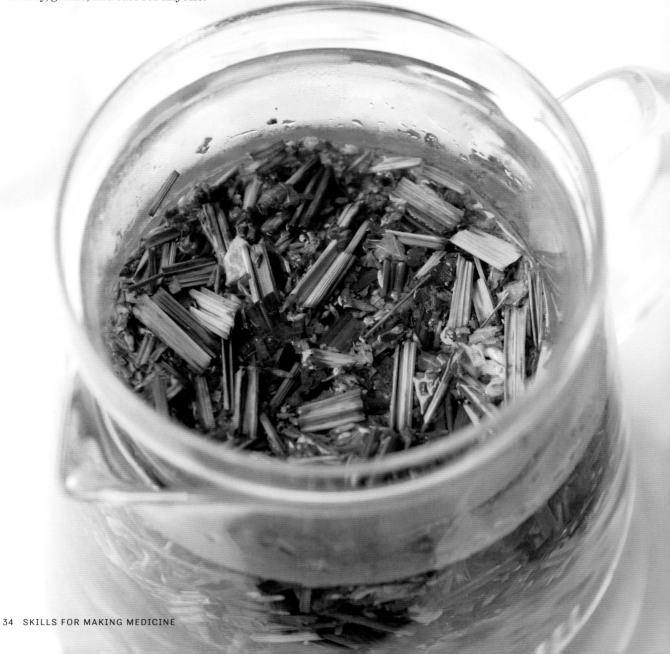

TEA INFUSION

WHEN WE INFUSE HERBS, we *steep* them in water, typically hot water. Leaves, flowers, and aromatic plants — those that are delicate and offer their medicine easily — should be steeped. They may lose potency with simmering. Dried herbs usually lend themselves better to the water than fresh plants. French press pots, in-mug infusers, and teapots or travel mugs with stainless strainers for infusion work well for this. Feel free to play around with how much herb you use, how hot the water is, and how long it steeps — it all works, but you'll notice subtle differences in strength and flavor.

1 heaping teaspoon to 1 heaping tablespoon dried herb

8–16 ounces near-boiling water

Suggested tools: vessel, strainer/infuser, mug

1 Place your herb in the vessel, cover with hot water. If desired, cover the vessel as it steeps (which will hold the aromatics in, though this isn't absolutely necessary).

2 Strain and drink. The duration of steeping will depend on the plant. Unlike true tea, most herbs should be steeped at least 10–15 minutes and will tolerate much longer steeping times (even hours). High-mucilage herbs like marshmallow root and mineral-rich herbs like nettle can be steeped for 4–12 hours.

3 Refrigerate any extras for up to 1–3 days.

VARIATIONS

Fresh Herb Infusion: While most herbs infuse best dry, aromatic herbs like holy basil and lemon balm work well fresh, but you'll need more plant material and time. Unless you want a really light infusion, use a handful of herb per 16 ounces of water and infuse for 20 minutes. Refrigerate extras for 1–2 days.

Super Infusion: Use this method for mineral-rich herbs and supersafe tonics and when you want *strong* medicine. Steep 1 ounce by weight in a 32-ounce French press pot or mason jar for 4 hours or overnight. Strain and squeeze out as much liquid as possible. See page 78 for more.

Cautions: Only use plants from clean soil (super infusions extract heavy metals, too), and bacterial growth may occur with long-term countertop infusions. If you're concerned about bacteria, opt to decoct (page 36) instead or move your tea to the fridge once the water has cooled. Refrigerate extras for 1–2 days.

Water Infusion/Seltzer: This makes a very light, refreshing, and hydrating beverage highlighting the plant's flavorful aromatics. Steep approximately three large sprigs of fresh herb per liter of water or plain seltzer for 30 minutes. Refrigerate extras, drink within 6–12 hours. See page 97 for more.

TEA DECOCTION

WHEN WE DECOCT HERBS, we *simmer* them in water. This method works best for roots, bark, and mushrooms as well as herbs rich in minerals, polysaccharides, and carotenoids — basically tough plant parts and constituents that extract best with more heat over time. Again, feel free to play around with the exact quantity of plant material and how long you simmer it depending on how strong you like it.

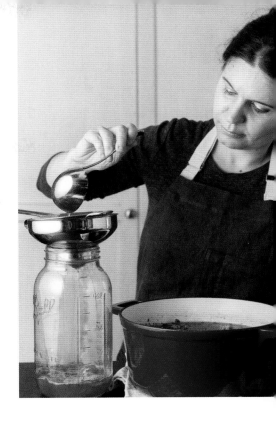

1 heaping teaspoon to 1 heaping tablespoon dried herb

8–16 ounces water

Suggested tools: pot, hand strainer, mug

1   Place herbs in the pot, bring to a boil, then reduce to a simmer.

2   Simmer for 20 minutes or to taste. (Decoct mushrooms for *hours,* even days.)

3   Strain and enjoy. Refrigerate extras and drink within 2–3 days.

Iced Tea, Two Ways

Iced tea tastes great in summertime! Here are two ways to do it.

Double Strength: Brew your tea as you would for a hot tea (see page 35 and above), but use *twice* the plant material. Strain your tea over ice cubes. Make sure to do this in a container that can handle heat and cold simultaneously — most ceramic and glass vessels will break, but tempered glass and stainless steel should hold up.

Chill It: If you've got time to plan ahead, brew your tea as you normally would, then transfer the chilled tea to the fridge until it's cold. Serve over ice.

Tea Ice Cubes: Add extra panache to your iced tea by freezing your favorite teas in ice cube trays to add to iced tea or purée into frozen drinks and smoothies. For more on herbal ice cubes, see pages 31 and 96.

VARIATIONS

Broth: Think outside the teapot! When you simmer ingredients in broth, you're essentially making a decoction. See pages 80, 81, and 153 for recipes and directions.

Thermos Cheat: The results are not quite as strong as an actual decoction, but you can do a long steep (1 or more hours) of many "decoction herbs" in a very well-insulated thermos. Convenient on the go.

A tincture is a liquid extract made with alcohol. Alcohol is as good, and sometimes better, for extracting most plant constituents as water, and it makes a far more concentrated product. Instead of drinking a whole cup of tea, you take just ⅛ to 1 teaspoon of tincture. Dilute your tincture in a little bit of water (or whatever drink you like) when you take it because the high alcohol content can burn your mouth. Alcohol extracts have a long shelf life — 5 to 10 years! — and they do a fine job preserving fresh plant properties that get lost in the drying process. They absorb rapidly into the body, bypassing digestion. But they *do* contain alcohol, which can be a problem for people who abstain for health or religious reasons.

CONCERNED ABOUT ALCOHOL?

In typical doses of 1 to 3 ml, you'll get very little alcohol effect from your herbal tincture. However, some people with alcohol issues (including addiction, allergy/sensitivity, special diets, and religious concerns) may want to avoid alcohol entirely. Instead of tinctures, turn to all the other forms of herbal remedies including glycerites (page 50), vinegar or oxymel (page 46), powders or capsules (page 56), and tea (page 35).

Tricky Tinctures

The alcohol proofs (percentages) offered in my recipes work as a general rule for most herbs. However, some herbs and constituents require a different treatment. See individual plant profiles for specific recommendations, but here are some general exceptions and considerations.

Resins: Resins repel water and require high-proof alcohol of 70 to 95 percent (151- to 190-proof) for optimal extraction. Pure resins include pine resin/pitch, boswellia, and myrrh. Pure resin tinctures are finicky in blends, sometimes precipitating out into a resin glob at the bottom of the bottle. High-resin herbs (which are not quite so finicky but still do best with relatively high alcohol extractions) include evergreen needles, poplar buds, and turmeric root.

Mushrooms: Polysaccharides (the complex starches in mushrooms that support the immune system) extract better via hot water decoction than in a typical tincture. You can cheat the system by doing a double-extraction tincture (page 42). This is ideal for mushrooms, which have an additional confounding factor of chitin fiber blocking the availability of many useful constituents; several hours of hot water extraction helps break that chitin down to release the mushroom's constituents.

Mucilage: Mucilage repels alcohol and extracts best via cold water, though hot water extracts also work. High-mucilage herbs include marshmallow and slippery elm. We usually use tea or powder rather than alcohol extracts of these herbs, though a low-alcohol (30 percent) tincture or syrup offers some benefits for formulation.

Minerals: Alcohol does not extract minerals, though a double-extraction tincture (page 42) would. Vinegar is a better solvent for minerals, but so is super-infused or decocted tea (pages 35 and 36) and food forms. Mineral-rich herbs include nettle leaf and oatstraw.

Tannins: Tannins provide astringent, tightening, and toning activities. They love to bind to alkaloids, minerals, and other constituents, precipitating out into chunks and making your tincture gloppy and less effective. Add 10 percent food grade glycerine to high-tannin plant tinctures (or formulas that include high-tannin plants) — such as most barks, bacopa, and yellow dock — to stabilize them and improve their shelf life. High-tannin tinctures and formulas still have a shorter shelf life, but the glycerine extends it from a few months to as long as a few years.

FRESH PLANT TINCTURE

IF YOU HAVE FRESH PLANT MATERIAL AVAILABLE, go with that for a tincture rather than using dried herbs. It's almost always better, and in some cases, it's really the only way to go. (See pages 27 and 28 for the short list of plants best used *dried*, as well as those you really *must* do fresh.)

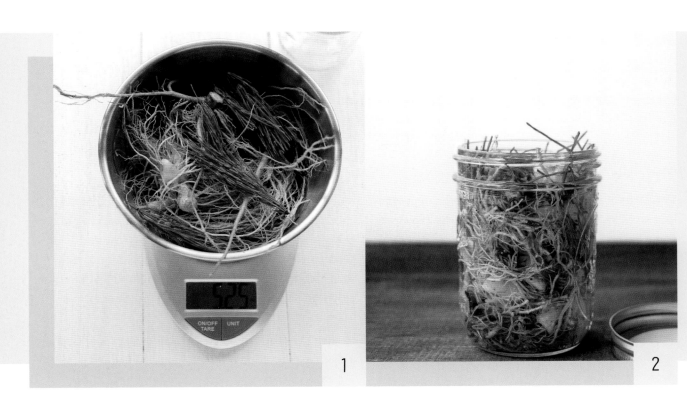

1

2

---

1 part by weight fresh herb

2 parts by volume 190-proof alcohol*

Jar with tight lid, scale, scissors or clippers

*NOTE: 190-proof vodka is sold in some states as ethanol or grain alcohol, though you can purchase food-grade organic grape and sugarcane ethanol online. Some states have banned 190-proof but offer 151-proof grain alcohol or vodka in stores, which will suffice. If this is not available, substitute 100-proof vodka, 80-proof vodka, or 80-proof brandy. The higher the proof, the stronger the extract.

1 Coarsely chop your plant material with clippers or scissors. Weigh it out.

2 *Shove* the material into the jar — for leaves and flowers, squeeze in as much as is humanly possible to get in there. For best results, use a jar that exactly fits what you need without extra space. See page 314 for reference.

I *love* making fresh plant tinctures. With minimal preparation time, you're rewarded with a fantastic extract, and you really experience your plant. High-proof alcohol sucks the water out of the plant and makes a better extract, but if you don't have access to it, see the note for alternatives.

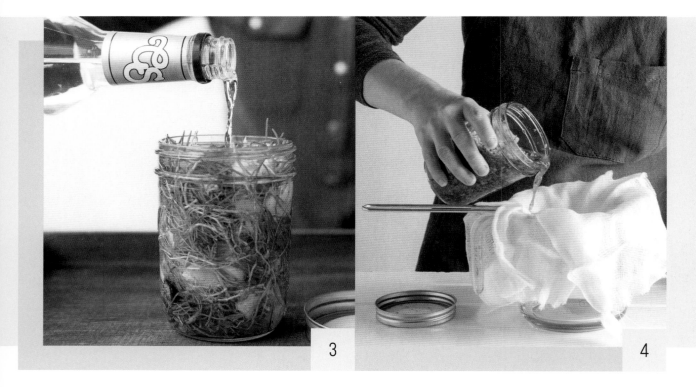

3 Cover to the tippy top of the jar with alcohol (even if this comes out to *slightly* more or less than the 1:2 ratio — it's more important to keep it covered). You may need to hold the plant material down as you fill the jar and use a knife or chopsticks to remove air bubbles. Put on the lid. No need to shake. Open the jar a few days later to top off the contents with a little more alcohol.

4 After at least 1 month, strain the mixture through a cloth. Squeeze out as much extract as you can with your hands. A potato ricer, wheatgrass juicer, or hydraulic tincture press will also work well here.

5 Pour into a dark glass bottle and store in a cool, dark, dry spot. The tincture will keep for 3–10 years.

DRIED PLANT TINCTURE

WE USUALLY TINCTURE DRIED PLANTS when fresh ones aren't available; for example, if you buy rather than grow them. For most plants, fresh is preferred but dried will do. However, a few plants are actually best tinctured when dried. Elderberry, elderflower, cherry bark, and alder bark have mild toxins and/or nauseating properties that are eliminated in the drying process. Many adaptogen roots, such as ashwagandha (shown here) are traditionally dried first to enhance potency.

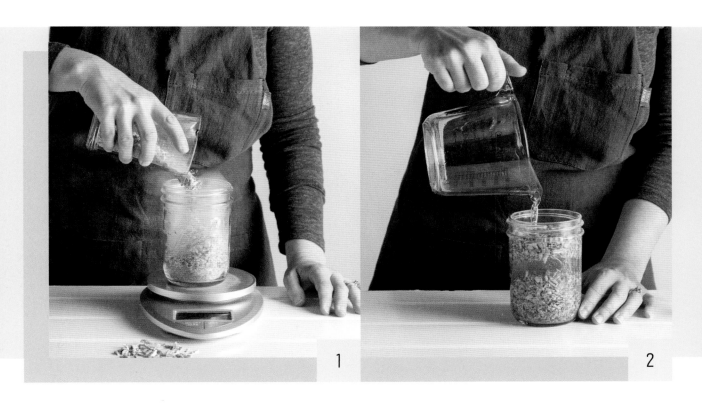

1 part by weight dried herb

5 parts by volume
100-proof vodka*

Jar with tight lid

*NOTE: Vodka, preferably 100-proof (50% alcohol), works well for most dried plants, but 80-proof brandy or vodka (40% alcohol) works in a pinch. Or mix 60 percent 190-proof ethanol with 40 percent filtered or distilled water to get approximately 60 percent alcohol in your finished tincture. As noted on page 37, use 10 percent food-grade vegetable glycerine with your alcohol for high-tannin plant material.

MAKING SENSE OF PROOF AND ALCOHOL PERCENTAGE

PROOF	% ALCOHOL	EXAMPLES	BEST FOR
190	95%	Ethanol (grain, grape, sugarcane)	Fresh plants, resins (preferred), diluting with water for other % alcohol
151	75%	Grain alcohol, vodka	Fresh plants, resins
100	50%	Vodka	Dried plants, acceptable for fresh plants
80	40%	Vodka, brandy	Topical liniments, acceptable for dried and fresh plants

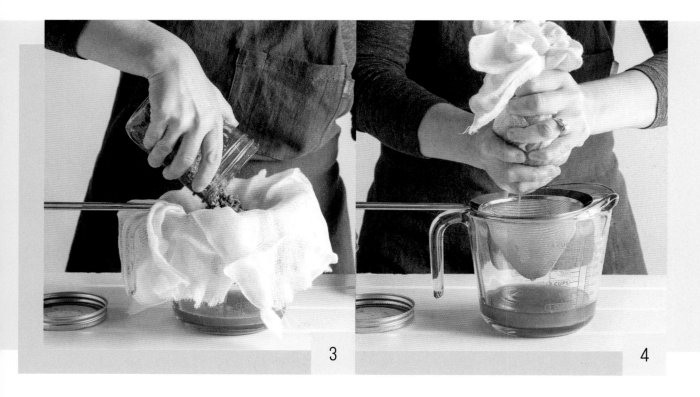

3

4

1 If desired, grind herb coarsely in a blender or crush with a mortar and pestle. This improves extraction but is not absolutely necessary. Place herb in the jar.

2 Cover herb with alcohol. Put on the lid and shake well. Shake regularly, every day or so.

3 After at least 1 month, strain the liquid through a cloth.

4 Squeeze out as much extract as you can with your hands. A potato ricer, wheatgrass juicer, or hydraulic tincture press will also work well here. Pour into a dark glass bottle and store in a cool, dark, dry spot. The tincture will keep for 3–10 years.

DOUBLE-EXTRACTION (DECOCTION) TINCTURE

THIS TINCTURE METHOD combines the decoction tea process with making a standard maceration tincture. It's useful for herbs and mushrooms that extract better in hot water but that you want to preserve and use like a tincture. This includes polysaccharide-rich mushrooms, mucilage-rich marshmallow, mineral-rich yellow dock, and allantoin-rich comfrey. Technically, you can use this method for any herb that you would decoct for tea, such as roots and barks, though these plants generally extract just as well in a standard fresh or dried herb tincture with *a lot* less effort.

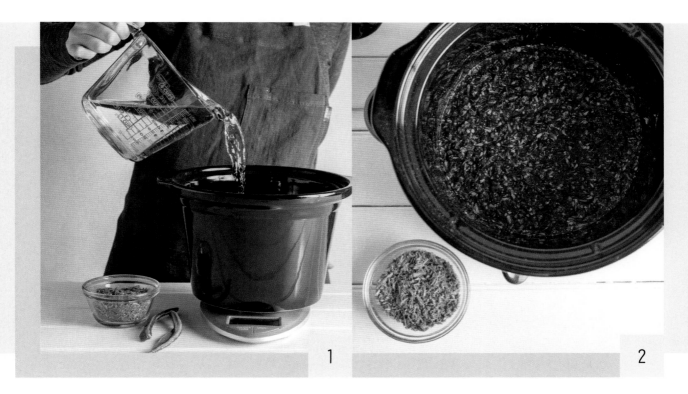

4 ounces dried plant or mushroom material*

About 12 ounces water (more if you plan to condense your "tea")

10 ounces 100-proof vodka

Quart jar with lid, metal strainer, 16-ounce or larger measuring cup, scale, pot with lid, large spoon; optional: grinder, cheesecloth, plant press

*OPTIONAL BUT PREFERRED: Grind your plant/mushroom material in a conventional or compact blender or coffee grinder until it's coarsely chopped or powdered.

1 Put your dried herbs in a large pot or slow cooker, and cover with water.

2 Simmer covered for at least 40 minutes. Mushrooms can be simmered for hours or days. Add more water as needed to keep everything covered.

For the double-extraction technique, some herbalists make their tincture first, strain the marc (which is tincture vocabulary for the dregs or leftover herb), decoct that, then add the tea to the tincture. Others make a separate decoction and tincture to blend together. Here, we make the decoction first, then add enough alcohol to ensure preservation and let it all macerate together as a tincture.

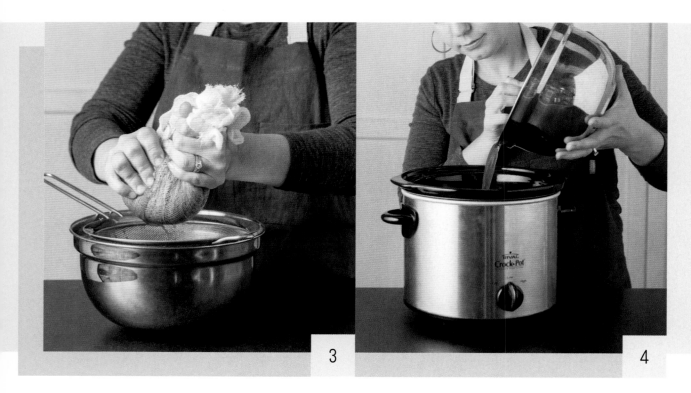

3   Strain the liquid to remove the herbs. Squeeze as much liquid out of the herbs as you can. (If you have one, a hydraulic tincture press, potato ricer, or wheatgrass juicer will work well.) Don't discard your strained herbs (a.k.a. marc). They will be used again in a later step.

4   Condense the liquid. You want 10 ounces of finished tea for your decoction tincture. If you have extra and would like to condense it, return the tea to the pot and simmer, uncovered, until liquid evaporates to get you to your 10-ounce goal.

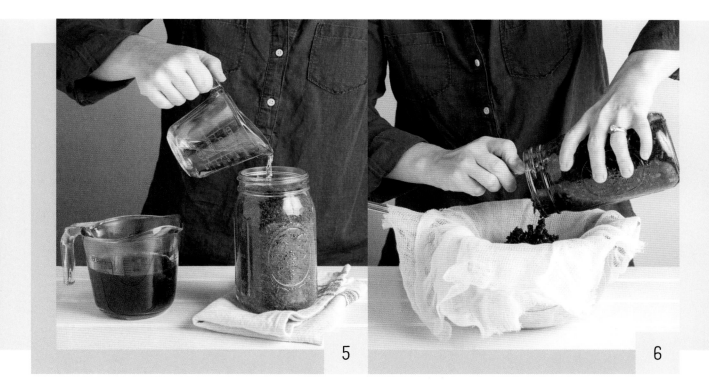

5

6

5   Put the marc into a quart mason jar. Pour in 10 ounces of decocted tea, then add 10 ounces of 100-proof vodka. Cap the jar tightly and shake.

6   Shake your jar every day or so. After a month, strain the contents, squeezing as much liquid out the herbs as you can. This is your finished tincture. It should be approximately 20–25 percent alcohol if made as directed, enough to keep it shelf stable for years. A typical dose is 1–2 ml, 1–3 times per day.

OTHER ALCOHOL PROOFS: Aim for approximately 20–30 percent alcohol or more to keep your finished product preserved yet still minimize alcohol's deleterious effects on mucilage and polysaccharides. (Herbs with constituents that tolerate alcohol can be made with 50–60 percent alcohol.) You'll need to calculate the percentage because most spirits are not 100 percent alcohol. To determine the percentage of alcohol in the spirits you're using, divide the proof in half (e.g., 100-proof vodka is 50 percent alcohol by volume).

I prefer using the highest proof spirits available because this allows me to use more of my decocted tea in the final product without compromising shelf stability.

DECOCTION TINCTURE CHEAT SHEET TO THE PROOFS

For the sake of simplicity, here's a cheat sheet to get 25 percent alcohol in your finished product. Note that you can use fresh plant material instead of dried, but you'll want to bump up your alcohol percentage a tad to compensate.

PROOF	% ALCOHOL IN SPIRIT	USE THIS MUCH WATER	USE THIS MUCH SPIRIT
151-proof vodka or grain alcohol	75% alcohol by volume	66.67% (⅔)	33.33% (⅓)
190-proof ethanol (made from grain, grapes, sugarcane, or corn)	95% alcohol by volume (treat it like 100%)	75%	25%
100-proof vodka	50% alcohol by volume	50%	50%
80-proof vodka or brandy	40% alcohol by volume	~35%	~65%

Liniment

A liniment is simply an alcohol extract (tincture) that you plan to apply topically. Liniments have a long shelf life, disinfect, and absorb into the skin quickly. They're quite versatile! Use them straight, apply as a spray, dilute them in water, shake them vigorously with an herbal oil (to improve glide and reduce alcohol irritation), use them as "waters" in a cream, and add a small amount to hydrosols to preserve them. You use a tincture as a liniment so that you have one product with multiple purposes. If you know you'll *only* use it topically, you may opt to use a lesser concentration of alcohol (25 to 40 percent) so that it's less irritating to the skin or use isopropyl "rubbing" alcohol, which costs *far* less but is toxic to consume. Popular plant choices for liniments include yarrow and St. John's wort.

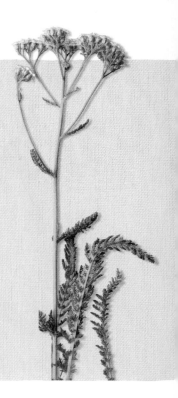

These shelf-stable liquid extracts can be used like tinctures, but the dose is a tad higher and they're not as potent or long lasting as tinctures. The recipes here include several alcohol-free options (glycerine, vinegar, oxymel honey, alcohol-free syrup) as well as sweet recipes that incorporate some alcohol (cordials, syrups with alcohol).

VINEGAR

VINEGAR IS RELATIVELY SHELF STABLE with decent extraction; it's not as potent as alcohol for most constituents, but it does well for alkaloid-rich plants (milky oat, berberines, lobelia) and is superior to alcohol for mineral-rich herbs (page 37). You can use vinegar topically as well (page 60). Vinegar lends its own healing properties: antiseptic, digestion enhancing, hypoglycemic. In culinary recipes, a splash of vinegar brightens flavor and can be used in salad dressing and marinades. Some people may not like or tolerate its sour flavor. Use apple cider vinegar (preferably raw) for medicinal vinegars; distilled white or apple cider for topical uses; high-quality clear vinegar (white wine, rice, champagne, organic distilled white) for colorful culinary recipes. Vinegars typically keep for at least a year. Fresh plant vinegars may not last as long as those made with dried herbs.

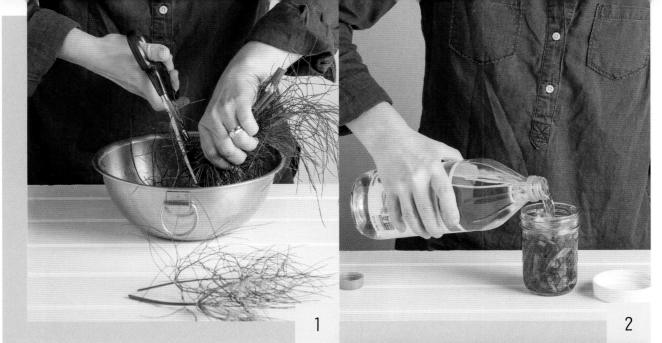
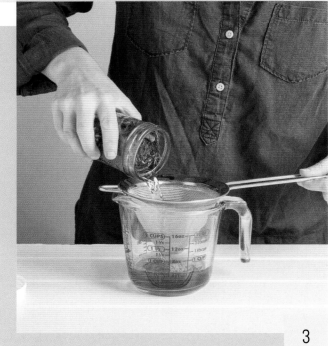

Fresh or dried plant material

Vinegar of choice

Jar with tight plastic lid

1 Coarsely chop fresh plant material, if using. Fill your jar loosely to the top with fresh plant material or approximately halfway with dried. (For medicinal tinctures, follow the fresh and dried plant tincture ratios on pages 38 and 40.)

2 Fill to the top with vinegar. Use a *plastic* lid (vinegar eats through metal, including mason jar lids, though completely lined lids might hold).

3 Shake regularly. Strain when the liquid tastes good, typically after 2–4 weeks.

VARIATION

Oxymel: To sweeten and smooth out your vinegar or make an alcohol-free "syrup," follow the instructions above using up to 50 percent honey (or to taste) combined with vinegar. The shelf life varies widely. Fresh plant oxymels may only keep for 3–6 months on the shelf though fire cider (page 236) lasts a year or more. Dried plant oxymels last longer. Store in the fridge or freezer to prolong shelf life.

HONEY

HONEY'S NOT A GREAT SOLVENT, but it *is* delicious! Honey makes a lightly medicinal extract that can be enjoyed simply for pleasure — by the spoonful, added to hot water for instant tea, and in dressings, dips, and marinades. Honey itself eases coughs and sore throats, even better when combined with herbs. Fresh plants taste great in herbal honey but are more prone to fermentation and spoilage because of the water present in them. The cooked method works better here (and can also be used for dried) to quickly extract the herbs in honey and help evaporate the excess moisture. However, you will lose the benefits of raw honey if you cook it.

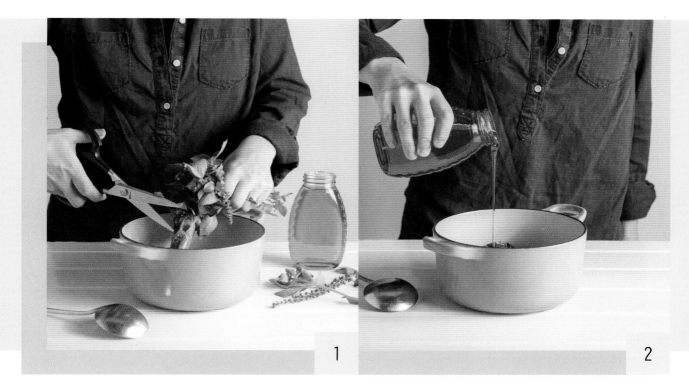

1
2

¼ cup chopped fresh
herbs or ⅛ cup dried

1 cup honey

Pot with lid, metal
strainer, heat-safe
pouring vessel, spoon,
jar with lid

NOTES: Honey boils at 160°F (71°C), which can be tricky to stay below with most cooking equipment. If you have a yogurt maker, you can leave your honey in that for about a day. You can also place it in a jar in the car on a warm day. Fresh plant honeys should be left uncovered to allow the moisture to evaporate.

Raw honey kept at or below 95°F (35°C) will retain its benefits.

Honey's heavy and is sold by weight, not volume. Its weight:volume ratio is approximately 2:3. So if you buy a 32-ounce jar of honey, the actual volume it will fill is approximately 20 ounces. Something to keep in mind if you want to fill a specific number of jars of a particular volume size.

You will lose the bit of honey that clings to your vessels and strained herbs. To avoid wasting it, pour hot water into your pot with the herb dregs, stir to dissolve the honey residue, then strain the dregs again. Enjoy this sweet tea hot or iced.

VARIATIONS

Raw Honey: This retains raw honey's health benefits. Best for dried herb due to moisture/spoilage with fresh plants, though you can use fresh and monitor for fermentation or mold. Cover your plant material with honey. Turn your jar every day or so (it's too thick to shake). Strain after 2–4 weeks.

Electuary: Sometimes used stirred into tea or taken by the spoonful. Powder dried herbs and mix with enough honey to make a thick paste. Enjoy ½–1 teaspoon as desired. This will keep for a year or far longer.

Honey-Alcohol Syrup: Add alcohol to your raw honey extract (fresh or dried plant material) to make a shelf-stable syrup. See page 52.

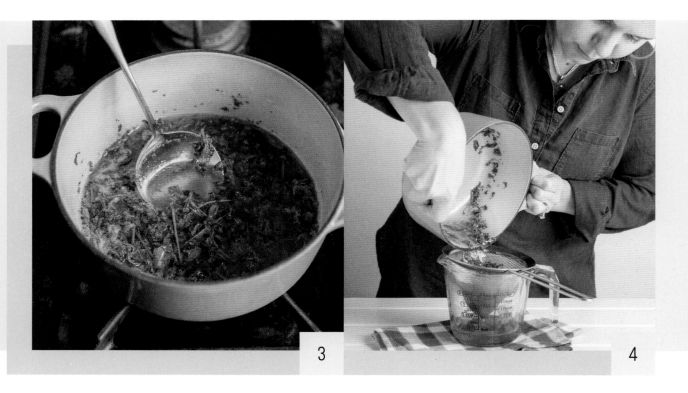

1 Coarsely chop fresh herbs (if using) or put dried herbs into the pot.

2 Cover herbs with honey.

3 Gently bring to a simmer, stirring regularly. Keep on as low a setting as possible. Once the honey begins to simmer, shut the heat off. Do not let the honey boil. Let it cool. Repeat the process at least two more times. You can do this the same day, or cover the honey once it's cooled and extend the process over several days.

4 After your last heating (when the herbed honey tastes good), strain it while it's still warm and pour into your jar. Once cool, check its viscosity. If it's watery, store it in the fridge and use it within a month. If it's as thick or thicker than the original honey, this should be shelf stable for at least a year. Crystallization is fine, but watch for any signs of mold or fermentation.

GLYCERITE

SWEET, SUGAR-FREE, AND ALCOHOL-FREE, glycerine's a popular substitute for alcohol extracts, particularly for children and recovering alcoholics. Glycerine soothes irritation and improves the flavor of blends, too. Consider it for throat sprays, bitters, flavor extracts, and as a "water" in creams. It keeps relatively well on the shelf. Glycerine does not kill germs like alcohol and vinegar, it simply maintains the current germ status, preventing further or future microbial growth. Downsides? Food-grade glycerine costs more than alcohol, yet it's not as potent or shelf stable, and you need to take a bigger dose. Use clean, sanitized equipment. Dried herbs will have a longer shelf life. *Well-made* glycerites can keep for a year or longer. If you want to be safe, you can store it in the fridge or freezer. I love this "sealed simmer" glycerite technique I learned from Thomas Easley and Steven Horne, which is done in a day. It's *excellent* for aromatic herbs.

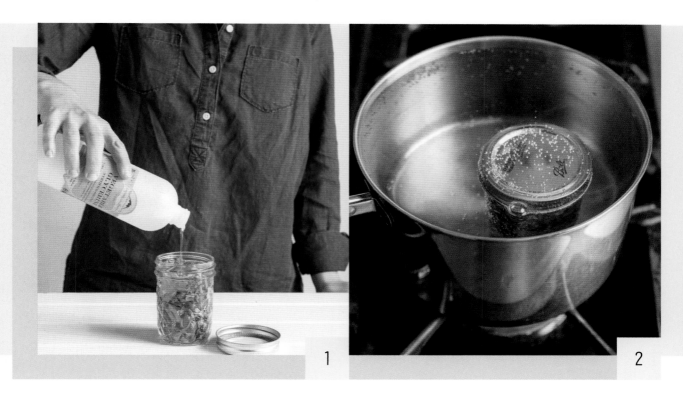

1

2

1 part dried herb or 2 parts fresh by weight

5 parts glycerine (70/30 glycerine/water for dried plants, 100 percent glycerine for fresh)

Canning jar with canning lid, pot that fits the jar, strainer, large glass measuring cup, jar-lifter tongs (optional)

VARIATIONS

Macerated Glycerite: Using the same ratios as on page 50, fill your jar to the brim, shake regularly or keep herbs submerged with a glass fermentation weight, and let it macerate as you would a tincture, straining after 2–4 weeks. Macerated rose petal glycerite is *delightful* (page 119).

Glycerine Transfer: If you'd like to remove the alcohol and water from a tincture to turn it into a glycerite, simmer equal parts (e.g., 1 ounce tincture plus 1 ounce glycerine) in a double boiler, uncovered, until all the water and alcohol have evaporated, leaving you with 1 ounce of glycerine extract in the pot. You will lose aromatics via this process but you may have a stronger extract of other constituents versus a standard glycerite.

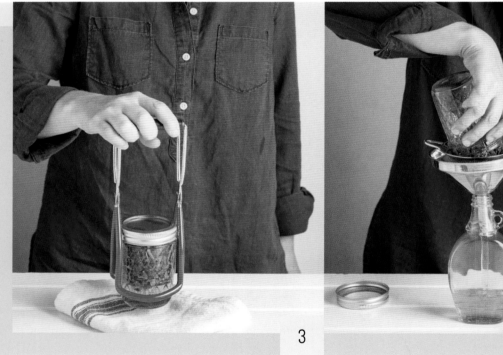

3

4

1 Cover your herb with glycerine (or glycerine/water), leaving approximately 1-inch headspace in the jar.

2 Screw on the canning lid. Place in the pot, cover completely with water, bring to boil, then reduce to a simmer. Simmer for 15 minutes or longer.

3 Remove the jar from the water bath with a canning jar lifter.

4 Let the jar cool completely before straining.

SHELF-STABLE SYRUP

SYRUPS ARE TRADITIONALLY made by making a strong tea, then dissolving a *lot* of sugar into it (see simmered syrup, right). I prefer *this* method, which makes a stronger, more shelf-stable recipe using less refined sugar thanks to the addition of alcohol. Syrups are typically taken by the teaspoon.

> Chopped fresh herb or dried plant material
>
> Honey (preferably raw)
>
> 100-proof vodka
>
> Jar with lid, strainer, measuring cup

1 Loosely fill your jar with fresh herb (half full for dried).

2 Cover with a combination of 50 percent honey, 50 percent vodka. (Because 100-proof vodka is 40–50 percent alcohol, your final syrup will be approximately 20–25 percent alcohol by volume.) Shake vigorously to combine.

3 Shake periodically and strain after 2–4 weeks.

NOTE: Substitute glycerine for honey to make this sugar-free. To make this shelf stable, aim for 25% alcohol in the finished product (see page 45).

VARIATIONS

Honey, Glycerite, Oxymel: All three of these remedies (pages 48, 50, and 47) have a syrup-like consistency, good shelf life, and similar dose range and can easily be used as an alcohol-free "syrup" substitute.

SIMMERED SYRUP

THIS IS THE CLASSIC METHOD for making a syrup. Although the shelf-stable syrup (left) lasts longer and tends to work better for many herbs, simmered syrup is great for extracting minerals, mucilage, and polysaccharides, which you don't get as much of with the shelf-stable macerated syrup. Syrups will last longest if you use refined white sugar, though raw sugar, glycerine, molasses, or honey could be substituted with varying preservative properties. Blackstrap molasses works well in nutritive syrups, but it's not very preservative and will need to be refrigerated and consumed within 1 to 2 weeks.

> Chopped fresh herb or dried plant material
>
> Sugar, honey, molasses, maple syrup, or glycerine

1 Make a double- to quadruple-strength tea via decoction (see page 42), then strain. For decoction-friendly herbs (roots, mushrooms), you can condense your syrup further by simmering the strained tea uncovered to the desired volume, which will make a stronger syrup. (For herbs that are best infused, simply steep your double- to quadruple-strength tea rather than decoct it. Though not "simmered," you can still use it to make a syrup.)

2 Measure your final liquid "tea" and add an equal amount of sugar, honey, molasses, maple syrup, or glycerine. While it's still warm, stir to combine.

3 Bottle and refrigerate. It is not shelf stable. Sugar- and glycerine-based syrups should keep for several months refrigerated. Honey should last for approximately a month in the fridge; molasses- and maple syrup–based syrups for 1 to 2 weeks. Freeze extras for longer storage.

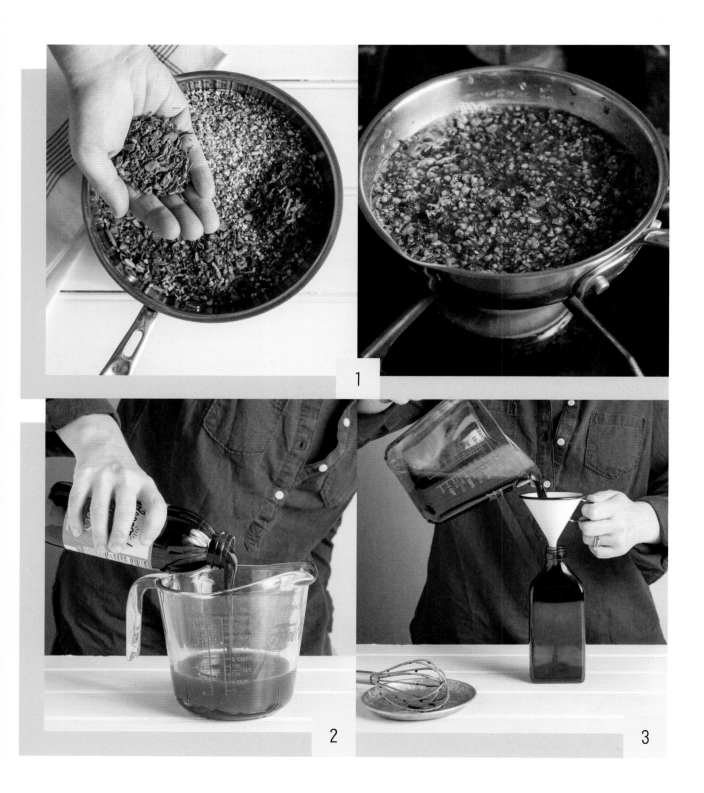

CORDIAL

MORE TREAT THAN MEDICINE, cordials offer a fun way to enjoy healing herbs. Digestive cordials (see bitters on page 134, Sweet Fennel Liquor, page 146) are popular, but you can also make heart tonics (Linden-Honey Cordial, page 231), aphrodisiac elixirs, or bedtime nightcaps. Sip them from a shot or cordial glass after a meal, add a splash to seltzer, or incorporate them into homemade cocktails. Cordials keep for several years on the shelf, but they lose color, flavor, and potency over time. Use your imagination and play around with the recipe!

Fresh herbs, dried herbs, and/or fruit

Simple syrup (see note), honey, or maple syrup

High-quality 80-proof vodka, brandy, or other spirit

Jar with lid, strainer, measuring cup

---

1 Loosely fill jar with chopped fresh herbs and/or fruit (half full for dried herbs).

2 Cover with a combination that is one-third simple syrup and two-thirds vodka/spirits. Shake well.

3 Shake daily and taste regularly. Strain as soon as the mixture tastes good, which may be the case in as little time as a day — letting it steep longer may actually hamper the flavor by letting it get too strong. Fresh fruit and herbs are usually best within 1–3 days. Dried herbs can stay in the infusion for as long as you like before you strain it.

NOTE: Simple syrup can be made by simmering 2 cups sugar in 1 cup water until dissolved. This keeps for several months in the fridge. You can infuse herbs into the simple syrup as if you were making a tea, or use tea in place of water. Herbal simple syrups should be refrigerated or frozen.

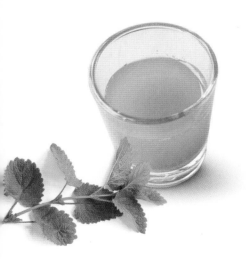

Herb powders can be used in a myriad of ways. Any herb that retains its properties dried (page 28) can be ground into a powder, but keep in mind that powders lose potency more quickly than a cut/sifted herb due to the increased surface area. You may find it impossible to grind dried herbs into a perfect powder with kitchen equipment. A compact or conventional blender or coffee grinder should work for leaves and flowers. Sift the ground herbs through a fine-mesh metal strainer or flour sifter to get a better powder. A suribachi, a grooved mortar and pestle meant for powders and pastes, also works. Roots and barks usually call for fancier tools. Unfortunately, *really* good powdering equipment costs too much for the home herbalist ($10,000 for a well-made hammer mill), but stainless steel Chinese grinders do a decent job and are a bit more economical ($100 to $200). Truth be told, the easiest way to work with powders is to buy them ready-made, but since the quality of powders on the market is so iffy, you may choose to make your own from herbs in your garden.

Cool Things You Can Do with Powder

Powders can easily be added to food and recipes. They're *much* more concentrated compared to cut/sifted dried and fresh herbs, so you get a lot of bang for your buck. Exact ratios vary widely depending on the density of the herb, but 1 teaspoon of powder equals approximately 2 grams or five capsules, ¼ cup dried cut and sifted herb, or 1 cup fresh. Ideal for safe, tonic, relatively tasty, and nutritious herbs. Besides powdered spices and cocoa/cacao, other popular powdered herbs include nettle leaf, marshmallow root or leaf, fennel seed, hawthorn berries, mushrooms (for cooked recipes only), maca, cayenne (just a pinch!), and ashwagandha root.

- Stir into water or juice and drink. Not amazing, but nice for people who hate tea and don't want alcohol.

- Stir into oatmeal, hummus, smoothies, soup broth, applesauce, yogurt, baked goods, casseroles, stir-fries, and other dishes.

- Stir into animal feed or baby food.

- Mix into honey to make a paste (which is called an electuary).

- Stir into hot milk (dairy, rice, soy, nut, seed, or other), sweeten with honey or maple syrup.

- Blend with a nut butter and honey, roll into balls, then roll in cocoa/cacao powder, toasted coconut, or sesame seeds — yummy medicinal energy snack!

- Blend with melted chocolate, dates, chopped nuts, seeds, and/or and other ingredients to make herbal chocolate truffles, fudge, and other treats.

CAPSULES

YOU CAN EASILY MAKE YOUR OWN HERB PILLS at home by putting powder into capsules. You'll get more bang for your buck with other powder techniques (see variations), teas, and tinctures, yet capsules work well for convenience and herbs you just don't want to taste. Store them in a glass jar with a tight lid in a cool, dark, dry spot for up to a year. "00" capsules hold 300 to 500 mg of herb. "0" capsules hold less, "000" capsules hold more. If you use a capsule machine, make sure the machine size matches your capsule size. But the exact amount of milligrams of herb per pill varies according to powder density and how tightly you pack the capsules. To discern your exact dose, put a kitchen scale in "gram" mode, zero it out with 10 empty capsules, remove those, and then weigh 10 full capsules. Divide the grams by 10, and you'll have your approximate quantity of herb per pill (1 g = 1,000 mg).

Ground herb

Empty capsules ("00")

Small, shallow bowl or capsule machine

To make a formula, measure your herbs by weight, then stir or grind together so they're well mixed.

To make capsules by hand, place your powder in a small, shallow bowl. Pull apart an empty capsule. Scoop the powder into both sides, then snap the capsule shut. (Tedious for large quantities but easy if you just need a few.)

To use a capsule machine, load the machine with the empty halves of the capsules. Sprinkle the powder over the side of the capsule machine with the larger half of the capsule evenly, using the scraper and tamper to push it over all of them and to push it down to get more in. Once the capsules on that side of the machine are full, remove any extra herb powder, and follow the manufacturer directions to snap them together. (You don't fill the small capsule half when using a capsule machine.)

VARIATIONS

Lozenges and Pastilles: No capsule machine needed! Great for "chill pills," bitter pastilles, and sore throat lozenges. Use your herb powders to make a dough/paste with honey/glycerine and water (add marshmallow root powder to help the mixture stick together if needed). Roll it into a long, thin "log." Slice it into small pieces (roll into balls if desired). Make sure they're a comfortable size to suck on or swallow. Dry in a dehydrator. If desired, sprinkle the pieces with herb powder or powdered sugar so they don't stick to each other. There are plenty of recipes available online.

Essential oils immediately come to mind when you see the word "aromatherapy," but the art of plant aromas can be so much more than that. You attain the benefits of aromatherapy when you brush by an herb in your garden or rub and inhale a potted plant in your windowsill. Essential oils are *highly* concentrated aromatherapy extracts, and while they can be excellent, potent therapeutic healing agents, you can make effective, safer aromatherapy remedies in your own kitchen. It's not practical to make essential oils at home due to the equipment and humungous amount of plant material needed. Lavender, which produces essential oil easily, requires approximately *16 pounds* of buds (each pound's the size of a throw pillow) to make 1 *ounce* of oil. Meanwhile, you need *1 ton* of rose petals to steam distill 1 ounce, which is why true, pure rose essential oil runs $600 to $1,000 a

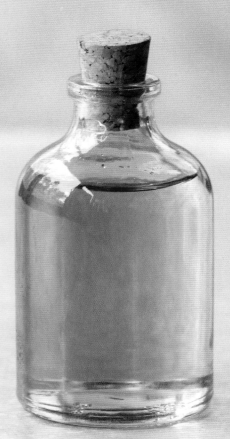

bottle. So, what can a home herbalist do? Plenty! Enjoy these tips, including several borrowed from the vivacious herbal aromatherapist Jessica LaBrie.

- **Steam:** Bring water to a boil, add herbs, remove from heat, cover. Let steep for a few minutes. Then open the lid, lean over the water, and cover yourself with a towel. Make sure the water has cooled enough so that the steam won't burn your skin.
- **Hydrosols:** Hydrosols extract distilled water with a few drops of essential oil, making a lightly aromatic remedy that you can use in food and elixirs, for topical application, and for aromatherapy. Directions on page 58.
- **Aromatic alcohol extracts:** Basically, you make a tincture (page 37), with the goal of aromatherapy. Many aromatics extract nicely in alcohol. You can strain aromatic tinctures within a few hours to 1 week (as opposed to the usual month of maceration) — they often smell better with a short maceration. Use aromatic tinctures as sprays or perfume, or add them to hydrosols to make them more shelf stable and add complexity to the aroma.
- **Glycerites:** Glycerine extracts (macerated or simmered still) do a lovely job capturing the aromatics of a plant, and you can use the glycerite internally or externally. Directions on page 50, Rose Glycerite on page 119. Holy basil makes a *divine* glycerite.
- **Tea, infused waters:** Drinking a cup of tea or infused waters provides aromatherapy inside and out! See pages 35–36 for recipes. Short shelf life, though.
- **Baths, soaks:** Aromatherapy while you relax! You'll absorb healing properties through your skin and inhale them simultaneously. Directions on page 60.

HYDROSOL

HYDROSOLS, ALSO CALLED FLOWER WATERS, can be made from any plant material that retains its aromatics when simmered, which includes roses and mint-family herbs. Lavender and holy basil hydrosols smell *amazing*. A hydrosol contains distilled water and a small amount of essential oil from your plant material. You can make them with fresh (preferred) or good-quality dried herb. Hydrosols are technically shelf stable, but they have no preservative properties and often go bad after a few weeks or months. To improve the shelf life, store them in the fridge or freezer or add an aromatic tincture to bring it to 10 to 20 percent alcohol. This hydrosol recipe uses everyday kitchen equipment, but if you're *really* gung ho, you can buy a copper distillation still online ($300 to $2,000) to make your own hydrosol and/or essential oil. Use hydrosols internally, externally, in cooking, as a toner, in creams, as aromatherapy sprays, and so on.

4+ cups fresh or dried plant material

Distilled or filtered water

Ice

1 gallon or larger pot with lid (no holes), heat-safe bowl or large glass measuring cup, metal mixing bowl, canning jar lid or clean brick, turkey baster or small ladle, 4- to 8-ounce bottle for finished hydrosol

1 Place your empty bowl or measuring jar in the middle of the pot surrounded by 2–3 inches of water. If your bowl is heavy enough not to float, place it on top of the outer circle of a mason jar lid. If it floats around, place it on a clean brick so it stays put in the middle. Outside your bowl, in the water, place your plant material.

2 Put the lid on the pot upside down. Place ice on the top — you can put it right on the lid or fill a large metal mixing bowl with ice. The greater the surface area of ice on the lid, the better.

3 Gently bring the water to a simmer. Keep the heat high enough so that steam rises to the top but not to the point where the water reaches a rolling boil (which could degrade your aromatics). The steam contains distilled water plus plant aromatics. As it hits the cold lid, it condenses back into a liquid, drips down, and collects in the bowl/measuring cup.

Let this simmer for about 2 hours. Replace ice/remove water from the top of the lid as needed (use a turkey baster or ladle if needed).

4 Remove ice and lid. Gently remove the hydrosol from the bowl/measuring cup. You can scoop the liquid out of the bowl with a small ladle or turkey baster or *carefully* (with mitts or towels over your hands — it's hot!), without letting the plant material slip into the hydrosol, remove the bowl to pour out its contents into a bottle.

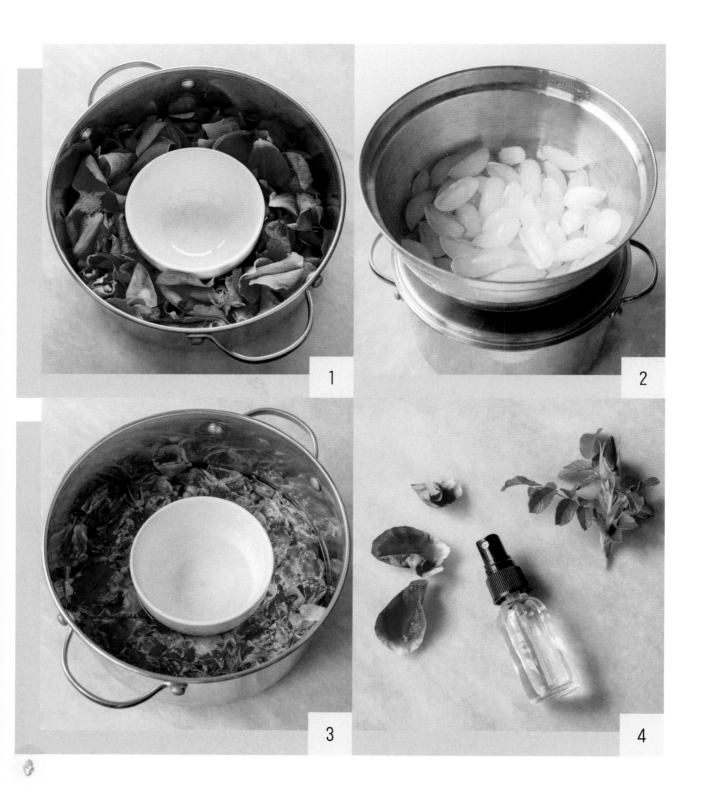

Your largest organ, your skin, stretches across your entire body. It protects you, manufactures vitamin D, interprets the world, holds you together, and acts as a semipermeable barrier, letting some things in and keeping others out. The art of applying herbs to the skin can be wielded in many ways. Most obviously, herbs help address topical issues like cuts, burns, bruises, rashes, wrinkles, hemorrhoids, and general skin care. But these remedies can go deeper. They relieve pain, relax the nerves, lift mood, speed healing, and improve blood vessel integrity. Herbalist Maurice Mességué inspired us to use topical herbs more broadly. He lived in France, where it's illegal for an herbalist to dispense remedies like tinctures (the domain of an apothecary), so he successfully relied on herbal baths and foot soaks to address all manner of health concerns. We focus on topical herbs for topical concerns in this book, but feel free to broaden your scope.

Topical Crossover Remedies

Many herbal remedies we take internally can *also* be adapted for topical use.

Tea = Bath, Soak Compress: Make a *strong* (double- to quadruple-strength) tea to add to the bath, use as a foot soak, or compress. Page 34

Tincture = Liniment: Add to herbal oils and creams; use solo on cuts, scrapes, and wounds; apply as a bug spray. Long shelf life, preservative, sinks into the skin quickly. Page 37

Vinegar: Used similarly to a liniment, but easier on sensitive skin. Vinegar also makes a nice facial toner, sunburn remedy, and base for poison ivy treatments. Page 46

Glycerine: Another water-soluble remedy that can be used in creams, sprays, and other herbal preparations. Glycerine helps soothe and soften the skin. Page 50

Honey: Raw honey naturally cleans wounds and promotes healing. Page 48

Hydrosol: Water-based light aromatherapy spray for use solo, with tinctures, and in creams. They go bad easily if not combined with alcohol/tincture/liniment. Page 58

POULTICE

THE SIMPLEST OF TOPICAL PREPARATIONS, no solvents are involved. Use vet wrap, bandage, gauze, or other cloth to hold it in place if needed. Adhesive bandages work for small areas, maxi pads (secured with cloth) in a pinch. Popular poultices include fresh plantain leaf for bee stings, yarrow leaf for wounds, and aloe for burns.

- Mashed fresh plant material or dried herb powders
- Water or other liquid (if needed) to moisten dried herbs
- Cloth or wrap (if needed) to hold poultice in place

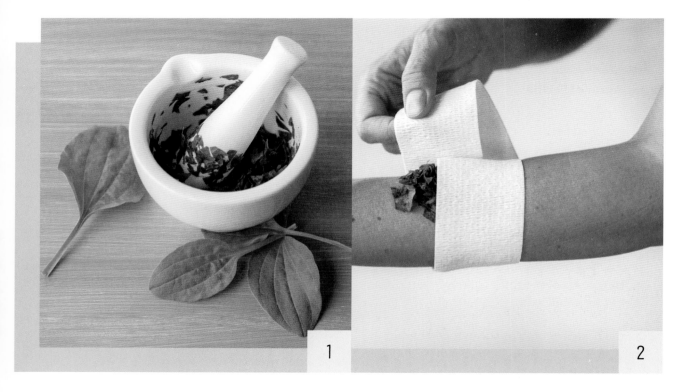

1

2

1 Chew fresh plant material or mash it with a mortar and pestle. Moisten dried herb powders with clean water, vinegar, honey, or an appropriate liniment/tincture to make a paste.

2 Apply poultice to the affected area. If needed, cover and wrap to hold it in place. Replace every 30–120 minutes as needed. Gently irrigate the area with saline solution or a diluted liniment between dressings.

VARIATIONS

Herb Pack Compress: Instead of placing the herb directly on the skin, get it good and moist, wrap it into a cloth pack, such as muslin cloth or a tea bag, then wrap that against the area.

Tea Compress: Make a strong tea, strain, and add salt if needed to make it saline (½ teaspoon per cup of boiled water/tea). Use hot or cold. Soak a cloth or disposable material, wring loosely, then place it on the area. Repeat as needed. Use cotton balls for small areas, such as when using calendula-goldenseal-salt tea for conjunctivitis.

INFUSED OIL

HERBALISTS OFTEN EXTRACT HERBS IN OIL to use topically. Rub it into the skin or use it to make a salve, ointment, cream, or oil-liniment rub. Oil's not a great solvent or preservative. It's apt to go bad easily, especially if you use fresh plant material. But we like oil because it glides easily over the skin, soothing and moisturizing as it slowly penetrates. I prefer this alcohol-intermediary technique (à la Michael Moore) for most herbs. It comes together quickly, and the alcohol improves extraction and shelf life.

7 ounces dried herb

½ ounce alcohol (190- to 100-proof)

8 ounces olive or other oil

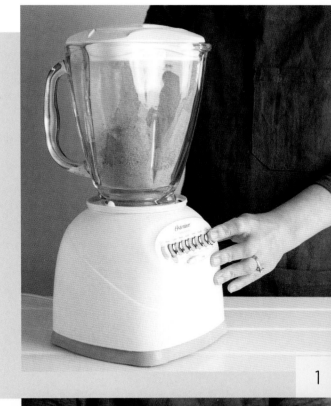

1   Coarsely grind your herb in a blender.

2   Add alcohol. Stir, blend, or shake to mix thoroughly. The consistency resembles damp potting soil. Cover tightly in the blender or a jar. Let sit for about a day.

3   In the blender, combine the prepped herb with oil. Cover and blend until the blender gets warm, about 5 minutes.

4   Strain through cheesecloth or muslin, squeezing out as much oil as you can.

5   If the strained oil contains a lot of herb dust, run it through a coffee filter. This slow process may take a few hours and require several filter changes.

6   Store the finished oil in a tight-lidded glass bottle in a cool, dark, dry spot. It should keep for about a year, possibly longer. Avoid rubber droppers except for short-term use — oil eventually eats through the rubber.

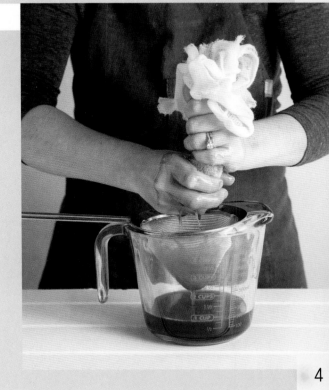

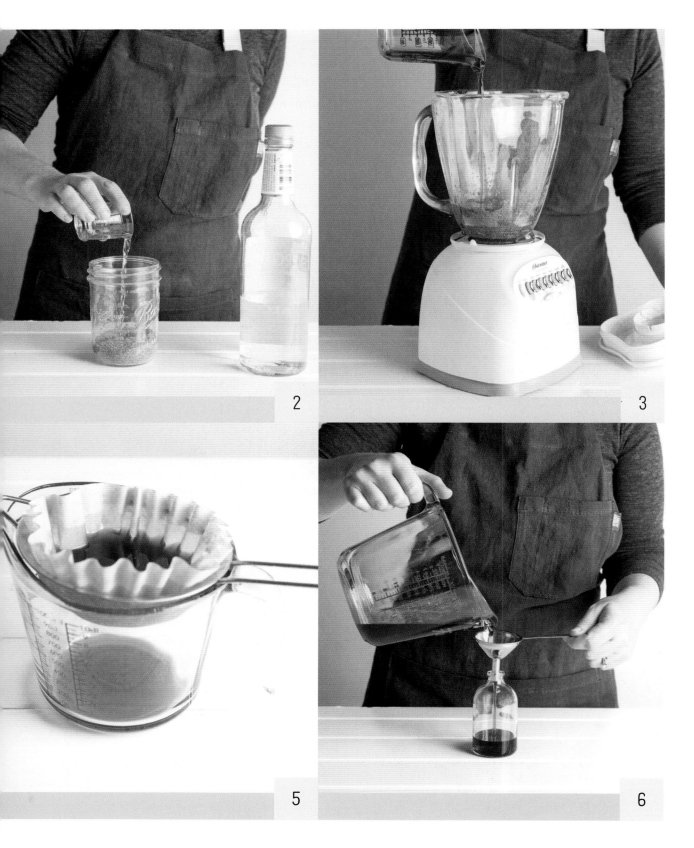

2

3

5

6

VARIATIONS

Macerate: This standard oil technique is also my least favorite because it extracts less and is most likely to spoil, but it's superior for herbs like St. John's wort that are best extracted fresh. Wilt juicy herbs first. Loosely fill the jar with fresh or dried herb, cover with oil. Shake or stir every day (especially important with fresh herb) or keep the herb submerged with a glass fermentation weight. For fresh herb, you can put a cheesecloth lid on to allow moisture to escape, just be sure to stir it regularly or ensure that it stays completely submerged. Strain after 2 weeks. This should last for a few months to a year, possibly longer.

Heat Method: Use this method for plants that extract well via decoction, including calendula, thuja, cayenne, and licorice. Coarsely grind 1 ounce dried herb, cover with 8 ounces oil. Gently bring the mixture to approximately 90–115°F (35–46°C) by heating it in a double boiler, slow cooker, or yogurt maker or by keeping it inside a greenhouse or car for several hours to several days, then strain. If using fresh herbs, leave uncovered (or cover with cheesecloth) to help the moisture evaporate.

Calendula Combo: For calendula, begin with the alcohol-intermediary method (page 62). After blending, pour all the slop into a jar and use the heat method before straining. You can use any method to make calendula oil, but this one comes out the best.

Liniment/Oil Blend: Dual action! Better shelf life! Mix an herb-infused oil approximately 1:1 with an herbal liniment. It will separate. Shake vigorously and apply as needed. Creams (page 66) also blend both oil- and water-soluble ingredients.

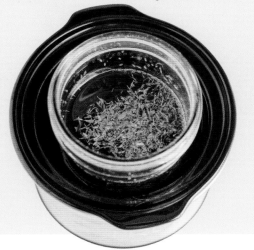

SALVE

TO MAKE A SALVE, simply melt beeswax into oil. Salves keep longer, are less messy, and stay put on the skin better than an oil. Wrap beeswax in a clean, sturdy cloth, then whack it with a hammer on a solid surface to break it into smaller pieces so it melts faster. If you don't have a scale, measure by displacement: Pour 4 ounces of oils into a glass measuring cup, then add beeswax until the total volume reaches 5 ounces. If you don't have a double boiler, simply use a metal mixing bowl over a pot of water. I love my stainless steel gravy ladle, which makes pouring into jars and tubes a breeze, but a glass measuring cup works. Salves keep for approximately a year. Multiply or divide this recipe as needed.

1 ounce beeswax

4 ounces herb-infused oil(s)

Additions: 15+ drops essential oils, 1 teaspoon vitamin E oil, 5 drops flower essence

Double boiler (see tip above), spoon, glass measuring cup, scale, jars or tubes, gravy ladle

1 Melt beeswax in the double boiler.

2 Add herb-infused oils. Stir until it's all liquid and combined. Remove from heat and stir in any additional ingredients (essential oils, and so on) to the base. Or you can add the essential oil directly to the empty salve containers, which allows you to mix up the "flavors."

3 Pour the base into the heat-safe jars or tubes. The salve settles and shrinks a bit as it cools.

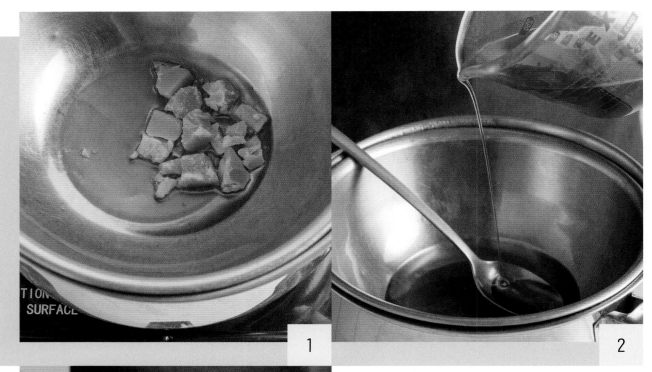

1

2

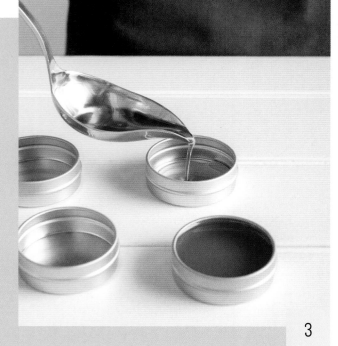

3

VARIATIONS

Lip Balm: The only difference between a lip balm and salve is your intention. Use the same 1:4 beeswax:oil ratio, using plain or herb-infused oils. My favorite: 1½ ounces coconut oil, 1½ ounces grapeseed oil, 1 ounce olive oil. Add 2–3 drops essential oil per empty lip balm tube for flavor before pouring in the base.

Ointment: A softer consistency than a salve, use approximately ½ ounce beeswax to 4 ounces oil, or to your preference.

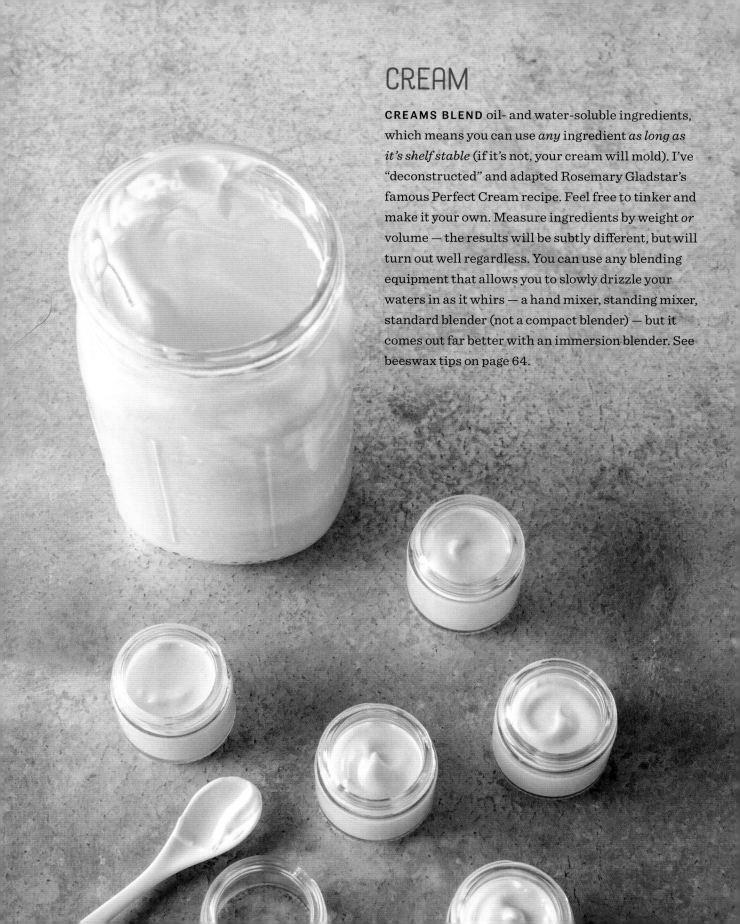

CREAM

CREAMS BLEND oil- and water-soluble ingredients, which means you can use *any* ingredient *as long as it's shelf stable* (if it's not, your cream will mold). I've "deconstructed" and adapted Rosemary Gladstar's famous Perfect Cream recipe. Feel free to tinker and make it your own. Measure ingredients by weight *or* volume — the results will be subtly different, but will turn out well regardless. You can use any blending equipment that allows you to slowly drizzle your waters in as it whirs — a hand mixer, standing mixer, standard blender (not a compact blender) — but it comes out far better with an immersion blender. See beeswax tips on page 64.

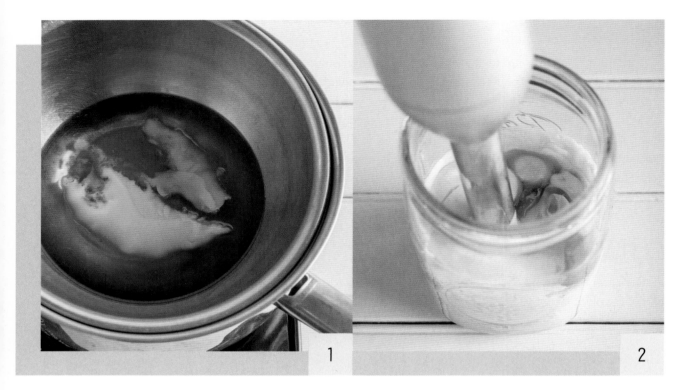

1

2

¾ ounce beeswax

6 ounces liquid oils (olive, grapeseed, herb-infused)

2½ ounces solid oils (coconut oil, cocoa butter, shea butter)

5½ ounces waters (distilled water, hydrosol, tincture, vanilla extract)

Additions: 15+ drops essential oil, vitamin E oil

Double boiler (see tip page 64), spoon, glass measuring cup, scale, jars, immersion blender, quart mason jar

1 Melt beeswax in the double boiler, then add liquid and solid oils. Stir until all melted and well combined. Pour into the container in which it will later be blended (e.g., mason jar). Let cool to room temperature (it's okay if it's a little warm to the touch), about an hour. The mixture will turn opaque with an ointmentlike consistency.

2 Measure your waters, adding any optional ingredients to this. Slowly pour waters into the wax mixture, blending with a mixing tool (e.g., an immersion blender). Stop from time to time to scrape down the sides of the pot or container, and continue blending until all the ingredients are thoroughly combined.

3 Scoop or pour the cream into jars. Pop them into the freezer for a few days or until you need a jar of cream (this prevents/slows cocoa butter forming granular bits). Let the cream thaw at room temperature. This is shelf stable for 6–12 months, but best kept frozen until you need it. If it separates over time, stir to recombine.

Dilute preparations like flower essences and homeopathic remedies diverge from other herbal remedies that rely on plant chemistry and more recognized modes of herbal action, providing something subtler and energetic that offers a different way to interact with the plants. Chemically speaking, there's little to nothing in these remedies except the "footprint" of the plant. Proponents believe they work by causing shifts in the vibrational energy of the person to encourage the body to heal itself. You can also view these remedies as a form of focused intention, almost like a prayer or spell, to help the universe help you. At the very least, they may act as placebos. I believe they hold their own special healing power and deserve a spot in your apothecary if you're willing to expand your concept of herbal medicine.

FLOWER ESSENCES

Flower essences are made with a plant's flowers (even if a different part of the plant is typically used for medicine), harvested at their peak just as they're opening. They're primarily used for balancing psychosocial-spiritual states, though they can also affect physical conditions. Rescue Remedy is the most famous flower essence, a blend of five flowers used to bring calm in cases of trauma, anxiety, panic, and shock. See page 312 for a quick list of flower essences by health concern and read plant profiles (page 246) for more details.

VARIATION

Low-Dose Tincture: Matthew Wood suggests using a regular tincture (page 37) like flower essences or homeopathic remedies. Simply take 1–3 drops as needed.

Fresh flowers

Water, distilled or filtered

Brandy

Scissors, 4-ounce bottle with cap, ½-ounce dropper bottle, funnel, small strainer, small clear glass bowl or cup

---

USAGE SUGGESTIONS:

- Take 1–5 drops of the stock or dosage bottle on the tongue one to three times per day, or as needed.
- Add to your drinking water, tea, beverages, animal water bowls.
- Add a few drops to tinctures, creams, salves, aromatherapy sprays.
- Place a drop or two on the skin.

---

1 On a clear, sunny day without much wind, carefully harvest a few flowers from your desired plant, preferably in the late morning. Place them in a glass bowl or cup filled with 2 ounces of water.

2 Place the glass in a sunny spot to sit for a few hours. The flowers float on top.

3 After a few hours have passed, bring the glass inside, strain the flowers, and fill your 4-ounce bottle halfway with the flower essence water. Fill the remaining half of the bottle with brandy (to preserve) and shake vigorously. This is your mother essence.

4 To make a stock bottle, fill a small bottle with 30–50 percent brandy, the rest water. Add 5 drops of mother essence. Shake vigorously. Use this stock bottle directly, add it to other recipes, or dilute it further into a dosage bottle.

5 To make a dosage bottle, once again, fill a small bottle with 30–50 percent brandy, the rest water. Add 3–5 drops each of stock essence of one to five different plants.

The Art of Formulation

When you first begin working with herbs, begin with "simples" (single herbs) to learn each plant one by one. Choose just one to five plants to learn at first. As you get to know each plant, you can practice the art of formulation — how to make better-tasting, more-effective remedies with careful blending of two or more herbs. Formulation also allows you to balance plant energetics so a formula isn't too hot, cold, dry, or damp. You don't need to follow any particular "rules" to blend your herbs. Simply use your intuition and try out the results in small batches.

Primary herb(s): Herbs with your main flavor or medicinal action.

Supportive herb(s): These provide additional useful benefits, buffer the strength or flavor of the primary herb(s), or provide a base note to ground the flavor. Other examples of supportive herbs include adaptogens, nervines, nutritives, and demulcents.

Synergist(s) and/or harmonizer(s): Synergist herbs kick up the flavor a notch and/or stimulate circulation, digestion, and other metabolic functions to better deliver the other herbs throughout the body. Spices, peppermint, and other flavorful herbs work well as synergists. Sweet-tasting herbs or honey harmonize a blend by integrating the flavors and actions so they work well together.

Good vibrations: These take your remedies beyond chemical medicine. If you'd like, add a few drops of flower essence, a sprinkle of flower petals, or aromatherapy herbs to your blend to heal on another level.

Don't get too caught up in labels, though. Simply play around, and also keep in mind that one herb can play more than one role. Start by combining just two herbs and note how the dynamics change: for example, catnip with spearmint, holy basil with lemon balm, nettle with peppermint, marshmallow with cinnamon, or oatstraw with Korean mint. Then go from there. Maybe you want to use dandelion as a digestive bitter for liver detoxification, but you don't love the flavor. Add a stick of cinnamon. Then try adding a cardamom pod or Korean mint. See how the flavor and action change as you tinker with the formula — use whatever tastes best and feels right for your body. Use the recipe blends in this book for inspiration. Keep in mind the best extraction method for individual herbs (described in the profiles on page 246) — for example, decoction versus infusion teas, fresh versus dried herbs — but rules can usually be broken.

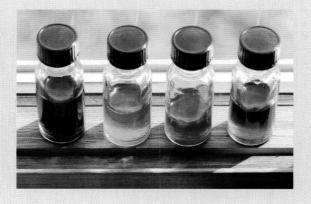

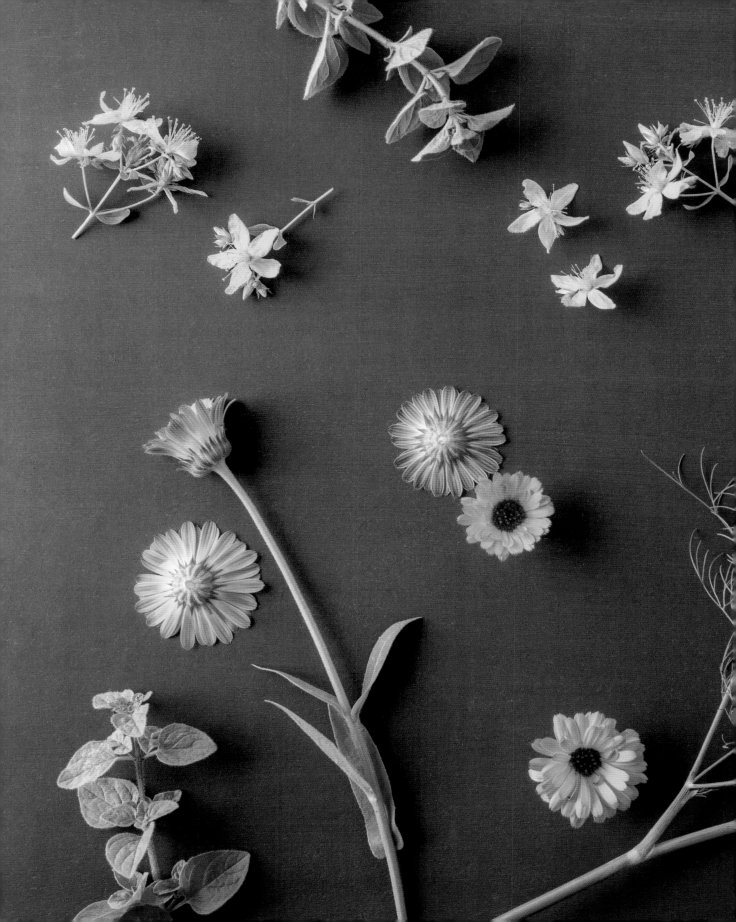

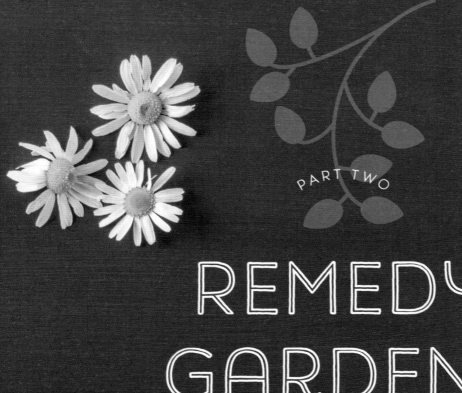

REMEDY
GARDENS

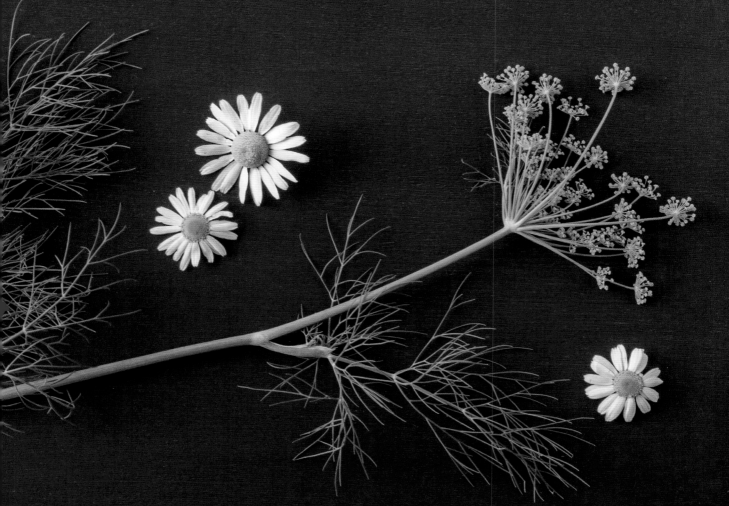

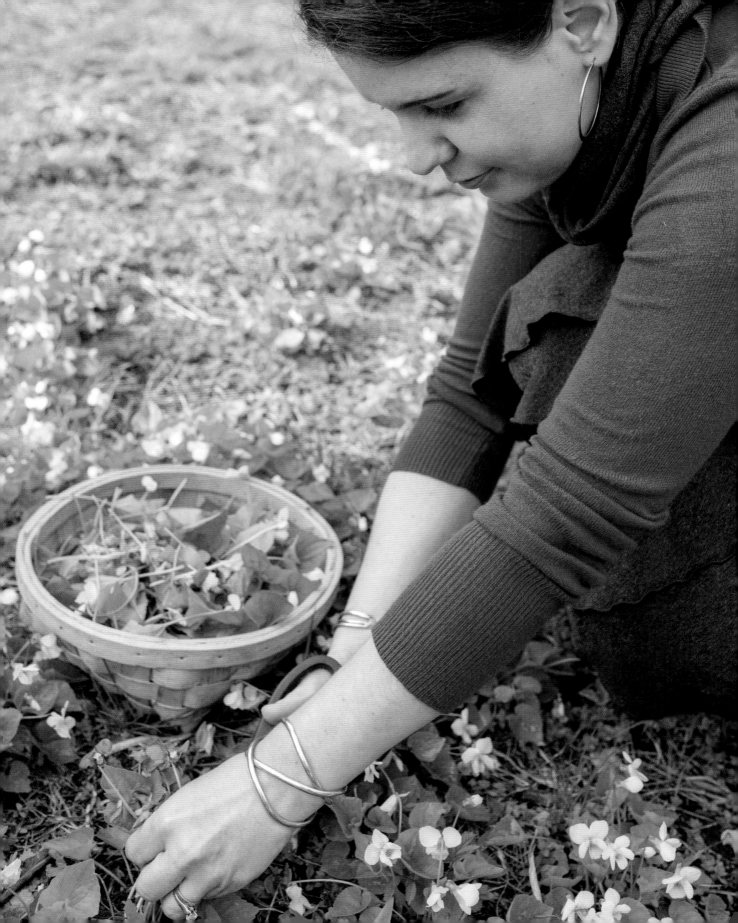

Daily Tonics

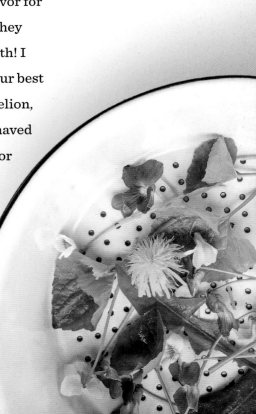

IF YOU'RE NOT SURE what herbs to plant in your garden, *these* gardens are a perfect place to start. Tonic herbs offer daily support for general well-being with foodlike safety. The herbs highlighted here provide nutrition, color, and delicious flavor for tea, food, and herbal remedies. In short, they bring joy to life and vibrance to your health! I use the term "garden" liberally. Most of our best nutritive plants — including nettle, dandelion, and wild raspberry — are common ill-behaved weeds that you're better off wildcrafting or letting naturalize on the edges of your yard rather than incorporating into your formal garden. Meanwhile, calendula, Korean mint, and lemongrass thrive in pampered beds, adding splashes of color and texture to your landscape.

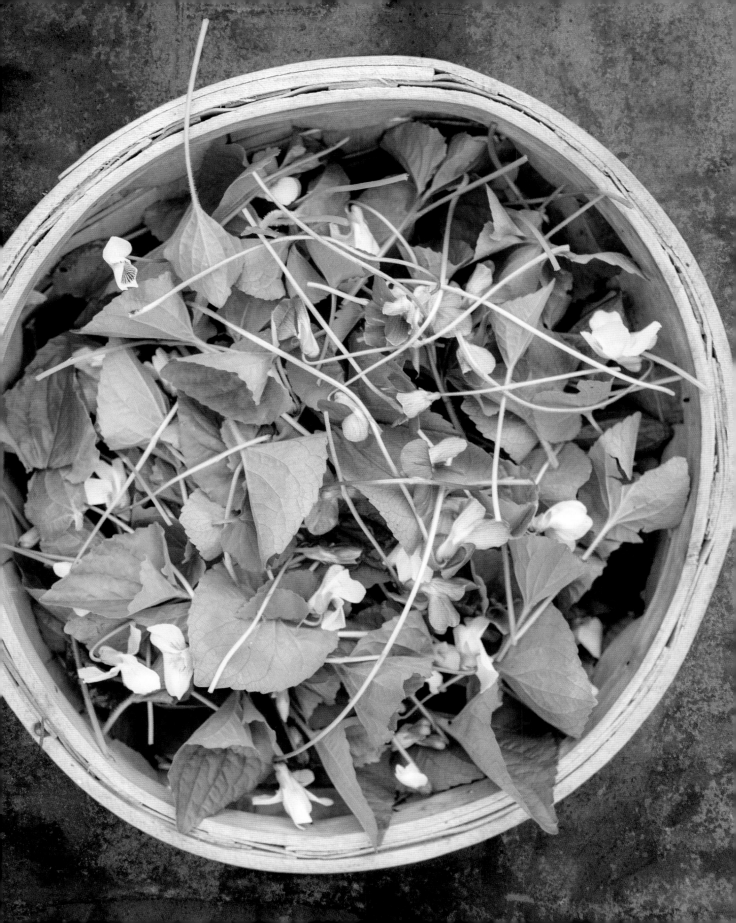

NUTRITIVE GARDEN

This garden features our most nutrient-dense herbs. Some can get weedy while others — like violet — are more garden-friendly, yet all could be included in a formal garden with careful attention to the weedier species. You may opt, as I do, to grow oats in their own plot (the previous year's chicken run or an unused new or old garden bed) and keep sprawling roses and stinging nettles in their own nooks. Any respectable gardener would be horrified to learn that you're intentionally planting something like nettle in your yard, but these are the kinds of wacky things herb gardeners do! With the exception of oatstraw and calendula, which are solely cultivated, the other herbs also grow wild. Other nutritive herbs you might want to try include dandelion, horsetail, burdock, raspberry leaf, chickweed, and red clover.

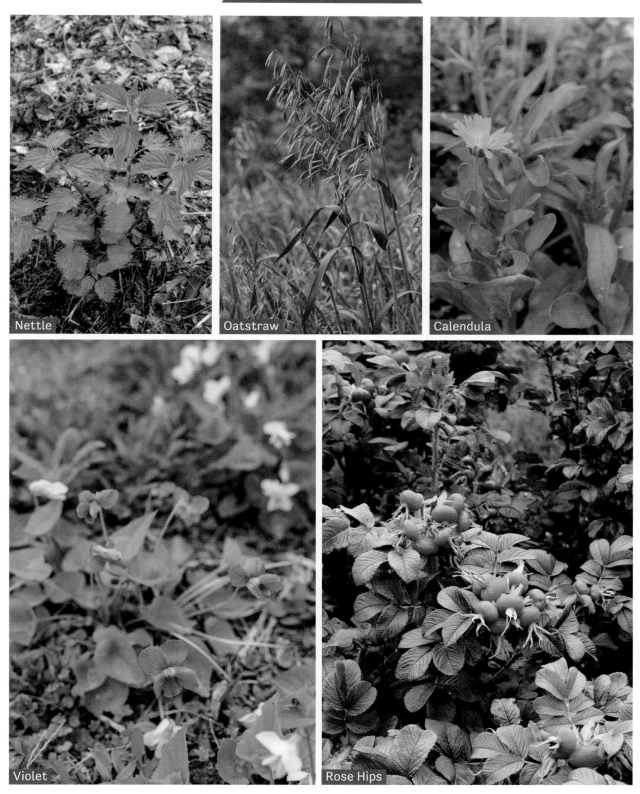

Nettle

Oatstraw

Calendula

Violet

Rose Hips

Nettle

Nettle leaves are one of our safest and most bioavailable calcium-dense plants on the planet, a verifiable safer-than-spinach super green. Cup for cup, strong nettle tea has more calcium than milk and contains additional supportive minerals like magnesium and silica, and many of its nutrients are more easily absorbed by the body than those from other sources. Go for super infusion, decoction, broth, food forms, or superfood powder. Nettle thrives in rich, moist soil and dappled sunlight, but it *stings* and spreads, so think carefully before you plant it. Also used for allergies and as a diuretic, see page 289 for more information.

Best in: tea, broth, food, vinegar, simmered syrup, glycerite

Oatstraw

Various parts of this cover crop cereal grain offer different medicinal activities. For nutrition, dry the green straw for an excellent, pleasant-tasting mineral-rich addition to tea and broth. Ounce for ounce, it boasts four times the vitamins and minerals of oatmeal, including calcium, magnesium, and silica, which support healthy hair, skin, nails, bones, and connective tissue. Sow seeds in fertile soil and full sun with consistent watering or rain, and keep in mind that this plant gets moderately tall. See page 290 for more information.

Best in: tea, broth, powder, vinegar

Calendula

With regular harvesting, calendula puts out showstopping blooms nonstop from early summer through fall in a pampered garden bed. Vivid yellow and orange blooms pack one hundred times the carotenoids of a sweet potato by weight, including beta-carotene, zeaxanthin, and lutein. Bring calendula's color pop from the garden to the kitchen. Sprinkle petals on salads, broth, and other dishes for color with minimal flavor. Calendula also supports skin, lymph, and immune health. See page 255 for more.

Best in: tea, broth, food

Violet

Cute, cheery violet blooms perk up the spring landscapes. Let it grow in the lawn, edge beds, and dot the garden. The leaves and flowers provide minerals, vitamin C, and beta-carotene. Unlike most (diuretic, drying) nutritives, violets moisten and soothe with their demulcent and mucilaginous properties. This gives tea a velvety mouthfeel and better suits people who tend to be dry. Violets lend a pleasant green flavor to tea, salad, and pesto all season long. See page 305 for violet's other uses.

Best in: tea, food (salad, pesto, smoothies), broth

Rose Hips

When it comes to vitamin C and bioflavonoids, nothing local compares with a sprawling hedge of rose hips. The fruits form in late summer and autumn. Use roses with a good-tasting hip, such as dog or rugosa roses. Best fresh, rose hips lose much of their vitamin C during drying, cooking, and storing, though bioflavonoids remain. The petals offer entirely different benefits. See page 296 for more.

Best in: jam (45 times more vitamin C than tea!), syrup, tea

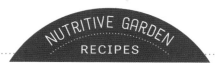
NETTLE-OAT SUPER INFUSION

SUPER INFUSING YOUR HERBS maximizes the mineral extraction from tonic herbs. One cup of nettle tea goes from having 40 to 80 mg of calcium per mug (for your standard infusion) to approximately 500 mg per mug! Drink this regularly as a bioavailable source of calcium, magnesium, potassium, and silica, which are particularly helpful for strong bones but also support everyday health. Measure your dried herbs on a scale.

0.6 ounce dried nettle leaf

0.4 ounce dried oatstraw

About 32 ounces boiling water

Suggested tools: quart-size French press (or a quart jar, large hand strainer, and clean cloth)

Add your herbs to a quart-size French press or jar, then cover them with boiling water, stirring to mix well. Let steep 4 or more hours, then strain, squeezing out as much liquid from the herbs as you can. Drink the tea over the course of 1–2 days.

Chai Base

This blend of common culinary spices perks up the flavor of many medicinal herbs, not only nettle and oatstraw but also dandelion root, burdock root, marshmallow, chaga, reishi, ashwagandha. Per 16 ounces of water/tea, use two cinnamon sticks (preferably one cassia, one Ceylon/sweet), two cardamom pods, seven cloves, and one star anise pod. Feel free to play around with other additions including one bay leaf, ¼ teaspoon licorice, ¼ teaspoon fennel, one slice of ginger, a pinch of nutmeg, one-quarter snipped vanilla bean or splash of vanilla extract. This tea will taste best if you simmer it, but long-term infusions will also bring out the flavors. In a pinch, sometimes I just use cinnamon sticks and cardamom. So yummy!

Safety Tips

Heavy metals: Nutritive herbs also bioaccumulate lead and heavy metals from the soil, which are also minerals (albeit not desirable ones). As minerals, heavy metals also extract more efficiently in a super infusion or decoction. Make sure your soil is not contaminated to prevent inadvertent exposure. Avoid growing or harvesting near old buildings and other potentially problematic sites, and consider getting a soil test.

Microbial growth: Steeping tea on the counter for several hours may increase the risk of bacterial growth, which is of particular concern if you have a compromised immune system. You may opt to move the tea to the fridge once it has reached room temperature to finish steeping there. For the least risk with excellent mineral extraction, decoct (simmer) the tea for 20 minutes instead.

NUTRI-TEA

MANY A NUTRITIVE TEA BLEND has been crafted on this theme: nutritious "green" herb(s) plus mint. It's tasty and easy. Feel free to play around with the ingredients.

1 tablespoon nettle leaf

1 tablespoon oatstraw

1 tablespoon peppermint and/or spearmint

Optional additions: red clover, horsetail, violet, raspberry leaf, lemon balm, oat tops, calendula, lady's mantle, rose petals

Steep the herbs in 16 ounces of hot water for at least 20 minutes, strain, and enjoy.

VARIATIONS

- 1 part nettle, 1 part peppermint
- 1 part nettle, 1 part peppermint, 1 part violet, 1 part marshmallow leaf, sprinkle of calendula petals
- 1 part nettle, 1 part lemon balm, 1 part oatstraw or tops, 1 part spearmint, 1 part peppermint, sprinkle of calendula petals
- 1 part oatstraw, 1 part Korean mint or lemongrass
- 1 part raspberry leaf, 1 part nettle leaf, 1 part mint

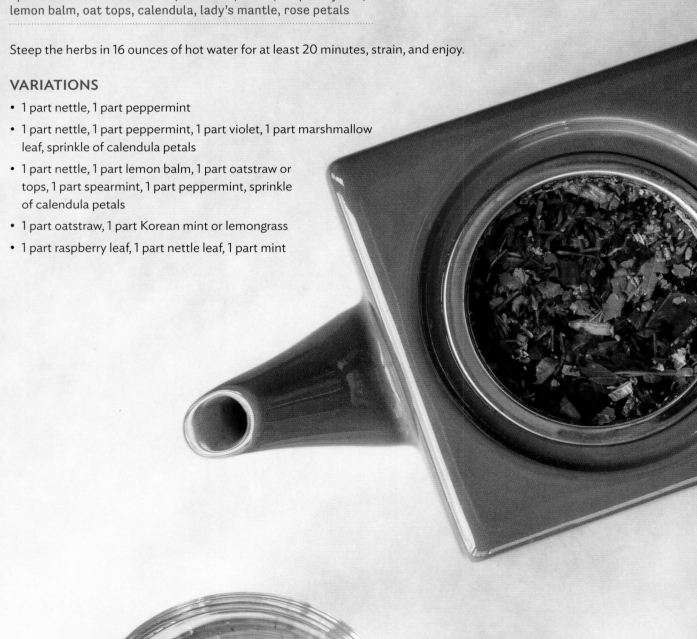

Nutri-Broth

Soup broth makes a fantastic delivery system for mineral- and carotenoid-rich herbs that extract well when simmered long term. Classics include calendula flowers (not too much, they get bitter), nettle leaf, oatstraw, horsetail, and/or burdock root. Add 1 to 3 tablespoons (or more) of total herbs, to taste, to a gallon of your standard broth ingredients — beef or chicken bones, veggies, salt, seasonings. Simmer for 30 minutes to all day.

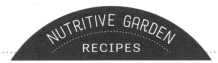

HERBAL NUTRI-BROTH WITH MUSHROOMS

THIS SIMPLE NOURISHING, IMMUNE-TONIC BROTH can be made with your favorite tasty nutritive herbs and whatever mushrooms you have on hand. Mushrooms support and modulate immune function — shiitake is my favorite for flavor and medicine — but you could certainly skip them if you prefer. Note that reishi and calendula can get bitter if you add too much.

1 chicken carcass

1–2 tablespoons dried nettle leaf

2 cups fresh mushrooms (shiitake, maitake, etc.) and ¼–½ cup dried mushroom (shiitake, reishi, turkey tails, chaga, etc.)

2 bay leaves

Salt to taste

Optional additions: turmeric, black pepper, calendula flowers, horsetail, oatstraw, violet leaves, splash of apple cider vinegar

Suggested tools: large stockpot, large strainer, half-gallon mason jars, freezer-safe containers

Simmer the ingredients in 1 gallon of water all day on the stove or in a slow cooker. Strain into mason jars or other heat-safe containers to cool. (Or take the strained broth, return it to the pot, and simmer uncovered until reduced to one-quarter of its volume to freeze in ice cube trays.) Then transfer to freezer-safe containers to store extras. Dose is 1 cup or 1–2 concentrated ice cubes 1–3 times per day plain or added to recipes.

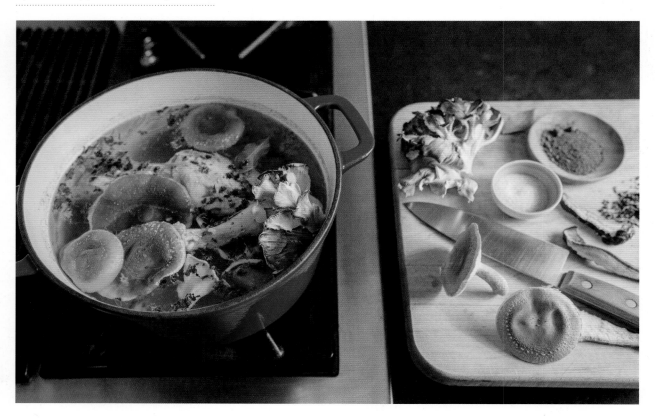

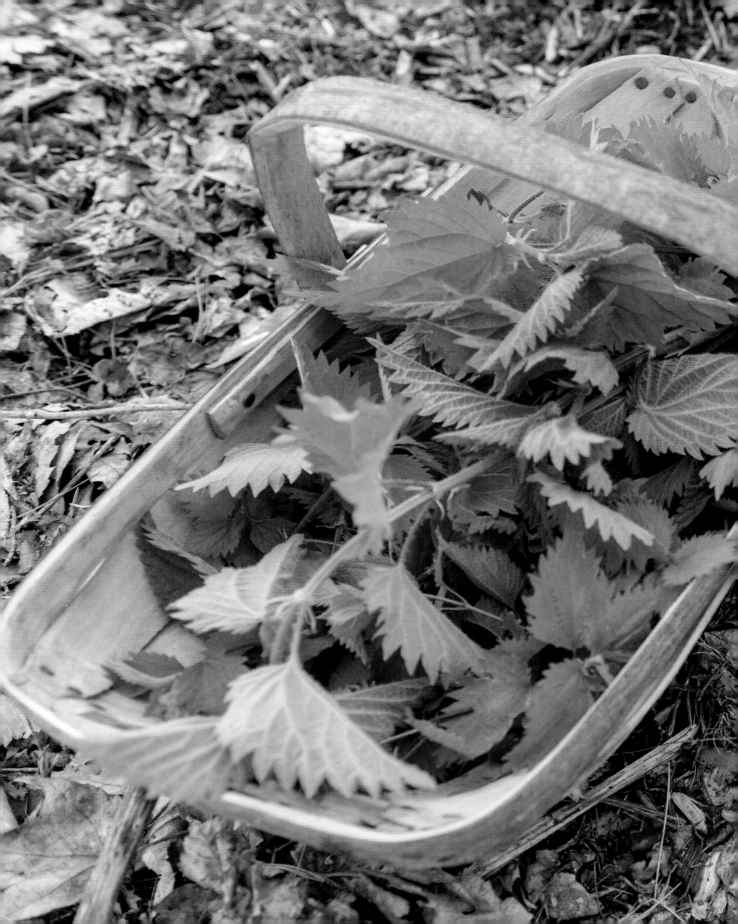

NUTRITIVE FORAGER

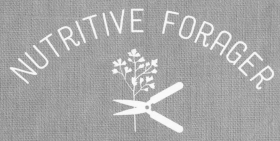

Most of our best nutritive herbs grow abundantly in the wild and get weedy in formal garden beds. Yet you'll want to keep them close by because they're so useful. Seek out wild stands of dandelion, nettle, burdock, horsetail, and violet near you or intentionally introduce them to locations in your yard where they can flourish without getting in your way or bullying out better-behaved garden plants. Other nutritive herbs you might want to try include raspberry, red clover, chickweed, rose hips, yellow dock.

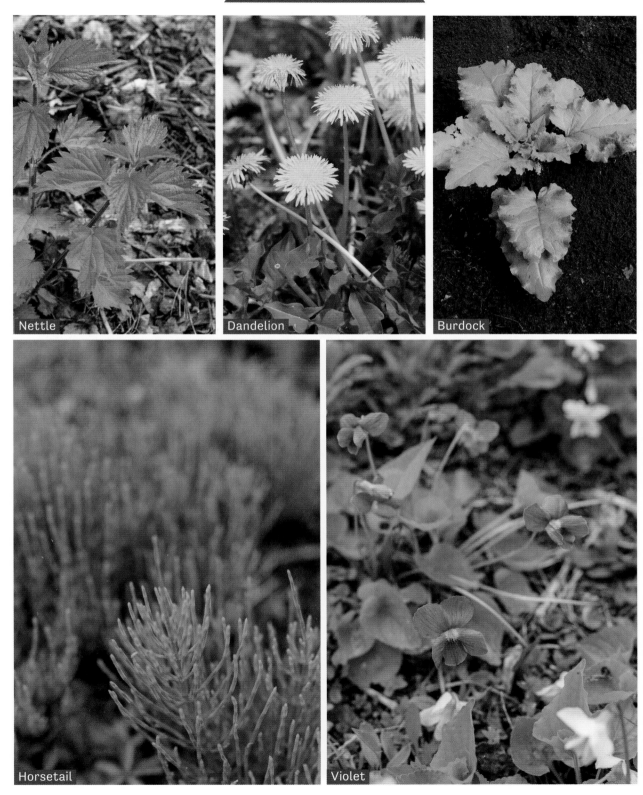

Nettle

Dandelion

Burdock

Horsetail

Violet

Nettle

Nettle leaves contain more bioavailable minerals in a safer-than-spinach package than almost any other plant on the planet. Calcium, magnesium, and potassium extracts best in super-infusion teas, decoction, broth, or superfood powder added to food to improve bone strength and nourish the body. However, the fire ant–like sting and weedy tendencies make it a good candidate for the *edges* of your yard with rich, moist soil in dappled or partial sunlight. See page 289 for nettle's many uses.

Best in: tea, broth, food, vinegar, simmered syrup, glycerite

Dandelion

All parts of dandelion offer nutritive benefits: various vitamins and minerals (notably calcium, potassium, and iron) in the leaves and roots, and carotenoids in the yellow petals. Dandelions also stimulate digestion, make you pee (diuretic), and encourage detoxification via the liver and kidneys. A cultivar of chicory called Italian dandelion provides tidy leaves in the garden. Use the bitter roots in tea, leaves in food. See page 262 for more on dandelion and chicory.

Best in: pesto (leaves), tea (roots), food (all parts), vinegar (all parts), simmered syrup

Burdock

Medicinally similar to dandelion, burdock root has a mild bittersweet flavor that's delicious in soup, broth, tea, and stir-fries. Compared to dandelion, burdock has more lymph-moving properties and is gentler and less diuretic. This biennial has huge leaves and produces tall thistlelike blooms in its second year, though it's the herb's roots below the soil that are harvested. Give it rich, damp soil on the edge of the woods, yard, or woodland path in dappled or partial sunlight where it can spread. See page 254 for more on burdock.

Best in: food (stir-fry), broth, tea, simmered syrup

Horsetail

This ancient water-loving weed thrives in damp soil and riverbeds. Gardeners *detest* it because it's impossible to eradicate, but it plays nice with others and offers more silica than any other herb. Silica helps strengthen bones, hair, skin, nails, and connective tissue. Horsetail also reduces arthritis inflammation and pain, heals the gut, and improves wound healing. For safety, harvest only from clean soil/water and process properly. See page 276 for more.

Best in: tea, broth, tincture, ointment, liniment

Violet

Violet leaves are a powerhouse of vitamins and minerals in a pleasant, mild format. Combine them with stronger-tasting nutritives to mellow their flavor, and nibble the fresh greens all season long. Compared with the other (more drying) nutritives, violet has pleasant moistening properties and a velvety, slightly mucilaginous mouthfeel. Welcome violets and heartease pansy into your lawn and garden. Their cheerful blooms brighten the spring landscape and garnish recipes. See page 305 for more.

Best in: food (salads), pesto, broth, tea, vinegar, edible flower/garnish

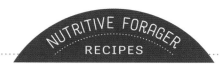
MULTIMINERAL VINEGAR

YOU'LL MAXIMIZE YOUR MINERAL EXTRACTION from herbs if you use them to make super infusions, decoctions, or broth or simply prepare the plants as food. That said, an herb-infused vinegar is vastly superior to a tincture or glycerite when it comes to minerals. Since you'll be consuming small amounts of the vinegar, you'll receive only a light dose of minerals, but delivering these nutrients alongside digestive bitters and ingesting vinegar improves your ability to absorb nutrients from your food. Use this vinegar in salad dressing or seltzer, or mix it with some water in a shot glass and drink it. Feel free to sweeten it with honey if you like. Use fresh or dried herbs, as available.

2 parts fresh or 1 part dried dandelion leaves

1 part dandelion root

1 part burdock root

1 part nettle leaf

Raw, organic apple cider vinegar

Optional additions: yellow dock root, violet leaves

Combine the herbs in a mason jar, filling it loosely with herbs. Cover with vinegar. Cap with a plastic lid (vinegar eats through metal) and let macerate for 2–4 weeks, shaking regularly. Strain and store in a cool, dark, dry spot for 6 months or more. It will keep in the fridge for longer. Enjoy up to 2 tablespoons per meal. (Brush or rinse your teeth afterward since the acidity of vinegar can damage tooth enamel.)

More Ways to Use Mineral-Rich Herbs

- Bone or veggie broth made with nettle, oatstraw, burdock, violet, and/or horsetail (page 80)
- Capsules made with dried, powdered nettle, horsetail, oatstraw, and/or dandelion leaf and root
- Salads with fresh violet and bits of dandelion leaves
- Chai Base (page 78) with nettle leaf, oatstraw, dandelion and/or burdock roots
- Infusion or super infusion with nettle, raspberry, oatstraw, violet leaves, and/or red clover blossoms, with peppermint, spearmint, Korean mint, or lemongrass for flavor
- Bitter Brew Coffee Substitute, page 158
- Nutri-Detox Tea, page 159
- Rose hip jam
- Horsetail tincture for bone strength

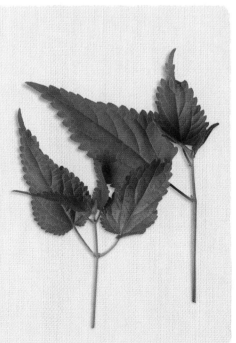

MINERAL-RICH "COFFEE" SYRUP

SIMMERING HELPS PULL MINERALS FROM THE HERBS QUICKLY, and molasses improves the flavor while providing additional iron, calcium, and magnesium. Together, the ingredients have a coffeelike flavor. Perfect for sweetening your morning beverage or enjoying by the spoonful. This recipe is made with dried herbs, but you could substitute fresh. Look at the back of the molasses bottle to find a good one that is rich in iron, calcium, and other minerals. Conventional molasses is weak.

¼ cup yellow dock

¼ cup dandelion root

¼ cup burdock root

¼ cup nettle leaf

2 cups water

About 1 cup blackstrap or organic molasses

Suggested tools: large saucepan, large spoon, large hand strainer, large glass measuring cup for liquid

Combine the herbs and water in a saucepan. Bring to a boil and let simmer for 30 minutes to 2 hours. Strain, squeezing out as much liquid as possible. Add an equal amount molasses. Store in the fridge and use within a week or freeze for longer storage. Enjoy by the tablespoon.

VARIATIONS

Stronger Syrup: Increase the water and herb content and simmer for 2 hours. Strain, then return the tea to the pot. Let it simmer uncovered until the liquid reduces to ¼ to ½ cup. Then add your molasses. This increases the mineral content.

Shelf-Stable Syrup: Combine your finished syrup with equal parts dandelion, burdock, and/or yellow dock tincture (so your finished product is 25 percent tea, 25 percent molasses, 50 percent tincture). The tincture(s) will provide digestive and detoxifying properties while making your syrup shelf stable.

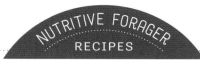
DANDELION-VIOLET WEED PESTO

MAKING PESTO gives you a potent nutritive herb punch that also tastes great. This is my favorite combination, but feel free to experiment with other nutritious weeds (chickweed, self-heal, lamb's-quarter, blanched nettles, sheep sorrel) and culinary herbs (garlic chives, chives, oregano, lemon balm, rosemary, parsley). If you're afraid dandelion will be too bitter, the other ingredients really work their magic smoothing it out.

1 bunch dandelion or Italian dandelion leaves

1–2 handfuls violet leaves

1–3 garlic cloves

1–3 ounces Parmesan

1 cup toasted salted/tamari pepita pumpkin seeds

½ lemon, juiced

¼ cup olive oil

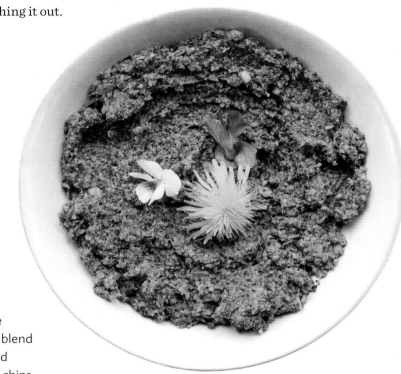

Suggested tools: food processor, processor-blender, or molcajete-style mortar and pestle

Coarsely chop your herbs and garlic. Combine everything except the lemon juice and oil and blend until diced or minced. Then add the liquids and purée until smooth. Serve with organic tortilla chips, crackers, and/or vegetable sticks. It tastes best fresh but will keep for a few days in a tightly sealed container in the fridge and can be stored for a longer period in the freezer.

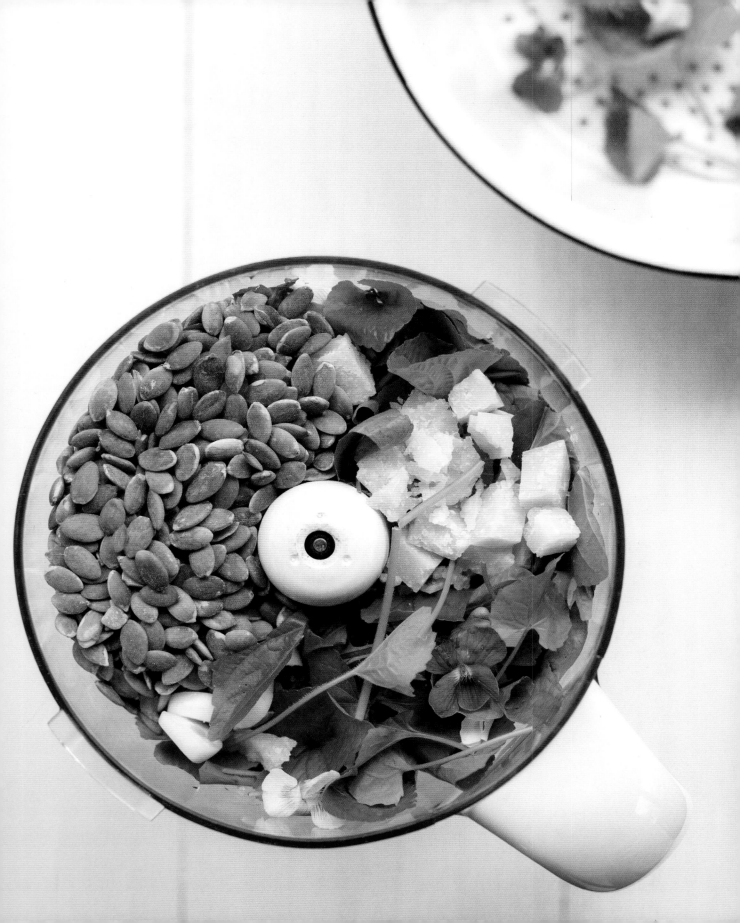

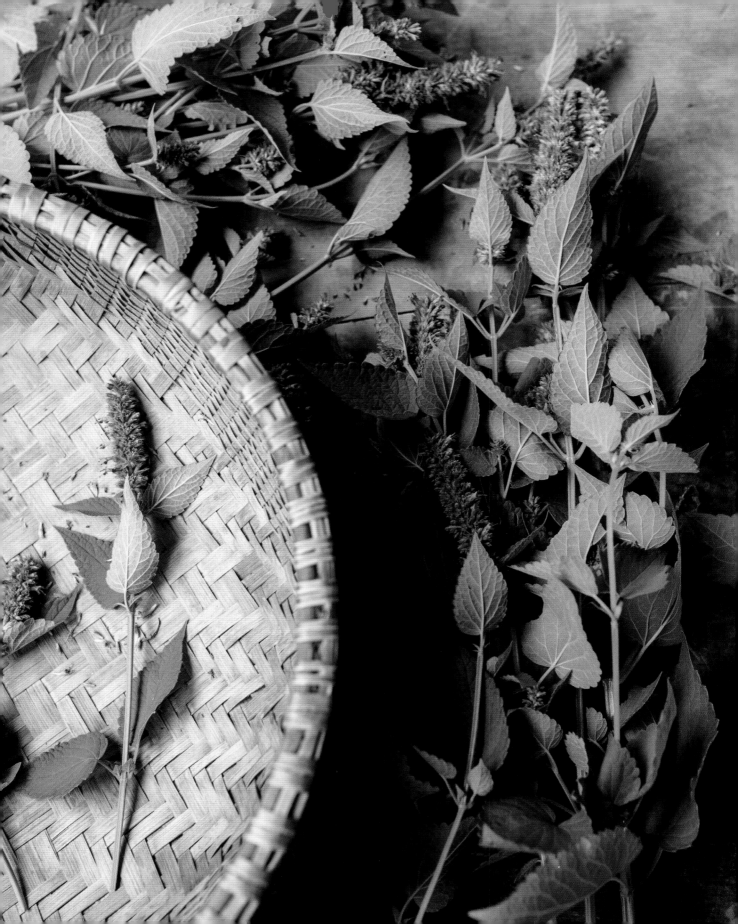

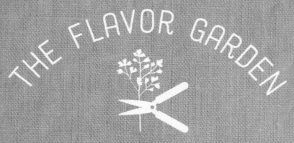

THE FLAVOR GARDEN

This garden brings joy to life with flavor, aroma, and color! While each plant possesses its own healing properties, we primarily use them in daily life because they taste and look good. Korean mint, anise hyssop, lemongrass, lemon verbena, mints, and calendula all do well in your pampered garden beds as culinary herbs — they need good soil and drainage, full sun, and regular watering. Treat most of these plants as annuals. They taste *fabulous* in beverages, from tea to bubbly. Other tasty herbs include stevia, holy basil, bee balm, lemon balm, chamomile, fennel, roses.

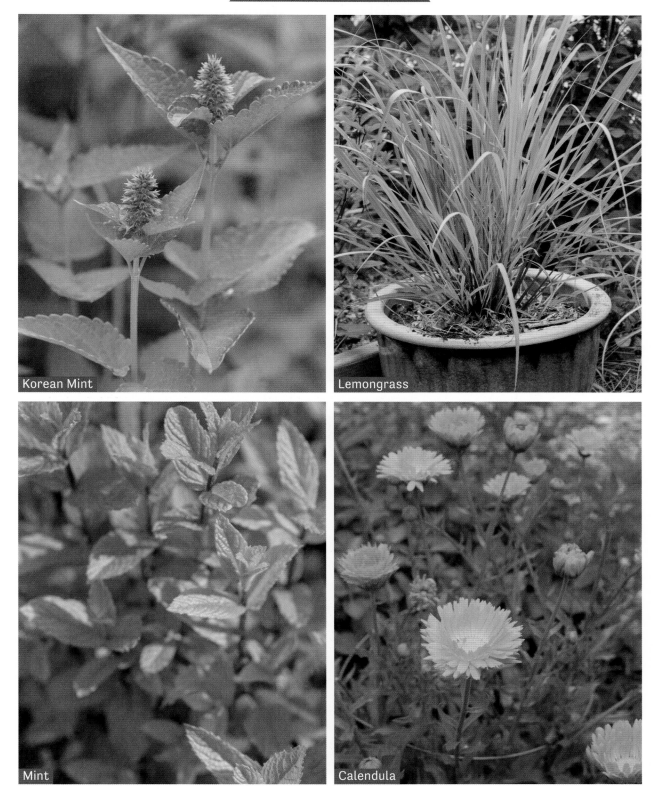

Korean Mint

Lemongrass

Mint

Calendula

Korean Mint

The beautiful, tall, purple blooms of Korean mint (and the closely related anise hyssop) brighten the late-summer garden. All parts taste like honey-anise-fennel, sometimes with a hint of mint. Korean mint is less minty than anise hyssop, but they're nearly indistinguishable and can be used interchangeably. They're delicious in seltzer — adding vanilla shifts the flavor to posh root beer (sugar-free!). Enjoy these short-lived perennials in teas, cordials, salads, and other recipes in place of fennel. Korean mint–infused honey pairs well with chive blossom vinegar and sesame oil for Asian dressings, marinades, and dipping sauces. See page 277 for more.

Best in: tea, water, seltzer, cordial, food, honey

Lemongrass and Lemon Verbena

The tender perennial tropical herb lemongrass has a delicious citrus aroma and flavor. You may recognize its zingy, bright flavor from Thai cuisine. I use the tightly wrapped stalks fresh or fresh-frozen to make cordials, seltzer/soda, curry paste, and broth. Dry and snip up the grassy tops for tea and potpourri; it keeps its flavor longer and better than any other lemony herb. Also consider lemon verbena, which hints at lemon cake, even more so when combined with vanilla. Dried verbena leaves lose their flavor within 6 to 9 months. Pack fresh leaves in sugar for a sweet verbena sprinkle. See page 281 for more information.

Best in: tea, water, seltzer/soda, cordials, broth, hydrosol

Mint

You'll thank yourself later if you plant your mints *outside* your formal garden beds, where they can roam free, or if you rein them in with a large pot. These "garden brutes" spread *rampantly* by root runners. In spite of mint's bad behavior, every respectable herbalist has it *somewhere* in the yard because it tastes so good. Go for peppermint/chocolate mint (a fave for tea and chocolate), spearmint (delish with lime, in tea blends, and in Mexican cooking), and/or apple mint (superb in seltzer/soda, with fruit, and in Asian, Mexican, Indian cuisine). Spread out your mints to prevent cross-breeding. See page 286 for more.

Best in: tea, seltzer/soda, food, tincture, glycerite, hydrosol

Calendula

Calendula isn't actually flavorful. As an accent, it brings a joyous burst of color to your recipes and garden. My favorite varieties glow orange so brightly they practically vibrate with color. Other varieties range from yellow to red-streaked. Sprinkle the bland fresh petals in salads, baked goods, scrambled eggs. Dried petals perk up tea blends and turn broth golden. If you *overdo* calendula (especially whole dried flowers), the flavor becomes bitter and vitamin-y. See page 255 for more.

Best in: food, tea, broth, ice cubes

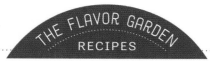
YUMMY TEAS

FIRST AND FOREMOST, all the herbs in this garden can be enjoyed as tea. Whether they are the stand-alone ingredient or used to boost the flavor, color, and joy of your blends, you'll quickly find these herbs indispensable in the tea pantry. Use these simple, tasty blends to get your imagination going. Unless specified, you can use 1 heaping tablespoon of the blend per 16-ounce mug and steep 10 minutes or longer.

Garden aromatics blend: 1 part each lemongrass, Korean mint, rose petals

Holy basil blend: 2 parts holy basil, 2 parts lemon balm, 1 part rose petals

Lemon cake tea: 1 part each lemongrass, lemon verbena, lemon balm (optional: ¼ vanilla bean, snipped into small pieces, or ¼ teaspoon vanilla extract)

Chocolate mint tea: 1 part each peppermint and/or chocolate mint with 1 part cacao nibs (best steeped 20–40 minutes; optional addition of vanilla, as described above)

Nettle-peppermint-marshmallow tea: see page 183

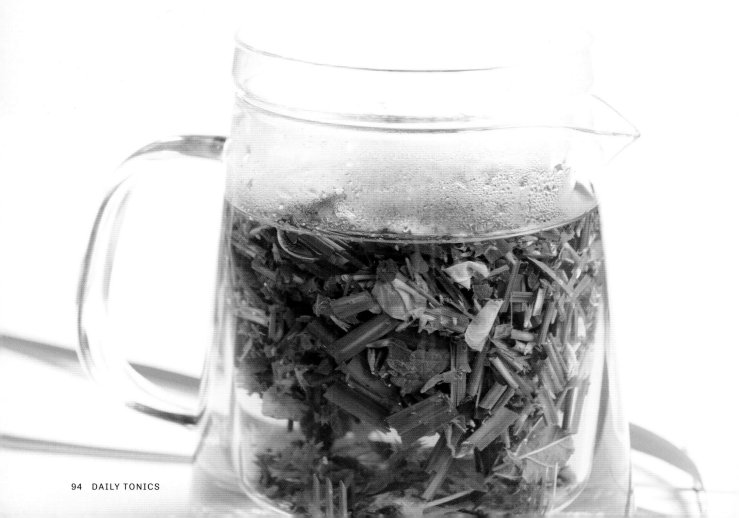

Tea Base Notes

Like base notes in aromatherapy and the bass of a song, some of our most beloved tea herbs have mild, bland flavors, which form the backbone of a blend, grounding and balancing flavorful herbs while offering supportive medicinal properties.

Nettle Leaf: Green, vegetal flavor. Mineral-rich. Page 289

Marshmallow Leaf, Flower, Root: Very mild, soft flavor (leaf and flower). Sweet, woody (roots). Velvety, soothing, mucilaginous mouthfeel. Pretty flowers. Page 283

Oatstraw: Haylike, slightly sweet, delicate. Mineral-rich. Page 290

Violet Leaf, Flower: Mild, green, slightly sweet flavor. Velvety mouthfeel. Rich in vitamins, minerals, mucilage. Pretty flowers. Page 305

Raspberry Leaf or Lady's Mantle: Mild, slightly astringent (tannic), similar to green or white tea without caffeine. Mineral-rich, tightens and tones tissues. Pages 294 and 278

Lemon Balm Leaf: Mildly tannic with a hint of citrus. Lifts mood, calms, improves focus. Page 280

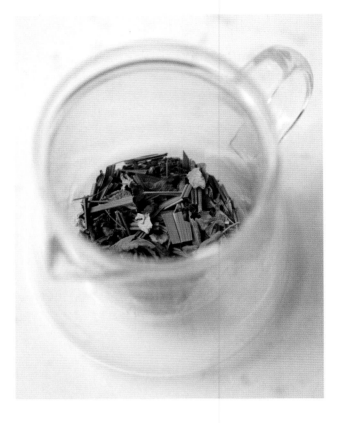

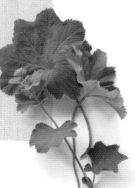

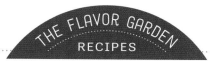
FLORAL ICE CUBES

THESE ICE CUBES ARE MORE FOR SHOW THAN FLAVOR. Serve water, punch, cocktails, and seltzer with extra panache that'll put a smile on your face and wow your guests. Supereasy to make!

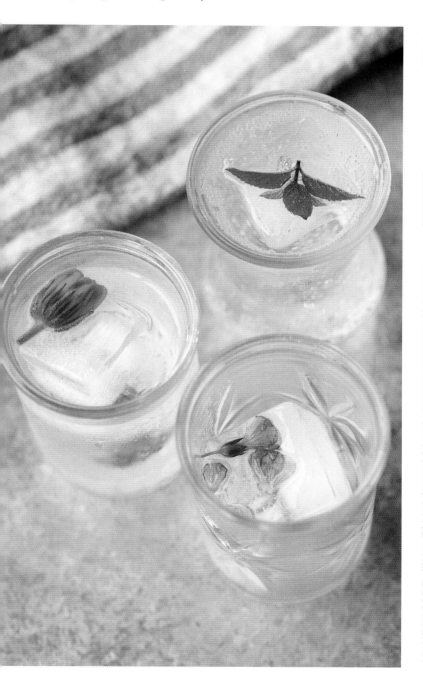

1–2 flowers per cube (or a couple petals)

Water

Suggested tools: ice cube tray

Place your herbs in the ice cube tray, cover with water, freeze. Pop out as desired.

TIP: If you want the herbs to stay centered in the cube, fill the tray only halfway with water, freeze, then fill the rest of the way, and freeze again.

Decorative Edible Flowers

- Mallow (bland)
- Violet (bland/sweet)
- Calendula (bland)
- Korean Mint (licorice-y)
- Fennel (licorice-y)
- Flax flowers (bland)
- Borage flowers (bland/cucumber)
- Bee balm (oregano-thyme/citrus)
- Peppermint (candy cane)
- Spearmint (Doublemint gum)
- Apple mint (mojito mint)
- New England aster (bland/resinous)
- Chamomile (apple-y)
- Purple basil (spicy basil)
- Hibiscus (tart)

INFUSED SELTZER, SODA, AND WATER

ONE OF MY FAVORITE WAYS to enjoy the flavorful herbs in summertime is to steep them fresh in sparkling or still water. This extracts their aromatics without many other constituents and the result is wonderfully enjoyable and refreshing to drink and beautiful to look at. Great for parties (posh, yummy, and calorie- and alcohol-free!) and as a conversation starter. If desired, add simple syrup or other liquid sweetener to taste to turn your seltzer into soda — I prefer them sugar-free. Use about two small sprigs for 16 ounces of water or three large sprigs for a liter. Use clear bottles and add eye-catching flowers — roses, violets, heartease pansy, Korean mint, calendula, mallow — for visual beauty. Drink the beverage within the day.

Rose blossom: steep at least 1-2 hours

Bronze fennel: steep 30+ minutes

Korean mint with a little vanilla extract: steep 15+ minutes

Holy basil: steep 5+ minutes

Lemongrass stalks: steep 30+ minutes

Apple mint: steep 10+ minutes

Spearmint or apple mint with lime wedge:
steep 5+ minutes

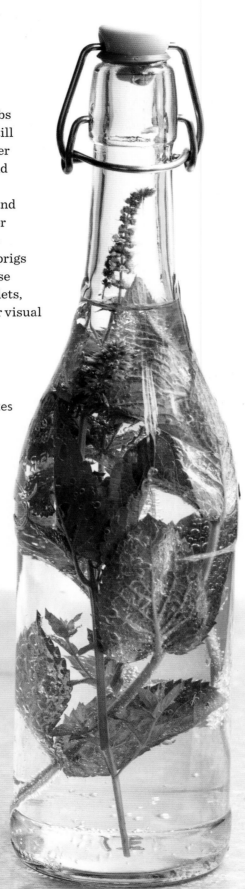
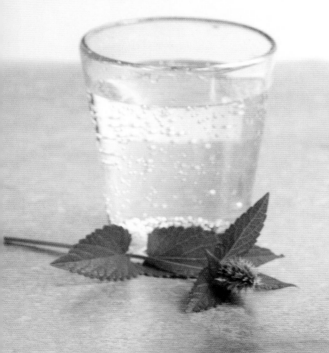

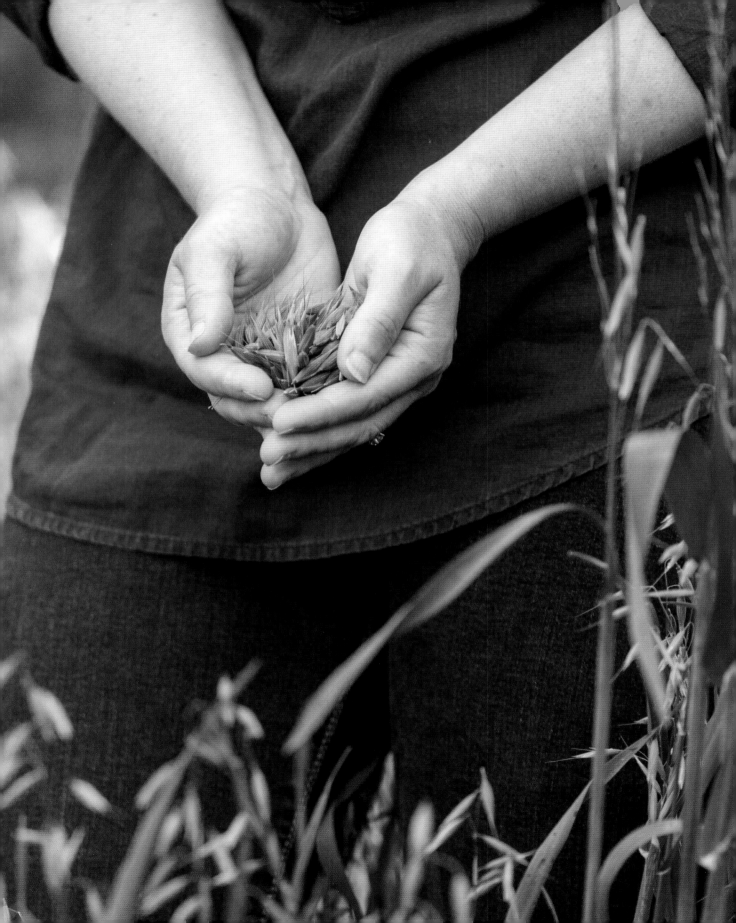

Energy and Relaxation

PLANTS HAVE A PROFOUND ability to affect our mood and energy levels. Many mood-enhancing herbs grow easily in the garden, and in several cases (including lemon balm, skullcap, milky oat seed, and St. John's wort), the fresh plant provides significantly more medicinal activity than the dried material does. Growing these herbs for making medicine will not only be empowering, save money, and help you connect with the plants, but also enable you to make a more powerful and effective remedy than you could buy in the store.

TYPES OF HERBS FOR ENERGY AND RELAXATION

You can grow many herbs in the garden that mildly boost energy, enhance focus, improve mood, nourish the nerves, and help you sleep. You could probably landscape your entire garden with these herbs — there are so many to choose from! Let's explore some of the common medicinal categories of herbs for energy and relaxation that you can grow in the garden.

Adaptogens

Generally speaking, adaptogens help the body adapt to stress so that you are not as strongly affected by it. They're generally mood boosting and provide varying levels of energy. Each one has its own perks, but these herbs are often used for longevity, vitality, libido, and cognitive well-being. The more strongly stimulating adaptogens such as ginseng, rhodiola, and eleuthero thrive in harsh climates, can be more challenging to grow in the everyday garden, and require several years until harvestable. If you're up for a challenge, though, and don't mind waiting so long to gather, you could consider growing them, along with codonopsis and schizandra, which are easier to grow but still take several years until ready for harvest.

In this book we'll focus on some of the calm-energy adaptogens that grow easily in the garden and can be harvested within one growing season. All of these plants act as nervines as well as adaptogens, and ease anxiety while providing deep energy. They include ashwagandha, gotu kola, and holy basil.

Nervines

Though some herbalists use the term "nervine" for any plant that affects the nervous system, in this case we are using it to refer to herbs that nourish, soothe, and rebuild the nervous system. Most are anxiolytic, which means they help relieve anxiety. They can be blended with stimulating adaptogens to encourage calmer energy or with sedatives to maintain calming effects with less sedation. There is a wide range of nervines that grow easily in the garden, though some of the trees may take several years before they're ready to harvest. Nervines include milky oat seed, lemon balm, and motherwort.

Sedatives

Think of sedatives for anxiety and insomnia. The level of sedation depends on the individual plant and on your personal reaction to it. For example, most people will find valerian and hops too sedating to take during the day, while plants like skullcap and passionflower could put some people to sleep at their desk but simply leave others in a pleasant, mellow mood. This is another category of medicinals with many garden-worthy herbs to offer. They include skullcap, passionflower, and valerian.

Antidepressants

Depression is a tricky condition to manage. Even though most of the herbal research on depression revolves around St. John's wort, no one herb is the quick answer for everyone. While this can be said for any condition, it's particularly true of depression. That said, adaptogens, nervines, and other mood-boosting herbs can be particularly useful. Just be aware that they can take several weeks or months to kick in, and it might take some trial and error to find

Crossover Herbs

Some nervines serve more than one function and cross categories.

Antidepressant nervines: St. John's wort, mimosa (tree)

Adaptogen nervines: ashwagandha, gotu kola, holy basil

Sedative nervines: skullcap, passionflower

the best plant for the individual. Antidepressants include St. John's wort, mimosa, and lemon balm.

Nootropics

Nootropics are "smart drugs." In the plant world, these are herbs (and mushrooms) that improve brain health, nerve function, cognition, and focus. Ginkgo tree leaves are well known, but many herbs actually work even better for a broader group of people. They include rosemary, gotu kola, and bacopa.

Calming Digestives

Because "fight or flight" stress and anxiety can shut down digestive system function, it's easy to have digestive issues related to your state of mind. Nervous indigestion, low stomach acid, colic, gas, pain, spasm, constipation, and some types of reflux are particularly common. Relaxing bitters both calm the nervous system while enhancing digestion, which can be very helpful, and most are easy to grow. Digestives are often consumed as tea and, as such, can be blended with even better-tasting carminative herbs that help relax both spasms and the mind. These include fennel, anise, Korean mint, peppermint, and spearmint. We'll discuss calming digestive herbs more in chapter 5. Top relaxing bitters include chamomile, lemon balm, and catnip.

Other Ways to Incorporate Herbs

Include aromatics: Scent has a powerful effect on the nervous system, and aromatic herbs can enhance the flavor of your blend. Holy basil, fresh lemon balm, roses, and, to some extent, chamomile lend a hand here. Mint invigorates while anise-flavored herbs like fennel, anise, anise hyssop, and Korean mint can be more soothing. Lemony flavors like lemongrass, lemon balm, and lemon verbena uplift. From the kitchen cabinet, adding a little vanilla bean or vanilla extract or a pinch of fresh-grated nutmeg will also soothe and uplift the spirits.

Flowers: Adding flowers to a blend gives a little something special to it, especially in loose tea blends. Just seeing those colorful little flowers lifts the spirits and makes the blend more special. Roses work very well here, though you could play with other edible and medicinal flowers such as mimosa, Korean mint, anise hyssop, lavender, or even plants otherwise unrelated to the nervous system like calendula. You can also explore the world of flower essences and the energetic, vibrational impacts of flowers in plant medicine. I add a few drops of flower essences to almost all of my tincture blends. See page 68 for more on flower essences.

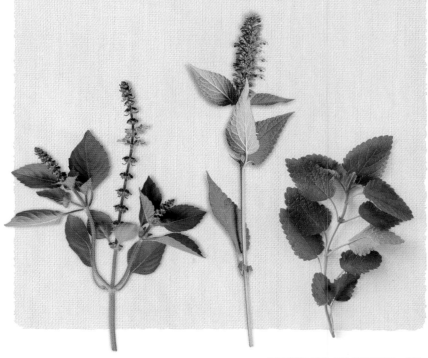

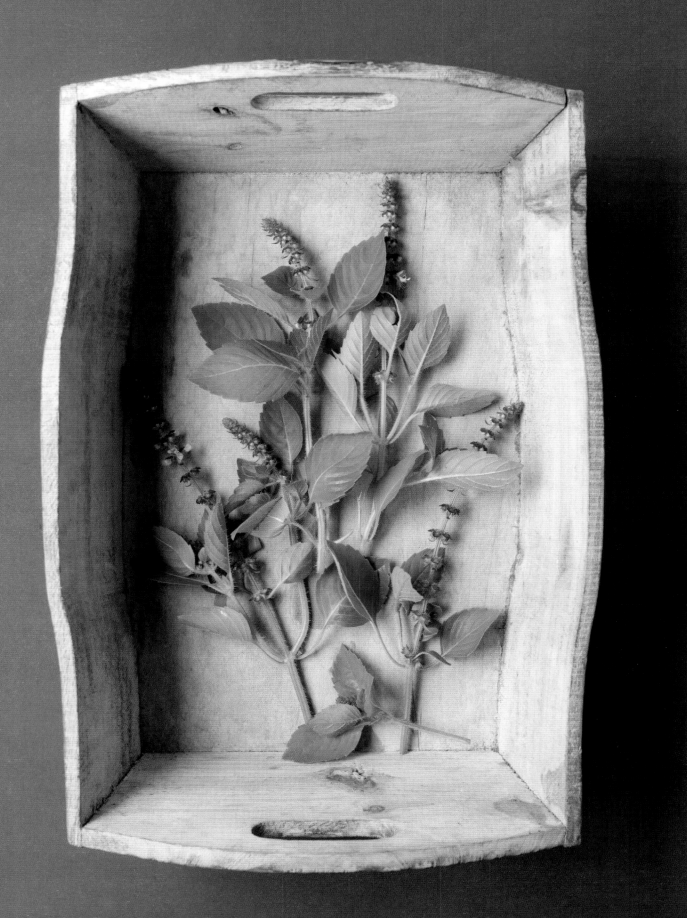

STRESS RELIEF

This garden contains adaptogens and a few nervines to help you better resist the negative effects of stress and attain deep, calm energy. They also boost mood and improve focus and cognitive function. You *could* grow all of these herbs in your standard garden bed. Holy basil, ashwagandha, and gotu kola are more garden-friendly, whereas oats and roses may do better in spots of their own. Other stress-relieving herbs include lemon balm, bacopa, lavender, blue vervain, and betony.

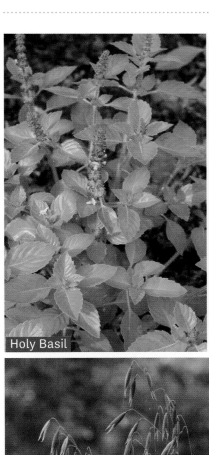

Holy Basil

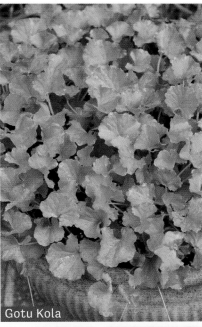

Gotu Kola

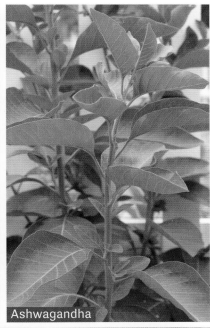

Ashwagandha

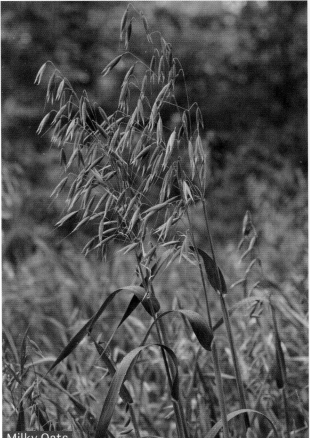

Milky Oats

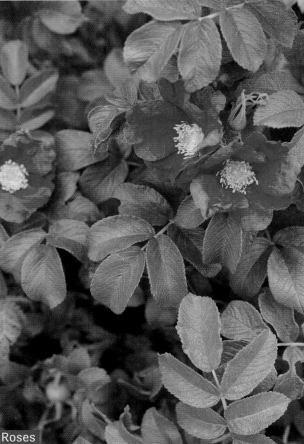

Roses

Holy Basil

This herb could easily be added to *any* of the Energy and Relaxation gardens — it's delightful and versatile. Also called tulsi, it's a calm-energy adaptogen-nervine that lifts mood, eases anxiety, improves focus, reduces blood sugar and stress-related food cravings, decreases inflammation, and more. A classic garden herb, it prefers full sun, hot weather, and good drainage. Treat it as a tender perennial; it won't survive frost. See page 274 for more information.

Best in: tea, tincture, vinegar, honey, capsule, glycerite, hydrosol, water, seltzer

Gotu Kola

This anxiety-relieving adaptogen offers *many* useful side benefits. As a nootropic, it heals nerves, improves memory, and protects cognition. As a vulnerary, it heals wounds and improves connective tissue systemically and on contact — in skin, gums, the gut, veins, and other parts of the body. Take high doses regularly over the long term to get the effects. This herbaceous, creeping Indian ground cover thrives in hot, sludgy conditions in dappled or partial sunlight, but it does fine in a well-tended container. See page 272 for more.

Best in: tincture, tea, powder, food

Ashwagandha

Yet another adaptogen from India, ashwagandha brings the strength of a stallion to those who take it regularly. A nervine-adaptogen, it eases anxiety, provides deep energy, improves libido, boosts thyroid function, decreases inflammation and pain, and modulates immune function. Treat it like tomatoes (its relative): good soil and drainage, full sun, plenty of warmth, no competition. It may exceed 4 feet in height. Unless you live in a hot climate, harvest the roots before frost in its first year. See page 247 for more.

Best in: tincture, tea, powder, milk, ghee, electuary, capsule

Milky Oats

Better known as a cover crop and cereal grain, oats can be harvested for medicinal purposes when immature. It's ready for just a few days when you squeeze the seed and milky latex spurts out. This "milk" contains alkaloids that restore and rebuild the nervous-adrenal system. Taken daily, it's like comfort food for your nerves. Dried, it loses potency but still serves as a source of minerals. Consider sowing oats in a new or resting garden bed. See page 290 for more.

Best in: fresh tincture, fresh vinegar, fresh glycerine

Roses

Use the petals or whole flowers of any good-tasting, nice-smelling, unsprayed rose, particularly damask, rugosa, cabbage, apothecary, wild, and heirloom species. Roses lift the spirits, gladden the heart, and help us work through grief and trauma. Focus on their aromatics, which extract best at cooler temps over time (bonus points for a sweet base). Most roses get "hedge-y" and swamp everything in thorns, so wildcraft or plant it along a wall or property edge. See page 296 for more.

Best in: glycerite, tea, water, seltzer, hydrosol, honey, oxymel, syrup

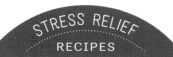
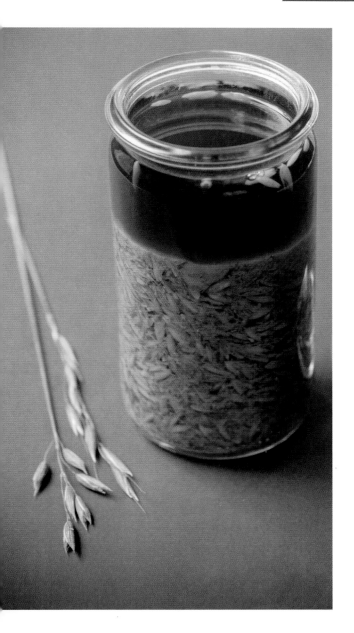

MILKY OATS TINCTURE

THIS TECHNIQUE IS ESSENTIALLY THE SAME as for a fresh tincture given on page 38, but whirring it in a blender better extracts the "milk." It will settle out in the bottle. Simply shake before dosing.

1 part by weight fresh milky oat seeds

2 parts by volume high-proof alcohol or apple cider vinegar

Combine the herbs and alcohol in a blender, and whir it together into a slurry. Pour it into a jar, cover, and shake periodically. Wait at least a month before straining. This is great in formulas but can also be taken solo, up to 1 teaspoon 3 times per day. (Do not use milky oats if you have a glutenlike reaction to oatmeal. Oats don't contain gluten, but they do have proteins with a similar structure.)

STRESS SUPPORT TINCTURE BLEND

HERBALISTS AND HERB ENTHUSIASTS often make individual tinctures that they can blend into a myriad of formulas as needed. This avoids issues of combining plants that may have different extraction methods (and it gives you more versatility to change your formula as desired). For example, lemon balm and milky oat seed extract best fresh in high-proof alcohol, while the preferred method of extracting dried ashwagandha is in lower-proof alcohol. Here's one sample blend that has a mix of adaptogens and nervines to improve mood, stress resistance, and brain function. Use glycerites instead of tinctures if you prefer a sweet-tasting alcohol-free blend. Play around and make your own custom blends. Bacopa, rosemary, and rose glycerite are worthy candidates. To make the following recipe in a 2-ounce bottle (six parts total filling 60 ml), each part would be about 10 ml.

2 parts ashwagandha tincture

1 part holy basil tincture

1 part Milky Oats Tincture (page 106)

1 part gotu kola tincture

1 part lemon balm tincture

Suggested tools: Mini-measure shot glass, small funnel, 2-ounce dropper bottle

Measure each part by volume and pour it into your bottle. The dose for this blend would be 2 squirts (roughly 2 ml or ½ teaspoon) 1–3 times per day. If after 2 weeks you feel like you need a bigger boost, bump up to 4 or 5 squirts (1 teaspoon) 1–2 times per day. Dilute the tincture in a small glass of water or juice and take with food.

More Ways to Use Stress-Busting Herbs

Holy rose water: Infuse cold water with fresh roses and holy basil in a pretty glass bottle. See page 97.

Holy basil tea: Delicious hot or iced, straight up or lightly sweetened. Enjoy it plain or with roses, lemon balm, peppermint, and/or green tea. Iced holy basil tea with honey and a pinch of salt makes a great energy drink alternative! See page 124 for more details.

Ashwagandha milk: Helps deliver ashwagandha to your fat-lined nervous system. Simmer ashwagandha roots or powder in whole milk, almond milk, or coconut milk, lightly sweetened with honey or maple syrup. For flavor, consider nutmeg, cardamom, and/or cinnamon to taste.

Ashwagandha chai: Use the Chai Base on page 78.

Ashwagandha powder creations: Simmer in steel-cut oats with ripe banana, cinnamon, and maple syrup; add to bone broth or smoothies; make Brainiac Bonbons (page 112); nice with chocolate; great as a tincture.

Alcohol-free fresh milky oats: Follow the instructions for a tincture with vinegar, vinegar/honey, or pure glycerine (pages 46 to 50). This may get funky after a few months, so keep refrigerated and store an abundance in the freezer to thaw as needed. Or purée in water and freeze in ice cube trays.

Rose glycerite: Divine calm! See page 119.

Gotu kola creations: Combine with holy basil and green tea. Add to salads. Sauté as a leafy green. Add fresh or powdered to smoothies. Tincture.

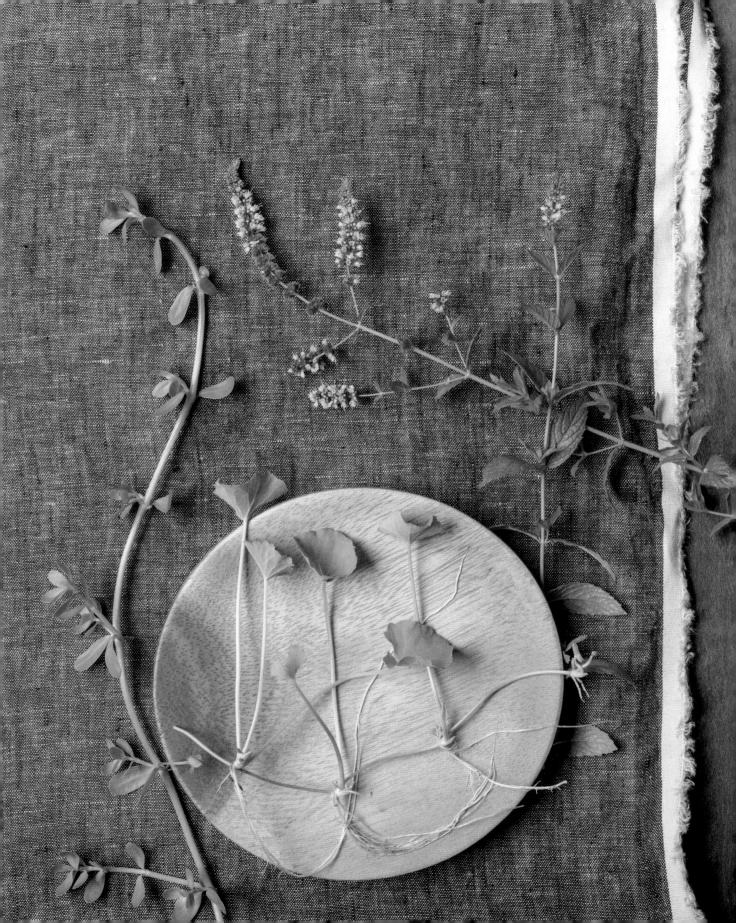

BRAIN BOOSTERS

Get ready to have your mind blown. You're probably already growing some of our best brain-boosting herbs in your garden. Human studies show that everyday mint-family herbs like lemon balm, rosemary, sage, peppermint, and spearmint perk up cognition, strengthen focus, and provide calming energy whether you inhale or ingest them. Add in some easy-to-grow nootropic (smart drug) herbs like gotu kola and bacopa, and you've got a cognitive cornucopia at your disposal. Other cognitive herbs include holy basil, ashwagandha, sage, and hawthorn.

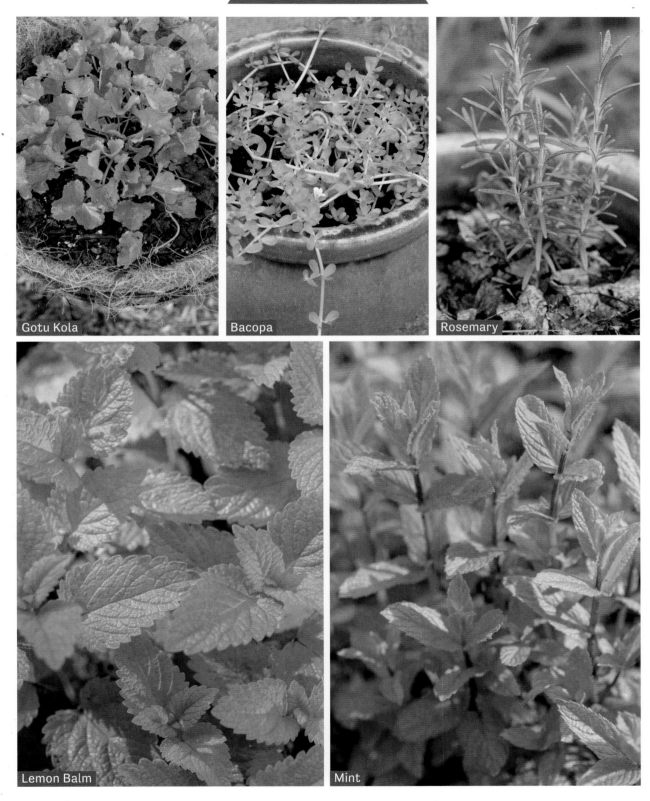

Gotu Kola

Bacopa

Rosemary

Lemon Balm

Mint

Gotu Kola

This creeping ground cover thrives in warm, rich, soggy soil in partial or dappled sunlight and tolerates well-tended containers. Ayurvedic practitioners have relied on gotu kola (sometimes called brahmi) as a brain tonic for thousands of years. Taking high doses long term helps the body adapt to stress, improves brain function, repairs and protects against nerve damage, boosts cognition and working memory, quells anxiety and hyperactivity, and enhances circulation. See page 272 for more.

Best in: food (salad, pesto, smoothies, sautéed), tea, tincture, capsule, powder, flower essence, broth

Bacopa

Another container-friendly herb from India, bacopa is also called brahmi and likes even wetter conditions than gotu kola. Bacopa also boasts a long history of use in Ayurveda. Studies on adults, children, and elders support its ability to calm and focus the mind, particularly in cases of memory and cognitive problems like delayed free recall and ADHD. It's quite bitter and astringent, like overbrewed black tea. See page 248 for more.

Best in: tincture, capsule, powder

Rosemary

You already know and love rosemary. Unlike gotu kola, this Mediterranean native prefers dry conditions and well-drained soil — perhaps in a terra-cotta pot. Greeks and Romans used "rosemary for remembrance," adding it to wedding bouquets and braiding it into their hair to inhale during exams. Inhaling its aroma makes people more alert and helps them score better on memory tests. In modern studies, consuming foodlike doses of 750 mg improved memory speed in older adults, yet higher doses worsened it. Use it in food and as a synergist. Dried works, but fresh is best. See page 297 for more.

Best in: food, tincture, tea, vinegar, powder, capsule, flower essence

Lemon Balm

Lemon balm quickly evokes a calm-alert state. In studies, just one dose increased cognition and relieved anxiety within 1 hour! It also improves word recognition, reduces anger and frustration, lifts the spirits, and aids sleep. I love it for children and adults who are too hyped up, overstimulated, or agitated to focus. Some people find it sedating in high doses, so play around to find your sweet spot. See page 280 for more.

Best in: tincture, glycerite, water, topically in cream or body oil, tea

Mint

Simply inhaling mint perks you up. Studies concur that peppermint's aroma boosts alertness and improves memory quality and speed. Spearmint extract doubled attention and concentration scores over 30 days, with some benefits seen in just 1 day. Add mint to tea and tincture blends to flavor and synergize them. Sip peppermint-infused water at your desk. Choose your location wisely when planting mint in the garden — this brute loves to take over. See page 286 for more.

Best in: tea, tincture, food, water, seltzer/soda, peppermint flower essence, glycerite, gum, essential oil

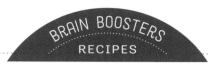
BRAIN-BOOSTING TINCTURE BLEND

YOU CAN PREPARE THIS from premade individual tinctures or make a combination fresh plant tincture (see the recipe on page 38). Feel free to play around with the formula and the ingredients to suit your individual needs.

2 parts gotu kola tincture

1 part bacopa tincture

1 part lemon balm tincture

½ part holy basil tincture

¼ part rosemary tincture

¼ part peppermint or spearmint tincture

If using premade individual tinctures, measure out each part by volume. For example, if each part is 1 ounce, your final tincture blend will be 5 ounces. Shake well to combine.

If making a combination blend from scratch, follow the instructions for a fresh plant tincture on page 38. If each part is an ounce by weight of fresh plant, make your tincture in a pint (16-ounce) jar.

Take 2–4 ml of your blend 1–3 times daily or as needed.

BRAINIAC BONBONS

These tasty energy balls are limited only by your imagination! Opt for good- or decent-tasting herbs (go easy on the bitter bacopa), and make sure the powder is ground superfine.

2 tablespoons nut butter (such as almond)

1 tablespoon honey or puréed date, or to taste

1 teaspoon powdered herb(s) (such as ashwagandha, hawthorn, gotu kola, holy basil)

Toasted sesame seeds or coconut flakes for rolling

Mix the nut butter, honey, and herbs thoroughly together. Feel free to add other ingredients, like chopped nuts or fruit. Roll into small balls. Then roll/dip them in the sesame seeds or coconut. If you're feeling particularly decadent, dip them in melted dark chocolate instead (chill the honey–nut butter balls first) and let cool on parchment paper or in mini baking cups. Enjoy one or two bonbons as a dose of herbs.

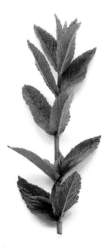

MINTY MEMORY TEA

THIS DELICIOUS TEA provides an instant boost and can be enjoyed as a daily tonic tea. Aim for 3- to 4-inch-long sprigs. Try it also as an infused water on hot summer days. You can use similar ratios of dried herbs, using 1 tablespoon total per 16-ounce mug.

3 sprigs fresh peppermint

3 sprigs fresh spearmint

3 sprigs fresh lemon balm

1 sprig fresh rosemary

Rub the sprigs to release their aroma. Combine the herbs in a 16-ounce mug, jar, or teapot, cover with hot or cold water, let steep 15 minutes. You don't necessarily need to strain out the fresh sprigs.

ROSEMARY-LEMON TEA

THIS FRESH, SURPRISINGLY TASTY TEA tastes equally great sipped at your desk as it does after a heavy meal. Not only does rosemary perk up and enliven the mind, but both rosemary and lemon cut grease and boost digestion.

1–2 sprigs fresh rosemary

1 lemon wedge

Steep for 5 minutes or longer in 8–16 ounces of hot water. No need to strain.

More Ways to Use Brain-Boosting Herbs

Rosemary seltzer: Toss a few sprigs into bubbly water.

Holy lemon water: Combine fresh sprigs of holy basil and lemon balm in seltzer or cold tap water.

Energy drink: Make an iced tea of holy basil and green tea with honey plus a pinch of salt.

Aromatherapy spray: Peppermint, rosemary, basil, and pine aromas all improve alertness. In a spray bottle, use a homemade hydrosol (page 58) or add 15 drops of the essential oil(s) to a 1:1 blend of vodka and water.

Flower essences: Use solo, add to other remedies, or make a room spray. Classic cognitive flower essences include peppermint, rosemary, cosmos, gotu kola, and sage. For more, see page 68.

Broth: Make a broth (page 81) featuring gotu kola, lion's mane mushrooms, shiitake mushroom, and perhaps a little ashwagandha, reishi, or chaga as a long-term brain tonic.

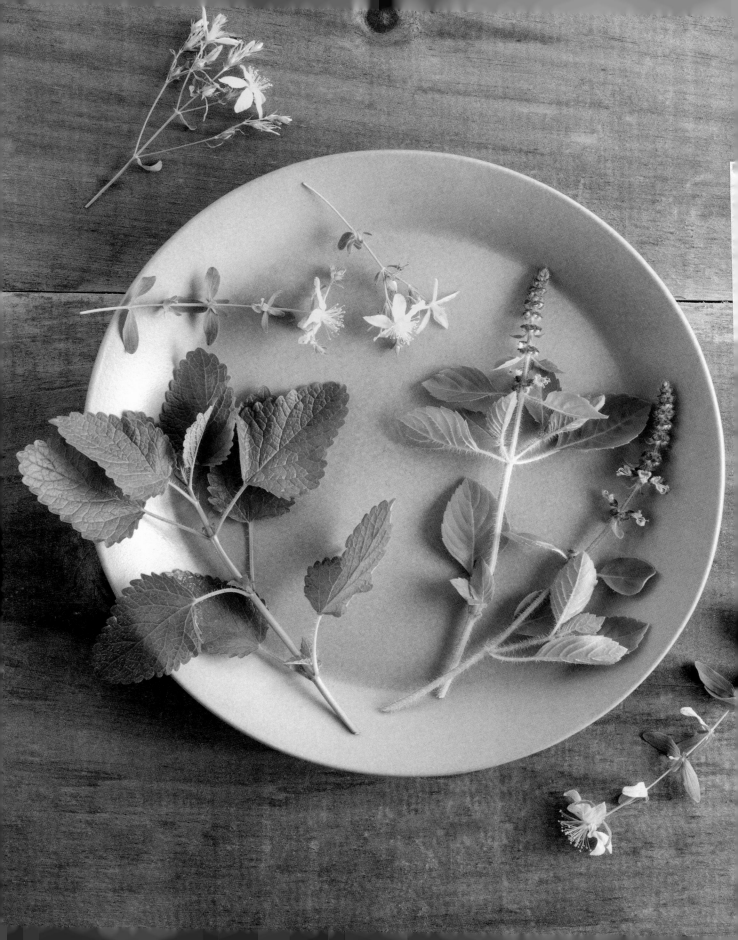

UPLIFT

Never underestimate the ability of a cup of tea to make the world feel right again. Simply spending time outdoors in your garden and brewing a mug (of anything) has been shown in studies to boost mood, make you friendlier, and improve your outlook on others. Although major depression can be tricky to alleviate, St. John's wort, mimosa, roses, holy basil, and lemon balm help lift your spirits. Other uplifting herbs include motherwort, ashwagandha, lemon verbena, and peppermint.

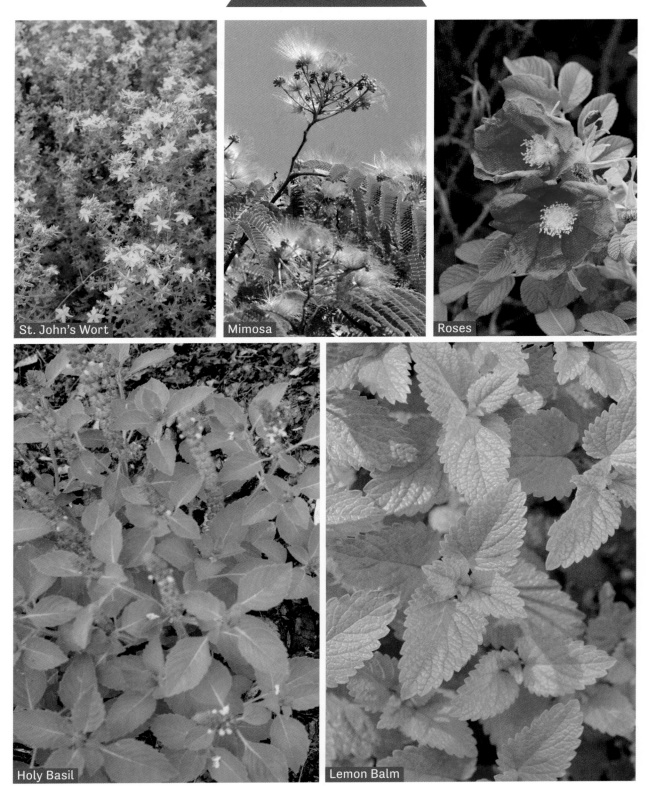

St. John's Wort

Mimosa

Roses

Holy Basil

Lemon Balm

St. John's Wort

This scrappy weed brings sun into your life. It blooms near summer solstice and the feast of St. John, thrives in sunny, dry spots, and is most potent after a hot, sunny week. Tincture the *fresh* buds and flowers, and refresh the batch every 1 to 3 years to ensure potency. Studies show that St. John's wort works almost as well as SSRI (selective serotonin reuptake inhibitor) medications like Prozac for depression (including seasonal affective disorder), and it may work even better when combined with lemon balm. Expect it to take 4 to 8 weeks of steady dosing to kick in. See page 299 for more, including herb-drug interactions.

Best in: tincture

Mimosa

Also known as the "tree of collective happiness," silk tree, and albizia, this graceful medium-sized tree is an attractive landscape specimen with adorable aromatic pink powder-puff flowers. Use the fresh or freshly dried bark (more potent) or blossoms. Mimosa makes you happy and calm and eases grief. In my clinical experience, it works faster and more reliably than St. John's wort for most people. However, it can be invasive in temperate climates and is not hardy below Zone 6. See page 285 for more information.

Best in: tincture, tea, possibly glycerite

Roses

Stop and sip the roses. Roses gladden the heart, ease heartbreak, lift the spirit, and remind workaholics to take a break and breathe. The sight, flavor, and scent of rose petals work their magic and make a lovely addition to blends. Choose any nice-scented, good-tasting rose. Unruly wild and heirloom species usually grow best as a hedge. Long, cool infusions best extract rose aroma. See page 296 for more.

Best in: glycerite, water, seltzer, honey, oxymel, syrup, flower essence, tea

Holy Basil

Holy basil (also known as tulsi) lifts mood and energy and clears brain fog while quelling anxiety. It fosters a Zen-like state of mind. Simply inhaling this potent aromatic brings a shift in consciousness. Be prepared to be blissed out. Some people even feel a bit high on tulsi. It blends well with other uplifting herbs and tastes pleasant. Grow it as you would culinary basil — it loves heat, sun, rich soil, regular water, and good drainage. See page 274 for more information.

Best in: tea, tincture, vinegar, honey, capsule, glycerite, hydrosol, oxymel, powder

Lemon Balm

This multifaceted, easy-to-grow herb could be added to almost any garden in this book, including every Energy and Relaxation garden. This calming nervine improves focus, gladdens the heart, and lifts the spirits. Best fresh or freshly dried, lemon balm supports and synergizes the herbs it's combined with, including St. John's wort or holy basil. This no-fuss herb grows easily and abundantly, thriving in part sun and rich soil. Best fresh. See page 280 for more.

Best in: tincture, tea, glycerite, water, seltzer, hydrosol, honey

LEMON–ST. JOHN'S WORT PICK-ME-UP

HERBS LIKE ST. JOHN'S WORT and lemon balm work best as fresh plant tinctures, and even better when combined — a tip I learned from David Winston. To ensure potency, refresh your batch every 1 to 3 years.

2½ ounces St. John's wort fresh buds and flowers

2½ ounces lemon balm fresh aerial parts

If you have premade tinctures, simply blend them 1:1 in a new bottle. To make a combination fresh plant tincture, follow the directions on page 38. Take 2 ml three times per day. It can take several weeks to fully kick in. Note that St. John's wort interacts with many medications.

Uplifting Simple Preparations

- Rose glycerite
- Mimosa bark tincture
- Lemon balm and holy basil tea, infused water, or seltzer
- Green tea with a fresh sprig of lemon balm, holy basil, or lemon verbena
- Peppermint and holy basil tea
- St. John's wort tincture (solo or with lemon balm)

HAPPY TEA

TURN TO THIS UPLIFTING, TASTY TEA for mild mood funks.

½ teaspoon lemon balm

½ teaspoon holy basil

½ teaspoon lemon verbena

½ teaspoon mimosa blossoms or bark (optional)

Sprinkle of rose petals

1 teaspoon honey

Steep the herbs in 16 ounces of hot water for 15–20 minutes. Strain, add honey, and enjoy 1–3 times per day.

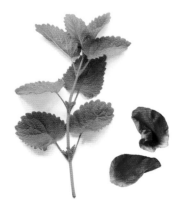

Rose Glycerite

Rose water (a hydrosol) gets all the attention, but I find rose glycerite far more useful and enjoyable. Simply steep rose petals in pure vegetable glycerine for a month or more. Magenta rugosa roses will eventually turn it a lovely shade of pink. Rose glycerite tastes heavenly — sweet, rosy, uplifting — and keeps a year or more on the shelf (unlike rose water). You can take it internally, add it to food and drink and also use it in skin care recipes. I keep a dropper bottle at my desk for a quick hit of happy sweet.

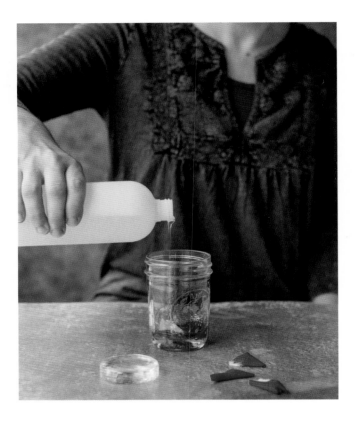

GOOD MOOD TINCTURE

THIS ST. JOHN'S WORT–FREE FORMULA is safer for people who are already taking medications alongside their herbs (still double-check with your pharmacist or herbalist, and keep your doctor in the loop). Regardless of whether or not you're taking medications, this formula is also broad spectrum for mood and often begins to work quickly. Still, be cautious introducing mimosa if you're on medications — there's very little safety data available, and you can skip it if you'd like to err on the side of caution.

2 ounce mimosa bark tincture (fresh or dried)

1 ounce holy basil tincture (fresh)

1 ounce lemon balm tincture (fresh)

1 ounce motherwort tincture (fresh)

1 ounce rose glycerite (optional)

If you have premade tinctures and glycerite, simply combine them and shake well. If not, combine the tincture ingredients in a 16-ounce jar following the instructions on page 38. Separately, make your Rose Glycerite (above), and add it, if desired, to the finished blend. Take 2–5 ml two times daily.

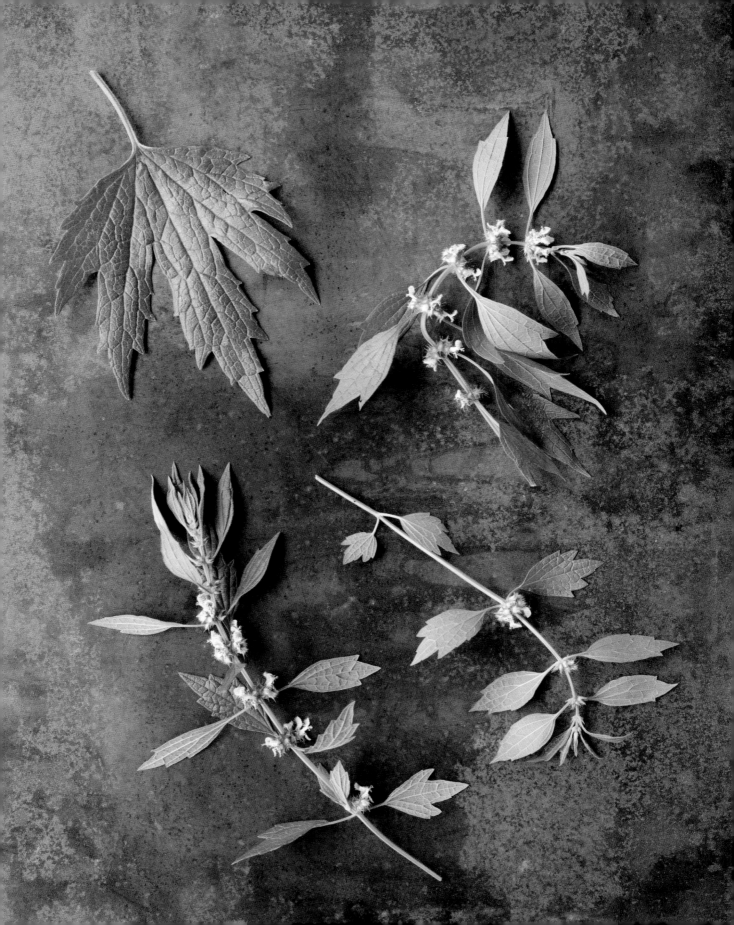

RELAX AND RESTORE

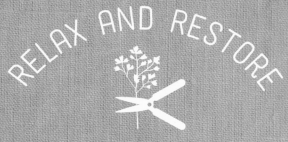

This garden contains mild sedatives, calm-energy adaptogens, and nervines. By day, motherwort, holy basil, skullcap, and lemon balm soothe frayed nerves, ease anxiety, and take the edge off of stress. By night, they can help you fall asleep more quickly and stay sleeping more deeply. The core herbs below are easy growers that reach 1 to 2 feet tall and have the appearance of classic herbs, perfect for growing in the general landscape or a standard garden bed. Other calming herbs include milky oat seed, passionflower, ashwagandha, linden, lavender, and rose.

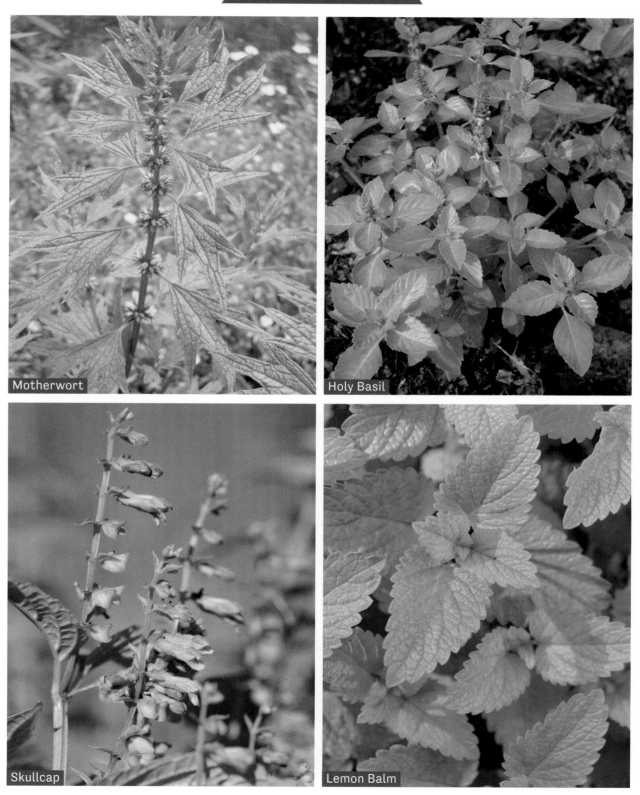

Motherwort

Holy Basil

Skullcap

Lemon Balm

Motherwort

This profoundly bitter mint-family herb offers love with better boundaries than its relatives. Use it daily or as needed for anxiety and panic attacks, especially when stress manifests in the heart with palpitations, tachycardia, and a tight chest. It softens those who feel overwhelmed, overworked, underappreciated, and on a rampage, as well as during life changes like perimenopause. It does best in good soil with moderate moisture. When happy, it reaches 5 feet tall and self-seeds rampantly. See page 287 for more information.

Best in: tincture, vinegar, oxymel, flower essence

Holy Basil

A delicious, delightful, aromatic herb, holy basil excels at relaxing the mind and body, improving cognition, and lifting the spirits. It also lowers blood sugar, modulates cortisol, decreases inflammation, improves digestion, and helps strengthen the immune system to protect you against common pathogens. Like culinary basil, holy basil thrives in a pampered garden bed. It adores full sun and hot weather, dying at the kiss of frost. Also called tulsi and sacred basil. See page 274 for more.

Best in: tea, tincture, vinegar, honey, capsule, glycerine, hydrosol, water, seltzer

Skullcap

Turn to this nervine-sedative for anxiety, stress, sleep, and pain. It's specific for those who are overly sensitive, easily irritated by touch, scent, light, or other stimuli. Skullcap turns the nerves down a notch. The strength of its sedative action varies person to person; in rare cases it aggravates depression and melancholy. A bit finicky to grow, it may thrive then die in the same spot from one year to another. It's always a gamble whether or not the perennial will come back or need to be planted anew. It prefers moist, rich soil. See page 300 for more.

Best in: tincture, tea, glycerite

Lemon Balm

This robust perennial emits a strong "Lemon Pledge" aroma that quickly dissipates once dried. Uplifting, cognition-enhancing, and mildly relaxing, lemon balm can be used day or night to ease depression and anxiety while increasing focus. It also boosts digestion and offers antiviral effects for herpes and possibly the flu. It prefers rich, slightly moist soil in partial shade but will grow almost anywhere. Best fresh or freshly dried. See page 280 for more.

Best in: fresh tincture, tea, glycerite, flower essence

Holy Basil Beverages

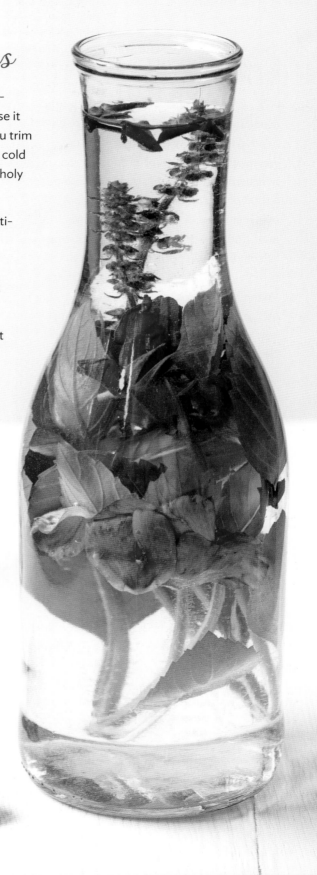

Holy basil's fabulous flavor and nerve-soothing, stress-busting properties make it a favorite beverage herb. Use it dried in tea. Fresh sprigs (including those blossoms you trim off to encourage growth) can be steeped in hot water, cold water, or seltzer. One of the great joys of summer! Try holy basil solo or consider these delightful garden blends.

Holy basil and lemon balm: calm energy, mood lift, anti-anxiety, great for workaholics to destress and before bedtime

Holy basil and rose: gladden the heart, ease stress, lift spirits

Holy basil and peppermint: invigorate the mind, boost energy, lift spirits

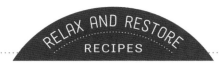
MELLOW ME GLYCERITE

CONSIDER THIS BLEND as a daily tonic or when you just need to chill out but still function during the day. It has calming, mildly energizing, heart-gladdening, and cognition-enhancing properties. While you could easily make this blend as a tincture (it would actually be a little stronger medicinally), as a glycerite it has a more pleasant, sweet flavor. Thank herbalist Steven Horne for this awesome, fast medicine-making technique! Feel free to skip an herb if you don't have it. For an 8-ounce mason jar, you'll want about 2 ounces of total prepped herbs by weight and 5 ounces by volume of glycerine . . . or you can just eyeball it.

2 parts fresh holy basil flowers or aerial parts, chopped

2 parts fresh milky oat seeds, whole

2 parts fresh lemon balm aerial parts, chopped

1 part skullcap or passionflower aerial parts, chopped (optional, for added sedation)

1 part rose petals

100 percent vegetable glycerine

Mason or canning jar with two-part canning lid

Combine the herbs in your jar, pack tightly but not quite to the top. Cover it with glycerine but leave a little headroom as you would for canning. Cap it and submerge it in a large pot of water. Bring to a boil and let simmer for 15 minutes. Allow to cool enough to handle before straining, squeezing as much liquid as possible. Store in a cool, dark, dry spot. Take ½–1 teaspoon (3–5 squirts) twice daily or as needed.

More Ways to Use Calming Herbs

Simple tinctures: All these plants make excellent simple (single-ingredient) tinctures, ideally from the fresh plant material, which is far more potent. Choose the one best suited for you or blend them into a formula. Fresh plant vinegars, oxymels, or glycerites can also be used. For calm energy, also consider ashwagandha or milky oat seed. For gentle sedation, try passionflower, blue vervain, or low-dose lavender.

Additional teas: Along with holy basil beverages, consider chamomile, lemon balm–mint, or linden tea.

Aromatherapy: Lavender or rose essential oil, hydrosol, glycerite, or potpourri helps bring things down a notch.

Flower essences: Blue vervain, dandelion, valerian, lavender, skullcap, lemon balm, betony, and others. Take a few drops on the tongue, add to water or tea, mix into tinctures, apply topically, or spray in the air. See page 68 (flower essence recipe) and individual plant profiles for more details.

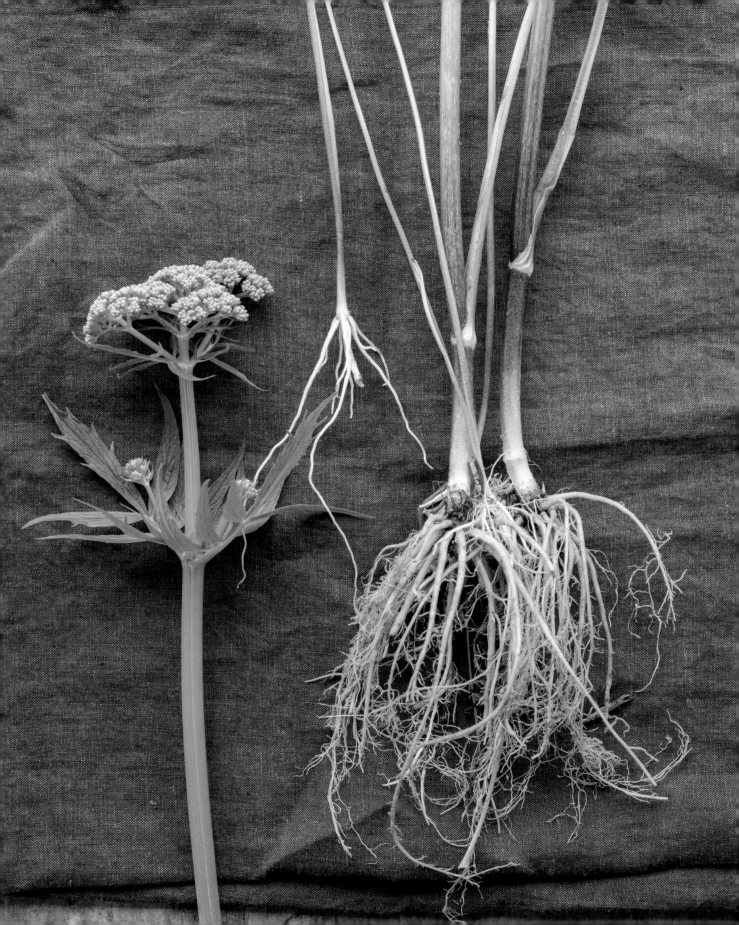

SLEEPY TIME

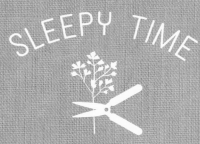

One in three Americans slacks on the recommended seven hours of sleep per night, and many can't sleep even if they try. Chronic insomnia is multi-factorial and sometimes tricky to fix, but valerian, skullcap, passionflower, and California poppy help point your body in the right direction — toward your bed! Dose yourself with these homegrown sedatives shortly before you hit the hay. Tinker around a bit — most people find one perfect plant that suits them better than any other, but blends work well, too. Other sleep herbs include lemon balm, chamomile, lavender, ashwagandha, linden, and magnolia bark.

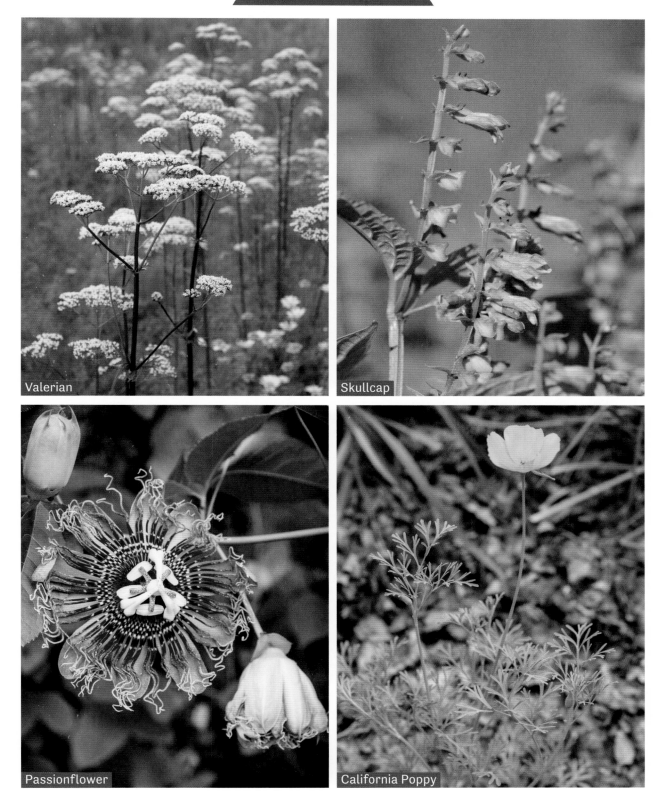

Valerian

Skullcap

Passionflower

California Poppy

Valerian

Even though valerian is the most studied and most famous herb for sleep, it's actually the least reliable for a broad group of people. Valerian suits anxious, thin-framed people who tend to be cold with taut muscles. For "valerian people," it loosens those muscles and improves sleep latency for a deeper, more restorative night's sleep. For others, it may not work at all, make them groggy or agitated, or overstimulate them. In the garden, valerian produces beautiful tall, pleasantly aromatic flowers that self-seed aggressively in good soil. Pull up the stinky roots in spring or fall for medicine. See page 304 for more.

Best in: fresh root tincture, flower essence, maybe tea (blech)

Skullcap

Think of skullcap when you can't get to sleep because *everything* gets on your nerves — from the stress of the day, a light outside the window, or a worry about tomorrow to a mosquito flying around the room or your bed partner's obnoxious breathing. Skullcap "caps your skull," nourishes your nerves, and brings your reactions down a notch so you can get some shut-eye. This creek-side wildflower can be hit or miss in the garden with alternating years of abundant, then puny, growth. It prefers rich soil and good moisture. Some years it comes back; some years it doesn't. Best fresh or freshly dried. Stock up your apothecary in good years. See page 300 for more.

Best in: tincture, tea, glycerite

Passionflower

Simply gazing into the otherworldly, mandala-like passionflower flower could lull you to sleep. In addition to its amazing beauty, intricacy, and sweet, calming aroma, passionflower may well be our most effective safe sedative and sleep aid. It works for almost anyone, quelling mind chatter to lull you into deep sleep. Although not as well studied as valerian, its effects in studies have been more profound, both as a simple herb and when combined with other sleep herbs. It's useful fresh or dried. See page 292 for more information.

Best in: tincture, tea, glycerite

California Poppy

Native Americans relied on poppy to induce sleep and mediate pain. Its safe, nonaddictive constituents produce a mild, tranquilizing effect. Think of it for people who wake in the middle of the night and can't go back to sleep, as well as those who struggle with spinning thoughts or pain that interferes with slumber. This Southwest native thrives in full sun and dryish soil. In cooler climates, seed it along a south-facing fence, wall, or hill. All parts can be used, but the roots are strongest. See page 256 for more information.

Best in: tincture, maybe vinegar or tea (not tasty)

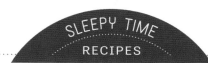
SLEEP TEA

SIMPLE AND EFFECTIVE, this pleasant-tasting blend works well for most people, even children. Passionflower's the heavy hitter here, with backup from skullcap. If it's too strong for you, bump up the lemon balm. Spearmint and honey bring the flavors together to make a tasty tea. Brew it in small, strong doses. You don't want it to make you get up and pee in the middle of the night.

½ teaspoon dried passionflower aerial parts

½ teaspoon dried skullcap aerial parts

½ teaspoon lemon balm leaf

½ teaspoon spearmint leaf

1 teaspoon honey

Steep the herbs in 4–6 ounces of hot water for 15–20 minutes. Strain, sweeten, and enjoy.

More Ways to Use Sleep-Inducing Herbs

- Chamomile tea, plain or with spearmint
- Lemon balm and holy basil tea, lightly sweetened with honey
- Ashwagandha honey milk
- Linden tea, for gentle calm
- Linden or linden–passionflower–lemon balm cordial
- Magnolia bark tincture, for those who wake early with a racing mind
- Passionflower and skullcap tincture blend
- Lavender essential oil or hydrosol, inhaled, as a dream pillow, or sprayed on the pillow
- Lavender or lemon balm cream, applied topically
- Valerian or lavender flower essence
- St. John's wort flower essence for when nightmares are a problem

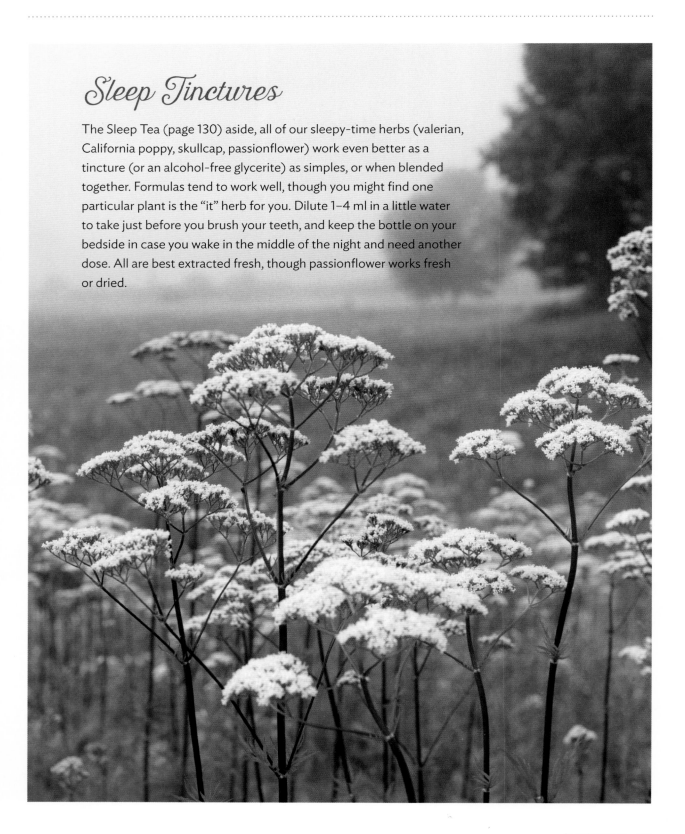

Sleep Tinctures

The Sleep Tea (page 130) aside, all of our sleepy-time herbs (valerian, California poppy, skullcap, passionflower) work even better as a tincture (or an alcohol-free glycerite) as simples, or when blended together. Formulas tend to work well, though you might find one particular plant is the "it" herb for you. Dilute 1–4 ml in a little water to take just before you brush your teeth, and keep the bottle on your bedside in case you wake in the middle of the night and need another dose. All are best extracted fresh, though passionflower works fresh or dried.

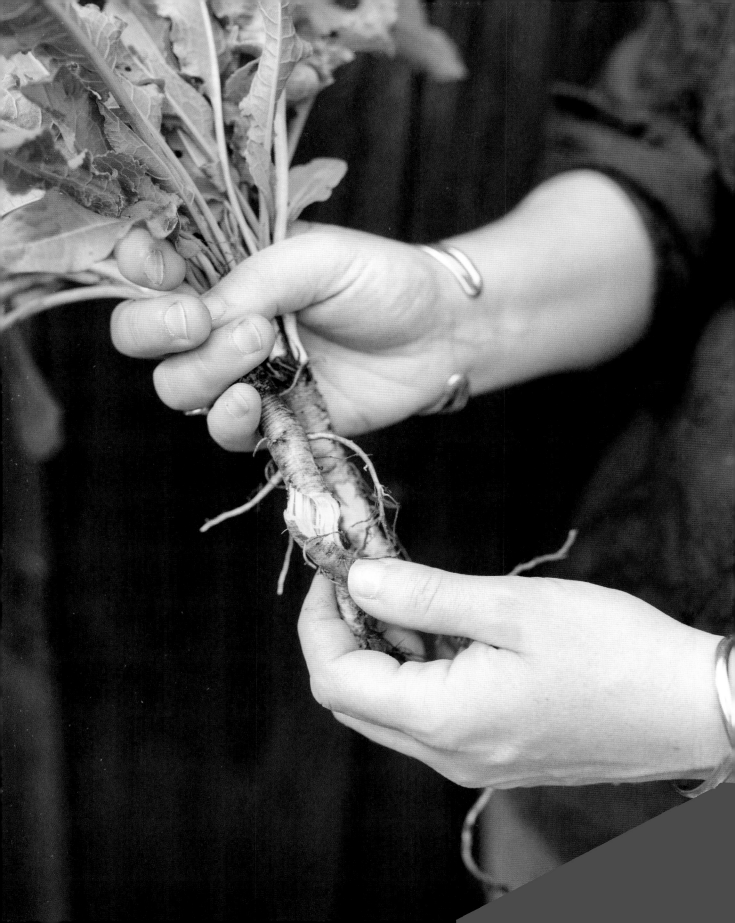

Digestion and Detoxification

FOR THOUSANDS OF YEARS, herbalists and holistic physicians have viewed digestion and detoxification as the most important body systems that affect overall health and well-being. Even seemingly unconnected conditions like reproductive hormone imbalance, autoimmune disease, and skin rashes and acne often relate back to the gastrointestinal tract (digestion) and the liver, colon, lymph, and kidneys (detoxification). Not only does their function have a profound impact on vitality versus disease, but they also respond readily to herbal remedies, many of which are easily cultivated or live in your backyard as "weeds."

TYPES OF HERBS FOR DIGESTION AND DETOXIFICATION

We turn to various categories of herbs to enhance the vitality of these body systems, but no class of herbs has the range of herbal bitters.

Bitters and Liver Movers

Simply put, "bitters" taste bitter. Thanks to bitter receptor sites on the tongue and throughout the body, bitter herbs turn on almost every aspect of the digestive process (the production of saliva, digestive enzymes, and stomach acid as well as the muscular contractions of peristalsis that move food through the digestive tract). Bitters also encourage liver-gallbladder detoxification ("cleaning" the blood, filtering out waste in the form of bile for elimination via the intestines). Their many other benefits range from regulating appetite (increasing hunger for healthy foods, decreasing sugar cravings, balancing blood sugar and insulin response, and improving satiety) to improving hormone function, metabolism, and excretion. When in doubt, try bitters. They include artichoke, dandelion, Oregon grape root, and catnip.

Carminatives

Carminatives complement bitters. In contrast to the generally "cooling" nature of bitters, carminatives tend to warm, yet both categories stimulate digestion. Carminatives are aromatic, flavorful, and rich in essential oils. Medicinally, they usually stimulate digestive juices, relax muscles, release spasms, dispel gas and bloating, ease pain, open the lungs, move stagnant mucus, and lift and/or calm mood. The mint and fennel families have many carminative species. Carminatives include peppermint, chamomile, lemon balm, and fennel.

Relaxing Bitters

Calming digestive herbs are often carminatives that also have a mild bitter flavor and not only stimulate digestive function but also calm the nerves. "Fight or flight" stress mode and anxiety shut down digestive system function, so it's easy to see how digestive issues relate to your state of mind. Nervous indigestion, low stomach acid, colic, gas, pain, spasms, constipation, and some types of reflux are particularly common. Herbs that relax the nervous system while simultaneously enhancing digestion can be very helpful here, and most are easy to grow. They're often consumed as tea. Calming digestives include chamomile, lemon balm, and catnip.

Demulcents

Demulcents soothe irritated, inflamed tissue and become somewhat (or significantly) mucilaginous in water or when mashed. You can tell — they feel slimy or velvety. High-mucilage plants may even attain a mucus-like consistency. We use demulcents for dry, irritated, hot, and inflamed states like reflux, gastritis, and leaky gut. Mucilage also helps feed beneficial gut flora; however, in some cases of

Crossover Herbs

You've probably noticed a lot of crossover herbs in these categories!

Calendula: bitter, vulnerary, lymph mover

Yarrow: bitter, carminative, antimicrobial, astringent

Plantain: demulcent, vulnerary, gentle astringent

Chamomile, Catnip, Lemon Balm: mild bitter, carminative

Burdock: mild bitter/liver mover, lymph mover

Bee Balm, Oregano, Thyme, Sage: carminative, antimicrobial

Elecampane: carminative, warming bitter, antimicrobial

small intestinal bacterial overgrowth (SIBO) and dysbiosis, too much mucilage may also feed pathogenic bacteria. (If high-mucilage plants make you gassy, stop using them and focus on lower-mucilage demulcents and other supports, such as bitters, carminatives, and antimicrobials. You may find the tea fine but the powder not.) Demulcents include marshmallow, plantain, and violet.

Vulneraries

These herbs complement demulcents nicely when you need to heal the gut. Vulnerary herbs heal wounds and irritated, inflamed connective tissue. Most famous for benefitting the skin, they're equally valuable for gut lining health and integrity, and some also soothe the lungs. They include calendula, gotu kola, and plantain.

Astringents

Astringent herbs contain tannins that tighten and tone boggy tissue by binding proteins in damaged tissue together, essentially knitting connective tissue more closely together. They can be useful when things are "leaky" like diarrhea, mild bleeding, or leaky gut. Note that diarrhea, bleeding, and severe gut issues often require medical attention first to ensure something more serious is not at play. For chronic,

everyday issues, astringents are wonderful. They usually have some degree of antimicrobial activity as well. Cinnamon is one of our most useful astringents. Garden-variety astringents include roses, plantain, and yarrow.

Antimicrobials

Antimicrobials help fight off pathogens, sometimes on contact (e.g., "bitter berberines") and a few more systemically (e.g., garlic). Fortunately, anything you ingest, in theory, has direct contact with the gut. We use antimicrobials in gut protocols where there is a chronic infection or dysbiosis (overgrowth of pathogenic bacteria). In acute cases antibiotics may also be necessary, but you might be surprised how well the herbs work, and they don't disrupt healthy gut flora as dramatically as antibiotics. We won't focus as directly on antimicrobials in our garden themes, but they're good to know. In your kitchen cabinet, you'll find cinnamon, cloves, and fresh ginger, which are also excellent for warding off infections. Some of our best gut antimicrobials from the garden include berberine-rich herbs, bee balm, elecampane, and garlic.

Diuretics and Kidney Tonics

Diuretic herbs make you pee more, which may not seem like a "benefit" except that this helps

flush out the kidneys, one of your primary detoxification organs, and may indirectly reduce blood pressure, edema (water retention), and arthritis pain as a result. Kidney tonics often contain soothing mucilage. Note that overt kidney conditions usually require immediate medical attention. For non-life-threatening edema and general kidney/detoxification support, consider parsley leaf, dandelion leaf, nettle leaf, or corn silk.

Lymph Movers

Your lymphatic system houses your immune system and also cleans the interstitial fluid around the blood vessels and cells. It's closely associated with your circulatory system but far slower, lacking a pump or its own muscular action to move things along. As you move your body with exercise, skin brushing, or massage, the pressure squeezes on lymph vessels, and valves keep things moving in the right direction. Lymphatic herbs (also called lymphagogues) improve the body's ability to move and filter the lymph. They include calendula, burdock, violet, alder and red clover.

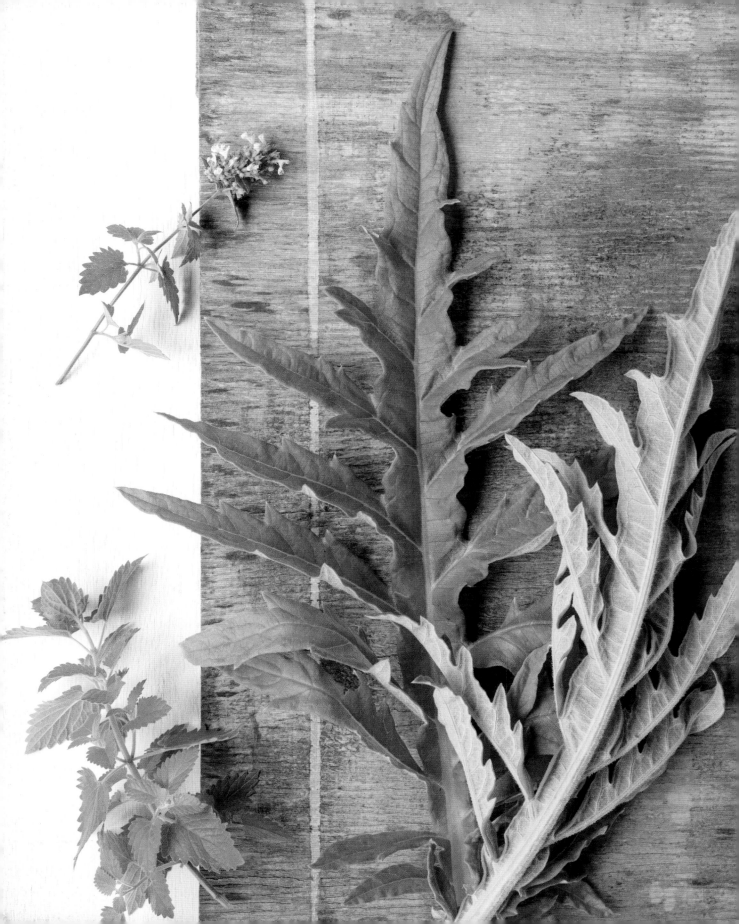

BITTER DIGESTIF

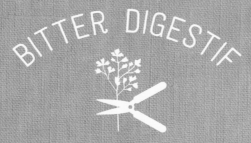

Where to start with a digestive garden? In truth, I could have written an entire *book* devoted to growing digestive herbs. You have so many at your disposal: for starters, almost every single culinary herb and tasty tea. In this Bitter Digestif garden, we focus on excellent bitter and carminative herbs: artichoke, dandelion, catnip, chamomile, and lemon balm. Poor digestion, gas, bloating, sluggish? Enjoy these herbs with, just before (apéritif), or just after (digestif) meals in teas, cordials, tinctures, or infused water or seltzers. They work best when you taste them and are the basis of historical European cocktail bitters. Other bitter herbs include chicory, burdock, elecampane, and berberine-rich herbs.

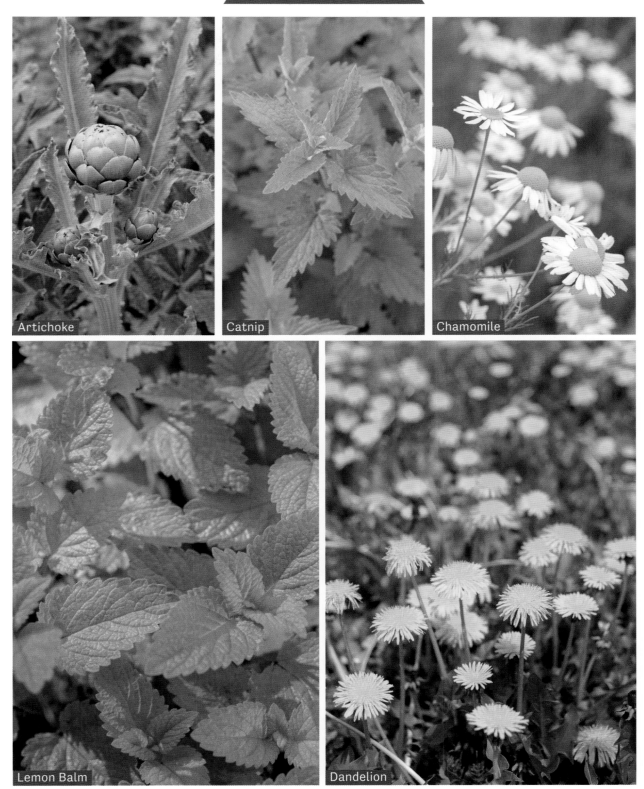

Artichoke

Catnip

Chamomile

Lemon Balm

Dandelion

Artichoke

Bitter is the artichoke plant, one of the oldest cultivated plants on the planet. Medicinally, turn to the intensely simple bitter leaves. As mentioned on page 134, bitter flavors turn on digestion, including peristalsis, digestive juices, and enzymes. This Mediterranean plant prefers heat, sun, and good well-drained soil. Balance the cold, bitter flavor with warming, tasty carminatives and a dash of something sweet. Too bitter for tea, the extract can be sprayed into your mouth or splashed in seltzer. See page 246 for more.

Best in: tincture, vinegar, oxymel, cordial

Catnip

Sure, it gets cats high, but there's so much more to catnip. Think of it as a cross between peppermint and chamomile. Mildly bitter, aromatic, carminative, and slightly calming, catnip's a supreme remedy for sluggish digestion, colic, gas, and bloating. It's quite popular for children. Especially consider it as a colic remedy for those who have allergic reactions to chamomile. It's palatable but not delicious — combine it with mint or holy basil to perk up the flavor. See page 257 for more.

Best in: tea, tincture, oxymel, glycerite, honey syrup

Chamomile

If you crave a digestive tea, look no further than world-renowned chamomile. Mildly bitter (especially with a long steep), carminative, and anti-inflammatory, chamomile enhances digestive juices and function; eases gas, bloating, and colic in babies and adults alike; and soothes off pathogenic gut bacteria including *Helicobacter pylori*. It also calms the mind and soothes fussy, whiny "babies of any age," aids sleep, and quells anxiety. Pinch off the young flowers of this self-seeding annual. Be aware that some people with daisy-family flower allergies may react to chamomile. If so, try catnip. See page 259 for more.

Best in: tea, glycerite, tincture

Lemon Balm

Like most mint-family herbs, lemon balm offers carminative, mildly bitter properties. It calms the nerves while improving digestion (perfect for nervous indigestion, gas, bloating, and IBS), though it's not as strong for gas and spasms as chamomile and catnip. Lemon balm has many other uses — mood, relaxation, focus, skin — and is so easy to grow, it deserves a spot in the garden. See page 280 for more information.

Best in: tea, fresh tincture, glycerite, oxymel, syrup, seltzer

Dandelion

Dandelion leaf and root act as simple bitters to enhance digestion. Use the leaves in culinary recipes like pesto (page 88) and sautéed greens, or sneak them into salads. The roots make a nice tincture, cordial, or tea, tasting a bit like weak unsweetened coffee or chocolate, especially when dry roasted. Dandelion also offers diuretic, detoxifying properties that benefit a wide range of conditions. Allow this weed to grow in unsprayed lawns and at the edges edges of your property in good soil with full sun. See page 262 for more information.

Best in: tea, tincture, food, glycerite, cordial, vinegar, oxymel

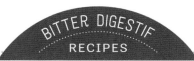
LEMON BALM-CATNIP GLYCERITE

CARMINATIVE, AROMATIC HERBS extract relatively well in glycerine, especially in this "simmered still" technique that borrows from water bath canning. Along with its sweet flavor, it's kid-friendly and alcohol-free. Watch for spoilage after a few months, though.

1¼ ounces fresh chopped catnip

1¼ ounces fresh chopped lemon balm

About 5 ounces glycerine

Suggested tools: 8-ounce mason jar with canning lid, pot of water with a lid that the mason jar fits in

Stuff herbs in your jar and cover with glycerine, leaving approximately 1 inch of headspace in the jar. Cover well but not super tight. Submerge in water, bring to a boil (covered), and let simmer 20 minutes. Let cool, remove, strain. Dose would be 1 teaspoon plain or added to seltzer, tea, or water.

VARIATIONS

Tincture: You can make this into a fresh tincture instead (directions on page 38), which will be shelf stable for years. Dose would be 1–2 ml.

Tincture/Glycerite: Do a 1:1 mix of glycerine and 100-proof vodka for your extract.

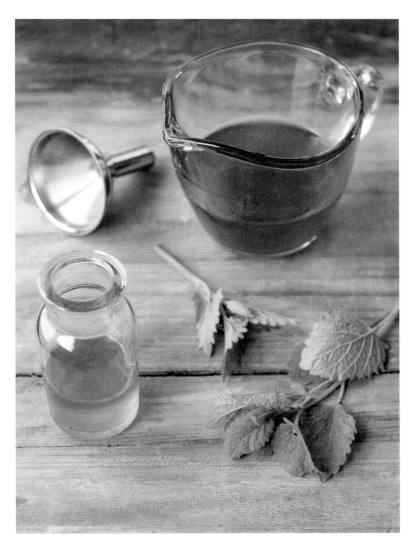

BITTERS SPRAY

A TRADITIONAL BITTERS FORMULA contains bitter-tasting herbs primarily, some carminative herbs to balance and flavor the blend, and a splash of something sweet. Check out Guido Masé and Jovial King's book *DIY Bitters* for a slew of recipe ideas, but here's one of my own to get you started. Bitters not only improve digestion but also regulate appetite and blood sugar.

2 parts lemon balm or catnip leaf tincture

2 parts dandelion root tincture

1 part artichoke leaf tincture

Glycerine, honey, or maple syrup

Optional additions:

Bitters: elecampane, burdock, berberines, citrus peel, grapefruit, evergreen needles, yarrow

Flavor/Carminatives: fennel seed, cinnamon stick, gingerroot, cardamom pod, Korean mint leaf, fenugreek, mint

Suggested tools: small glass spray bottle

If you have the premade tinctures, simply blend them together and add a splash of something sweet (honey, glycerine, or maple syrup). Or you can make this recipe as a combination fresh or dried plant tincture (see directions on pages 38 and 40, respectively) using 25 percent glycerine (or honey or maple syrup), 75 percent 100-proof vodka as your base. Keep a small amount of this remedy in a spray bottle and squeeze 1–5 spritzes into your mouth at mealtime or add a teaspoon to seltzer.

Bitter Berberines

Berberine-rich herbs include goldenseal, Oregon grape root, and barberry. These herbs taste intensely bitter due to the bright yellow alkaloid berberine present in the plants. You can use small doses as a basic digestive bitter, but they shine when you also need antimicrobial support. For this, they one-up the basic bitters mentioned above. Berberine has potent antifungal and antibacterial actions "on contact," which includes the digestive tract. Think of berberine-rich herbs for the stomach flu, dysbiosis, leaky gut, small intestinal bacterial overgrowth (SIBO), and chronic yeast infections. Berberines taste terrible, so stick with tinctures or capsules. Learn more on page 271.

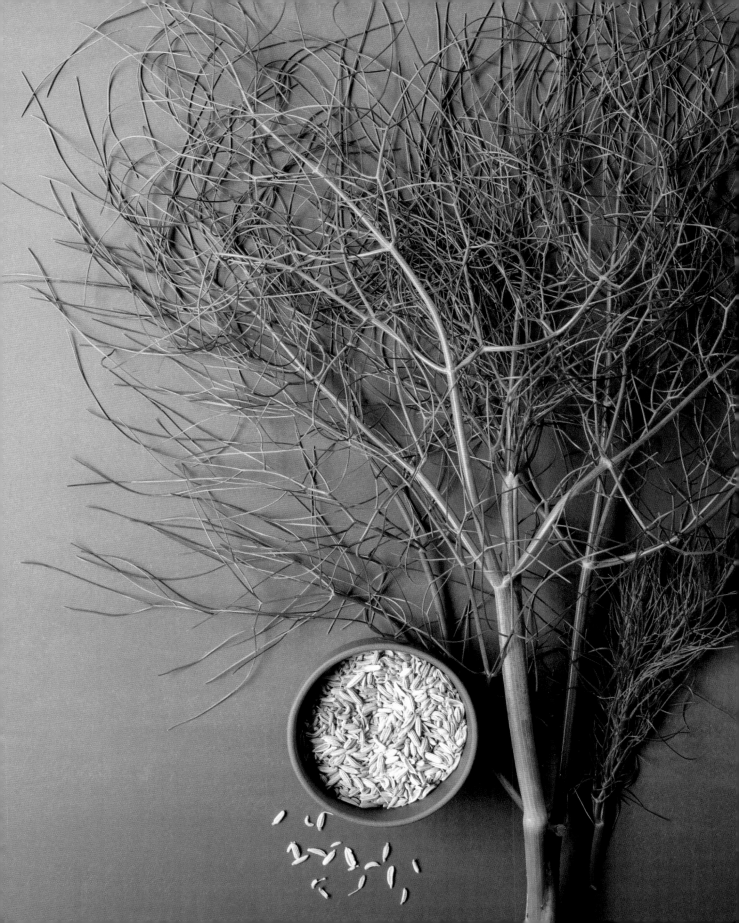

CARMINATIVES

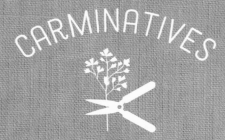

Carminatives are aromatic, often tasty herbs, rich in essential oils. For digestion, they offer a complementary action alongside bitters but can also be used solo. Fennel, mint, Korean mint, chamomile, and dill gently warm the body; relax muscle tension, spasm, gas, pain, and bloating; and enhance digestive function. Many aromatic carminatives also lift and calm the spirits and benefit many parts of the body, including the respiratory system. Almost *everything* in your culinary herb and spice cabinet is carminative. Classics include ginger, fennel, and cardamom. Enjoy these favorites from the garden. Other carminative herbs include lemon balm, catnip, holy basil, rosemary, and culinary seeds.

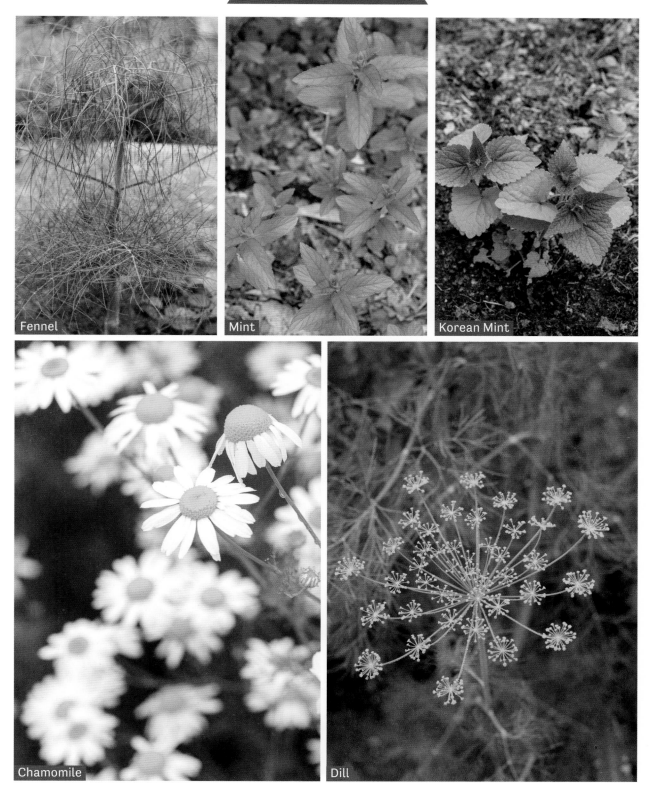

Fennel

Mint

Korean Mint

Chamomile

Dill

Fennel

Fennel's easy to grow, pretty, yummy, and sweet — what's not to love? Any fennel will do, but I prefer bronze fennel for its ferny fronds and seeds with its special purple hue and Good & Plenty flavor. The fronds and bulb provide plenty of flavor and will be easier to harvest in abundance, but the seeds are stronger. Fennel's not too fussy but prefers good soil and full sun. See page 267 for more.

Best in: seed — tea, honey, syrup; fronds — vinegar, glycerite, seltzer/soda, water; any part — tincture, cordial

Mint

Almost all aromatic mint-family herbs act as carminatives. True mints are no exception. Peppermint and chocolate mint (a variety of peppermint reminiscent of Andes candies) pack the punch of menthol — tasty, uplifting, and powerfully antispasmodic. They are great for gas, pain, bloating, IBS, and IBD. Menthol does, however, aggravate heartburn and reflux in some people. Spearmint, apple mint, and other mints tend to be milder. All are wonderful flavoring agents, though a bit unruly in the garden. See page 286 for growing tips.

Best in: tea, tincture, oxymel, glycerite, seltzer, water, capsule

Korean Mint

This lesser-known herb deserves a spot in your garden. It brings joy to life with its fennel-honey flavor, purple flowering stalks, and long harvest season. Medicinally, think of it as a cross between fennel and mint for digestion. Traditional Asian herbalists employ it to soothe sore throat and as a cold and flu remedy. It has mild uplifting, nervine properties. This short-lived, self-seeding perennial loves good soil. Use its close relative anise hyssop similarly, but Korean mint tastes better. See page 277 for more.

Best in: tea, glycerite, honey, seltzer/soda, cordial, syrup

Chamomile

It's bitter. It's carminative. It's calming. It's anti-inflammatory. It's mildly antimicrobial. When it comes to gut health, chamomile tea is an easy answer, classic for colic, gas, bloating, gut healing, sluggish digestion, and nervous indigestion in babies and adults alike. It's very safe, but use caution if you're allergic to daisy-family flowers (if so, try catnip instead). The longer you brew the flowers, the more bitter the taste becomes. Plant in well-drained soil in a sunny area. See page 259 for more.

Best in: tea, tincture, glycerite, flower essence

Dill

Dill and fennel are so closely related, you may need to smell them to tell them apart. If you grow them too closely together, they'll interbreed and self-seed a hodgepodge herb I call "fill." Like fennel, this carminative herb relieves intestinal spasms, gas, bloating, and indigestion; improves digestive function; and quells nausea. Use any part, the seeds being the strongest. The flower essence eases digestive and emotional upset and hypersensitivity triggered by stress overload. See page 263 for more.

Best in: food (pickles!), vinegar, tincture, glycerite, flower essence, tea

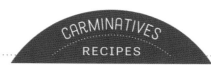

FENNEL AND KOREAN MINT SELTZER

THE SLIGHTLY SWEET, FRESH FLAVORS of fennel fronds and Korean mint sprigs in bubbly water make a *perfect* accompaniment to summertime meals. No need to add a sweetener unless you have a *really* sweet tooth. Together, the two herbs look stunning in the bottle. Supereasy, and glamorous enough for fancy parties.

3 medium-sized fennel fronds

2–3 large Korean mint (or anise hyssop) sprigs

1 liter plain seltzer

Suggested tools: Clear glass 1-liter pop-top bottle (I seek out specialty drinks in stores, buy and drink them, remove the label, and reuse. Also check out fermentation supply and well-stocked kitchen stores.)

Put the herbs into the empty bottle. (They'll be easier to remove later if you put them in stem-side-up.) Gently fill with plain seltzer water or club soda. Refrigerate for at least 30 minutes before serving and drink that day.

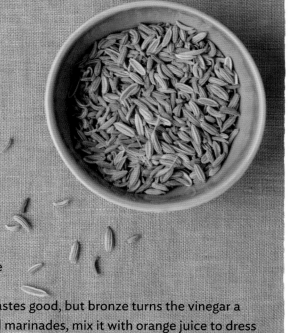

Fun with Fennel

Sweet Fennel Liquor

Sambuca lovers, try this garden-variety riff: Fill a jar one-third full with equal parts dried fennel seed and Korean mint leaves (optional: add another equal part whole star anise pods). Make a cordial (page 54) using 35 percent simple syrup and 65 percent good-quality 80-proof vodka. This liquor tastes great within 1 day, but it's fine to steep longer before straining. Sip straight or add a splash to seltzer.

Bronze Fennel Vinegar

Simply chop up fresh fennel fronds and make an infused vinegar (page 46) with any good-quality white vinegar (rice, champagne, organic white distilled — not conventional white distilled). Any fennel variety tastes good, but bronze turns the vinegar a stunning shade of red! Delicious in salad dressings and marinades, mix it with orange juice to dress beet salads. Sweet bronze fennel glycerite is also divine — and gorgeous purple.

Fennel Seed Chews

My go-to remedy for intense gas and spasms couldn't be easier (or cheaper). Simply chew on some fennel seeds. You can swallow or spit them out after they lose their flavor. Relief usually comes within 15 minutes. Dill, anise, cardamom, and caraway work similarly.

CHAMOMILE-MINT TEA

THIS SIMPLE TEA does the trick! Sip it at the end of a meal to help you digest. If you're not a chamomile person, substitute catnip leaf. While any mint will do, spearmint blends particularly well with chamomile. Chances are you can find mint or chamomile tea anywhere you go in the world, and either will do as a simple tea, too.

1 teaspoon dried chamomile blossoms

1 teaspoon spearmint or other mint of choice

Honey to taste (optional)

Steep the herbs in 12–16 ounces of hot water for 3–5 minutes (chamomile gets bitter if overbrewed; while helpful for digestion, most people find it unpalatable). Sweeten with honey, if desired.

QUICK DILL PICKLES

MY MOTHER'S RECIPE comes out perfectly, a favorite among family and friends. The pickles keep for a surprisingly long time in the fridge, but they *eventually* lose their crisp. My friends and I sip the pickle juice from a shot glass (with or without the accompanying shot of whiskey, something I learned from my little brother). These pickles and the juice improve digestion, ease indigestion, and mellow out nausea. Makes 6 pints.

4 pounds whole pickling cucumbers

3 tablespoons salt

3 cups apple cider vinegar

3 cups water

Seasonings Per Pint Jar

2 cloves garlic, peeled, halved

1 teaspoon yellow mustard seeds, whole

1 head fresh dill flower/seed heads

1½ teaspoons dill seed

3 black peppercorns, whole

1 hot pepper (optional)

Slice cucumbers (don't peel) into spears or circles. Loosely fill 6 clean, hot pint jars with them. Meanwhile, bring salt, vinegar, and water to a boil. Add seasonings to each jar, then fill with brine. Refrigerate for 2 weeks before eating. They will keep for several months, possibly years, in the fridge.

VARIATION

Canned pickles can be kept on the shelf until you open them, but the pickles become flaccid from cooking. Leave headspace in the jar and can via water bath. For spears, simmer for 7 minutes for quart jars, 5 minutes for pint. For whole pickles, go 20 or 10 minutes, respectively.

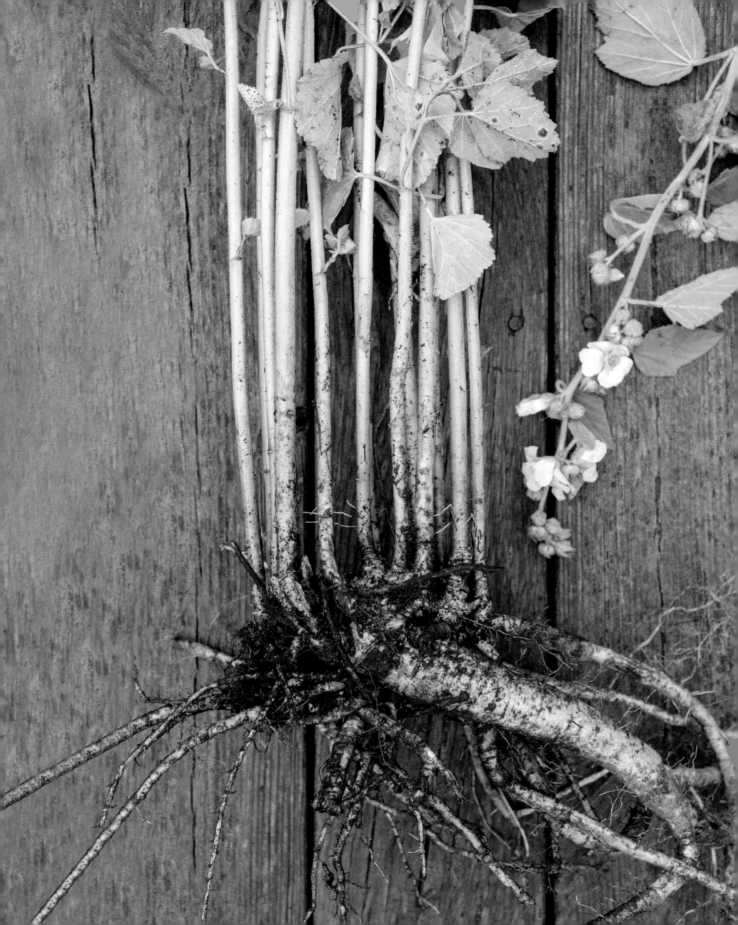

TUMMY SOOTHERS

The vulnerary (wound healing) and demulcent (soothing) herbs in this garden heal and soothe irritated, inflamed, and damaged gut lining. Think of marshmallow, plantain, calendula, roses, and meadowsweet to relieve reflux and heartburn, ulcers, gastritis, leaky gut, Crohn's, colitis, other forms of inflammatory bowel disease (IBD), and irritable bowel syndrome (IBS); to settle an upset stomach; and to speed recuperation after food poisoning. Add carminatives for flavor and additional support. These herbs shine in tea, broth, powder, or food, *not* in tincture form. Other gut-soothing herbs include fennel, chickweed, inner aloe gel, and alder bark.

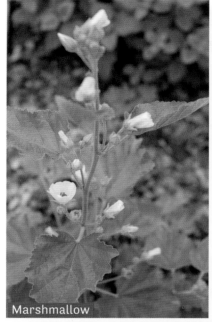

Marshmallow

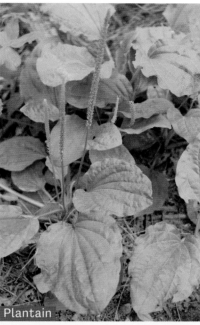

Plantain

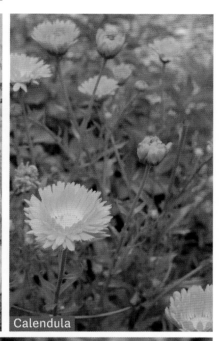

Calendula

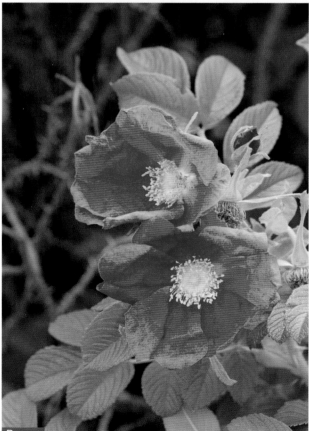

Roses

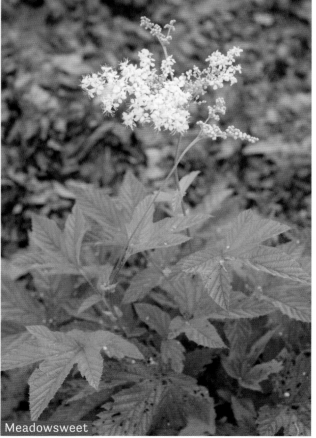

Meadowsweet

Marshmallow

The number one demulcent, mucilaginous herb from the garden, this attractive flowering herb tastes nice and grows easily. The root has serious slime — it gets mucous in water — while the milder leaves and flowers provide a velvety mouthfeel to teas. Amazingly soothing, healing, and gently laxative. Feel free to substitute the leaves and flowers of hollyhock and mallow species. The roots may not agree with people who have SIBO and FODMAP (fermentable oligosaccharides, disaccharides, monosaccharides, and polyols) reactions (gas, bloating, diarrhea). See page 283 for more.

Best in: tea, broth, powder, lozenge/pastille, syrup

Plantain

It's too easy to overlook this common weed of lawns, pavement cracks, and woodland plants. Plantain leaf makes a fantastic, underused ingredient in gut-healing teas, broths, and other soothing, healing recipes. This powerful vulnerary herb also mildly astringes and tones the gut and offers demulcent properties. People who can't handle marshmallow's mucilage often do better with plantain. The richer the soil, the bigger the leaves will grow. See page 293 for more.

Best in: tea, broth, food, powder, syrup

Calendula

Rather than a source of demulcent, mucilaginous activity, calendula is a powerhouse vulnerary with anti-inflammatory, mildly antimicrobial, and digestion-enhancing bitter properties. It's rich in beta-carotene, which turns into vitamin A as needed, improving immune health and mucosal tissue integrity. People who have daisy flower allergies beware: you might find the tea too bitter, but it's otherwise well tolerated, not to mention it's a beautiful garden flower. See page 255 for more.

Best in: tea, broth, powder, lozenge/pastille, food

Roses

Roses make an appearance in almost all my gut-healing tea blends. The colorful petals make you smile as you brew your tea — great for people with gut issues who are also stressed and moody (commonly concomitant). But rose is more than a pretty face. The flowers fight pathogenic bacteria yet encourage beneficial gut flora. They gently astringe leaky, irritated, and boggy gut lining and are safe to sip regularly for leaky gut, dysbiosis, and chronic diarrhea. See page 296 for more.

Best in: tea, powder, pastilles

Meadowsweet

Meadowsweet tastes sweet with hints of honey, cherry, wintergreen, and watermelon. It contains feeble aspirin-like constituents (salicin and methyl salicylate) that decrease inflammation, yet — unlike NSAID drugs and other "herbal aspirins" — it soothes and heals the gut lining rather than irritating it and decreases gut inflammation. Consider it for ulcers, gastritis, leaky gut, and inflammatory bowel disease. It does not aggravate SIBO or dysbiosis. See page 284 for more.

Best in: tea

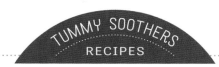

GUT-HEALING TUMMY TEA, TAKE ONE

I RELY ON THIS BASIC RECIPE for many of my clients with gut issues — it provides soothing mucilage, demulcent, and vulnerary gut-healing support. Perfect for ulcers, reflux, gastritis, heartburn, and leaky gut issues. Feel free to raid your spice cabinet for additional digestive support.

2 parts marshmallow root

1 part marshmallow leaf or flower

1 part plantain leaf

1 part fennel seed or Korean mint leaves (or to taste)

Sprinkle of rose petals

Optional additions (per cup): pinch of licorice root, 1–2 cinnamon sticks, 1–2 cardamom pods, 1 star anise pod, 3–5 clove buds

Suggested tools: French press pot or tea-infuser travel mug

Cover 2 heaping tablespoons of the herb mixture with hot water in a 32-ounce container. Let steep for several hours or overnight. Feel free to move to the fridge once it cools. Strain and drink over 1–2 days. (You can steep it for a shorter period of time — 15 minutes or so — but the mucilaginous herbs and the spices will be more potent with a long steep.)

GUT-HEALING TUMMY TEA, TAKE TWO

IF HIGH-MUCILAGE HERBS LIKE MARSHMALLOW don't agree with your gut, consider this SIBO/FODMAP-safe tea blend, inspired by herbalists Thomas Easley and Juliet Blankespoor. What it lacks in "slimers" it makes up for with anti-inflammatory and vulnerary properties — perfect for improving the integrity of the gut lining and healing damaged tissue.

1 part plantain leaf

1 part meadowsweet flowering tops

½–1 part calendula flower

Cover herbs with hot water. Steep for 15–30 minutes, strain, and drink.

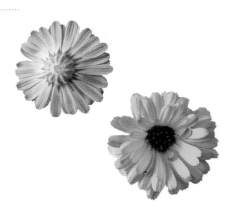

GUT-HEALING BROTH

THINK BEYOND THE TEAPOT. This broth recipe combines our healing herbs with the gut-healing benefits of bone broth. That said, you *can* skip the bones if you're vegetarian. I make broth with meat on the bone, saving my bones in the freezer for later use.

Bones: 1 chicken carcass (especially wings, back, and feet if you have them), 1 beef knuckle, or the bones of a few fish

1 tablespoon plantain leaf

¼ cup marshmallow root or leaf (if tolerated)

1 tablespoon calendula blossoms (if tolerated, slightly bitter)

Salt to taste

Optional additions: nettle leaf, burdock root, bay leaf, horsetail

Suggested tools: 1-gallon or larger stockpot, large fine-mesh metal strainer, widemouthed canning funnel

In the stockpot, cover your bones and herbs with 1 gallon of water. Bring to a gentle simmer, and keep simmering for several hours, preferably all day. Strain and discard the solids. Transfer to large mason jars and drink 1–4 cups daily as plain broth or as an ingredient in recipes.

VARIATIONS

Freeze: Fill freezer-safe mason jars (16- and 20-ounce widemouthed — quart jars are not freezer-safe) or plastic deli containers, leaving approximately 1 inch of headspace. To thaw, run a deli container under hot water to pop it out, then heat on the stove. Mason jars should thaw in the fridge for a few days.

Concentrated Ice Cubes: After straining your solids, return the broth to the pot to simmer uncovered until the liquid is reduced to approximately one-quarter the original volume. Let cool, pour into ice cube trays, and use one to two cubes per day. Simply plunk into a mug of hot water or recipes.

Gut Dysbiosis?

Digestive health issues — especially conditions like leaky gut, chronic diarrhea, irritable bowel syndrome (IBS), small intestinal bacterial overgrowth (SIBO), fermentable oligosaccharides, disaccharides, monosaccharides and polyols (FODMAP) food intolerance, and recurring ulcers — often involve gut dysbiosis. This broad term refers to an overgrowth of pathogenic bacteria and fungi, or an abundance of these "critters" where they don't belong (like the upper small intestine). Addressing dysbiosis is complicated and individual; however, certain natural approaches are often useful. This includes consuming probiotics or fermented foods to encourage beneficial bacteria while also introducing antimicrobial herbs. Backyard antimicrobials to consider include alder, berberines, bee balm, thyme, garlic, elecampane, yellow dock, and rose petals. Ginger, cinnamon, cloves, cardamom, and pau d'arco may help, too. I add the better-tasting ones to gut-healing teas and use the others in a tincture blend.

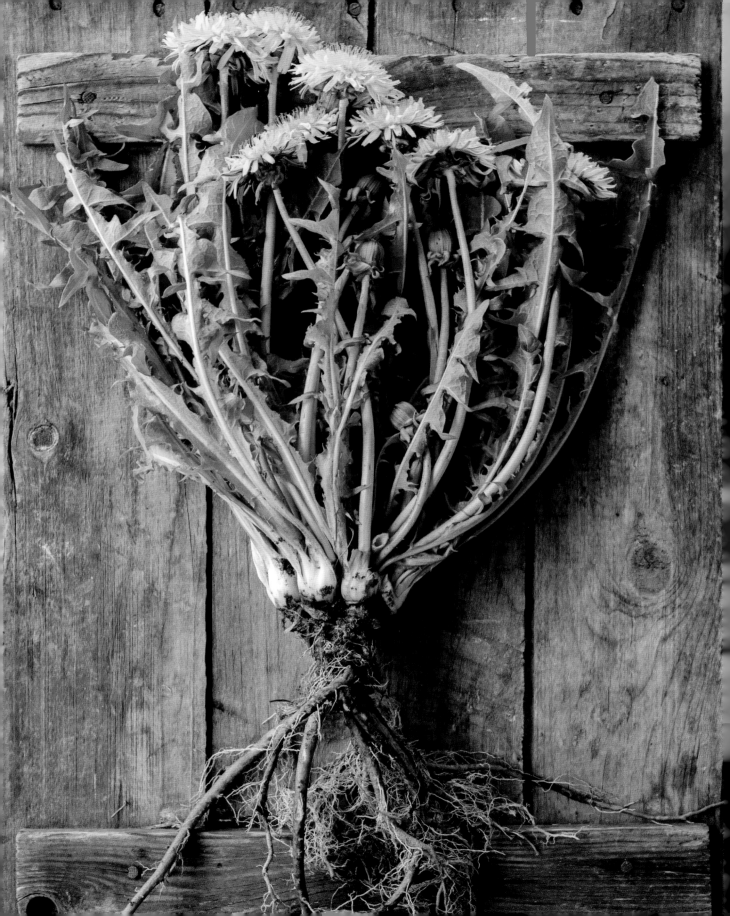

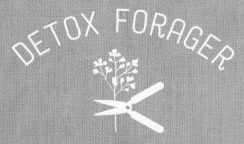

DETOX FORAGER

Look no farther than your backyard weeds like dandelion, burdock, violet, red clover, and yellow dock for detoxification.   These wild plants support your liver, kidneys, lymph, and colon in healthy elimination of day-to-day metabolic waste and toxins. These herbs are also called "alteratives" because they alter your body from an unbalanced to a vital state by encouraging the body's own natural cleansing systems. Think of them for general detoxification, skin eruptions (rashes, acne), sluggish digestion, and hormone wobbles. They're also rich in minerals. When wildcrafting, only harvest from clean land that has not been sprayed with chemicals and isn't loaded with heavy metals — avoid power lines, roadsides, railroad tracks, questionable waterways, and old dump sites. If the plants aren't growing in your backyard already, you may want to invite them in. Other detoxifying herbs include nettle, chicory, calendula, alder, and birch leaves.

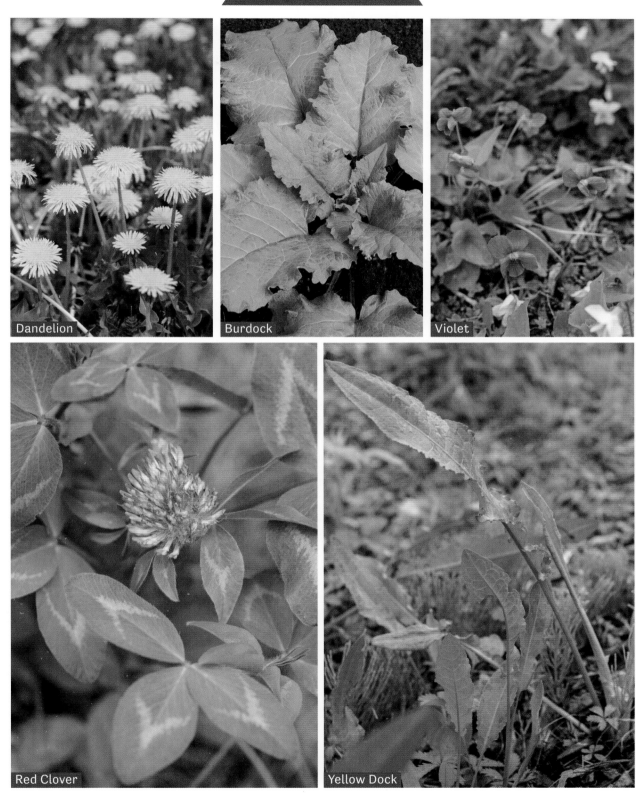

Dandelion

Burdock

Violet

Red Clover

Yellow Dock

Dandelion

Dandelion leaves have potent kidney tonic and diuretic actions (hence the French name *pissenlit*, or "piss the bed") while the roots are more liver specific. Nonetheless, both encourage detoxification via the liver and kidneys, taste bitter (bitters are good for digestion, page 134), and abound with minerals. Inulin fiber in the root feeds good gut bacteria. Let dandelion take over your lawn and eat what you pull from the garden. See page 262 for more.

Best in: tea, tincture, food (pesto), vinegar, syrup

Burdock

First you'll see this biennial's huge rhubarblike leaves and, in the second year, tall thistlelike purple flowers that stick to your clothes and inspired Velcro. Dig the sweet, earthy, mildly bitter roots in spring or fall before it puts up flower stalks. Burdock root encourages liver and lymph detoxification and is one of our safest, gentlest, yet still profound alteratives. Edible and medicinal, it's used for skin conditions and as a general tonic. See page 254 for more.

Best in: tea, tincture, food, broth, vinegar, flower essence

Violet

These cute flowers and tasty leaves lend a mild, fresh "green" flavor to tea, salad, and pesto. Rich in vitamins and minerals, violet gently boosts lymph detoxification, alleviates skin conditions, and dissolves noncancerous fatty cysts. It's easy and pretty enough to grow in the garden or let naturalize in the lawn. Unlike most of the other herbs listed here, it has a mild demulcent property that gives it a slightly slimy, velvety mouthfeel and helps moisten dried-out tissues. See page 305 for more.

Best in: tea, tincture, syrup, food (salad, pesto)

Red Clover

This popular cover crop loves to grow in sunny meadows, lawns, and along the edges of pathways. Pluck the flower tops in the morning and dry them promptly and thoroughly in a dehydrator or tincture fresh. Red clover aids lymph detoxification, contains a variety of minerals, and offers some phytoestrogens. This controversial old-time anticancer remedy may also ease hot flashes in perimenopause, strengthen bones, clear the skin, and relieve water retention and edema. See page 295 for more.

Best in: tea, tincture

Yellow Dock

With its big, leathery leaves and rusty-colored seed heads, yellow dock certainly looks like a wayside weed. Dig up the yellow-hued root in spring or fall. This bitter herb boosts liver detoxification and encourages healthy bowel movements for those with constipation without loosening things up too much. It also alleviates anemia (via iron content *and* liver action) and acne. See page 308 for more.

Best in: tea, tincture, oxymel, vinegar, syrup

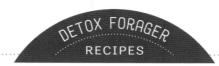

BITTER BREW COFFEE SUBSTITUTE

TRYING TO KICK COFFEE? These bitter, detoxifying roots won't satisfy your caffeine addiction, but the flavor bears resemblance to a cup of joe. Adding cream and sweetener dampens the detoxifying properties a bit, but it tastes great. Enjoy it "black" over ice, too.

1 heaping tablespoon dried burdock root

1 heaping tablespoon dried dandelion root

1 heaping tablespoon dried roasted chicory root

Optional additions: chaga, reishi, maca, cinnamon, ginger, cardamom, nutmeg, ashwagandha, yellow dock, cacao nibs

Suggested tools: pot, hand strainer, mug

Cover the herbs with 16 ounces or more of water and simmer for 20 minutes before straining. Enjoy as desired — black, iced, with dairy or plant-based milk or sweetener of choice. The Mineral-Rich "Coffee" Syrup (page 87) would be a nice addition. If you'd like to make a big batch, it will keep in the fridge for a few days. Freeze in ice cube trays and blend for a frosty "coffee" drink.

More Ways to Use Detoxifying Herbs

- Dandelion-Violet Weed Pesto, page 88
- Multimineral Vinegar, page 86
- Mineral-Rich "Coffee" Syrup, page 87
- Bitters Spray, page 141
- Dandelion, burdock, and ginger tincture or vinegar/oxymel blend
- Detox Chai: Add burdock, dandelion, and yellow dock to the Chai Base, page 78

NUTRI-DETOX TEA

MOST OF OUR GENTLE DETOXIFYING HERBS
are also nutritious. Here's a riff on the Nutri-Tea
on page 79 that's a little more geared toward
whole body detoxification.

1 teaspoon violet leaf and flower

1 teaspoon red clover

1 teaspoon nettle leaf

1 teaspoon mint of choice

1 teaspoon birch leaves (optional)

Sprinkle of calendula petals (optional)

Steep the herbs in 16 ounces of hot water for
20 minutes, strain, and enjoy.

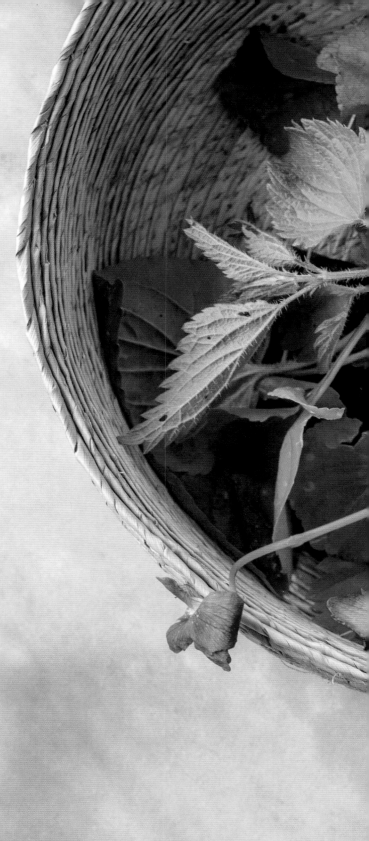

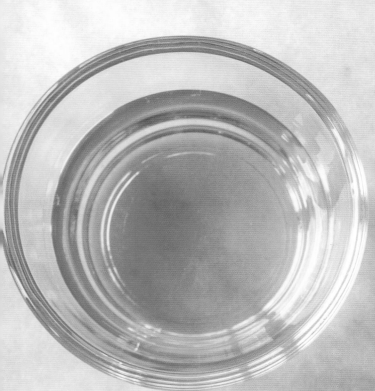

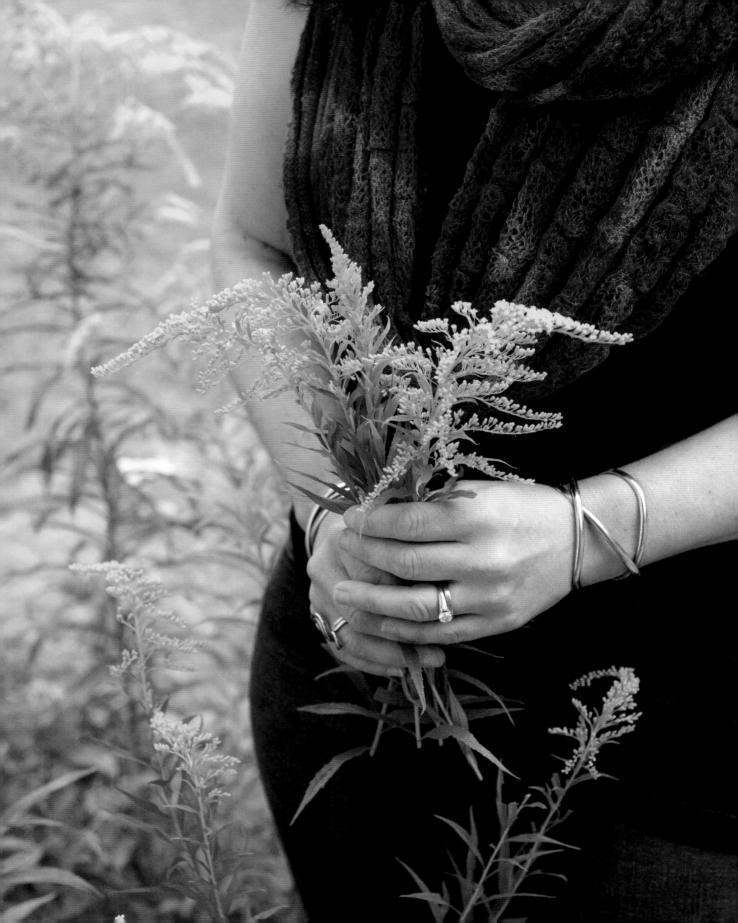

Immune and Respiratory

YOU MIGHT BE SURPRISED how many immune and respiratory tonic herbs you can grow in the garden. You can start with culinary-immune-respiratory herbs like oregano, bee balm, thyme, and sage, and then branch out to showier garden blooms like echinacea and elecampane, as well as lesser-known herbs like horehound and red root, and common wild species like goldenrod and alder.

TYPES OF HERBS FOR IMMUNE AND RESPIRATORY HEALTH

The herbs in this section fit into a couple different boxes depending on which herbal actions you need most for the condition at hand. Some remedies modulate (balance) immune function, which helps with chronic conditions and prevention, whereas others specifically stimulate the immune system and do their best at the onset of an acute infection. For the lungs, you'll want to think: Do you need to soothe inflamed, irritated tissue or dry and warm things up? Do you need to move mucus, reduce histamine, open the lungs, or provide more direct antimicrobial activity? You'll have more success if you choose the herbs that suit your particular needs best rather than think that one herb is the be-all, end-all immune remedy.

Immune Modulators

These remedies modulate — or balance — the immune system. Some herbalists might call this property "amphoteric" (able to regulate two seemingly opposite conditions) or a "trophorestorative" (restoring vital function). These herbs downregulate an overactive immune system (allergies, autoimmune disease) while strengthening weak immune function. These herbs (and mushrooms) work well to prevent

infections and even improve resistance to bigger issues like cancer. They work best when taken regularly as a tonic. They include medicinal mushrooms, astragalus, and ashwagandha.

Immune Stimulants

Turn to these herbs at the onset of an acute infection or if you know you're going to encounter situations (air travel, sick family members, big parties) that are likely to expose you to pathogens. These herbs either put your immune system into hyperdrive or they have more direct antiviral action. You might also consider our upcoming category of herbs: antimicrobials. Immune stimulants include echinacea, elecampane, and elderberry.

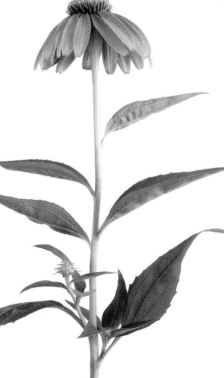

Antimicrobials

These herbs have direct antimicrobial activity, often on contact or indirectly by targeting specific areas of the body like the lungs or gut. They include oregano, bee balm, thyme, berberines, and elecampane.

Aromatics and Lung Tonics

These herbs support the lungs by breaking up mucus, opening the airways, and soothing irritated tissues. They include the previously mentioned antimicrobials as well as horehound, goldenrod, mullein, wild cherry bark, and elecampane.

Antihistamine

These herbs directly or indirectly reduce the histamine response, which notably eases allergy symptoms but can also be useful in chronic lung issues like asthma and supportive during acute infections. They include goldenrod, nettle, and berberines.

Demulcent (Soothers)

You might recall this category from our digestion section. Here, demulcent herbs soothe irritated, inflamed tissue. Some are more overtly mucilaginous (marshmallow root) while others are subtler in their slime factor. They include marshmallow, plantain, and mullein.

Medicinal Mushrooms

Mushrooms live in a kingdom all their own, completely unrelated to plants, but most herbalists consider them honorary "herbs" for all the amazing ways they aid health. Most prominently, complex starches called polysaccharides (including glucans) in all our edible and medicinal mushrooms strengthen and modulate immune function when consumed on a regular basis. Always cook your mushrooms, in order to free the beneficial constituents from the tight bonds with chitin (think crab shell) so you can absorb them, and to break down mildly toxic components in otherwise safe-to-eat mushrooms. They are best in food, broth (page 81), and decoction

tea (page 36), as well as decoction tincture extracts (page 42). You can forage for the following mushrooms or grow them in a shady, moist, temperate landscape.

Shiitake: Not wild but easy to cultivate on logs, shiitake tastes great and supports immune and brain health. Put them upside down in the sunlight for a few hours to boost their vitamin D content (you can do this with any tender edible mushroom). Eat fresh or dry for storage.

Maitake: Tastes like chicken when sautéed fresh. Maitake supports immune health.

Reishi: Though bitter and tough, this "mushroom of immortality" boasts calm-energy adaptogen properties, aids sleep, decreases inflammation, and supports immune, respiratory, and liver health. Other *Ganoderma* species, including hemlock reishi and artist's conk, have somewhat similar properties.

Turkey tails: Easily cultivated and foraged, turkey tail extracts are widely prescribed as adjunct cancer treatment in Asia and have the most human research of all mushrooms.

Chaga: This slow-growing sterile fungal growth (not technically a mushroom) is only wildcrafted but is becoming threatened. It tastes pleasant in tea and extracts and is more overtly energizing.

Lion's mane: One of our most delicious mushrooms (with a texture like crabmeat), lion's mane also has the unique ability to support nerve growth and repair, aiding mood and cognition. Use other *Hericium* species interchangeably.

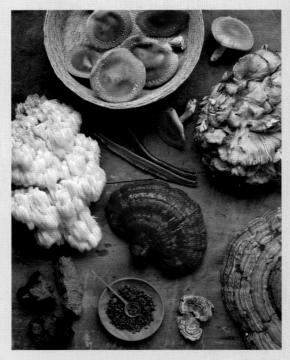

Clockwise from top left: shiitake, maitake, artist's conk, turkey tails, chaga ground and in chunks, lion's mane
Center: whole reishi mushroom and slices

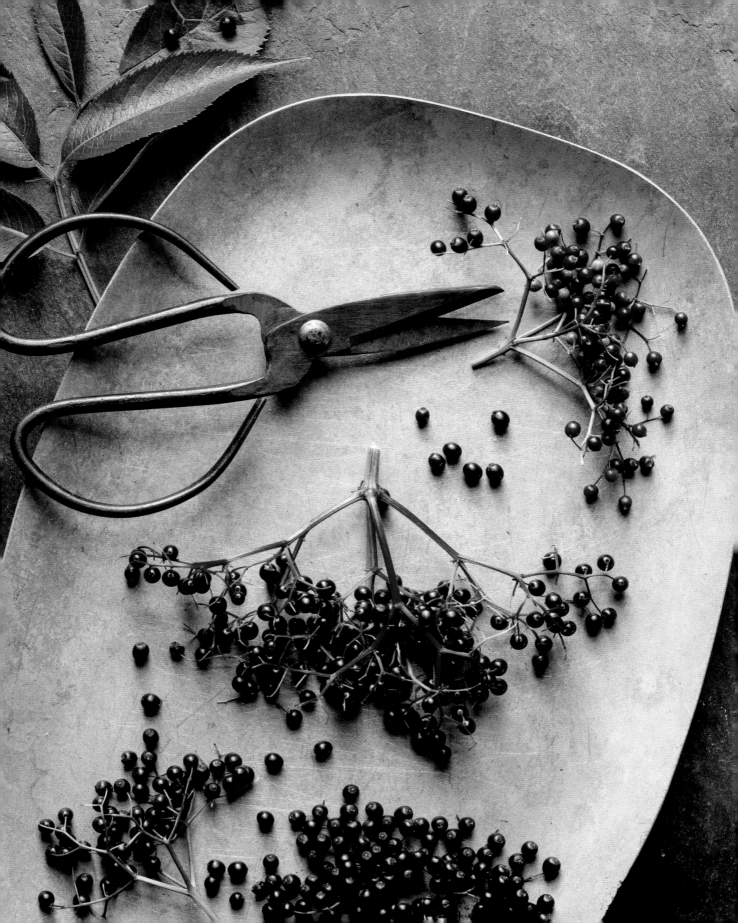

IMMUNE SOS

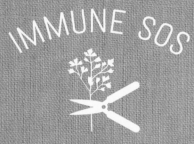

Turn to elder, echinacea, bee balm, and garlic for acute infections, starting with the very first inkling of an oncoming infection or if you know you're likely to be exposed or susceptible: for example, during air travel, when you're around a sick household member or coworker or in crowds at big parties, or when you're really run down from stress or short on sleep. Hit these herbs hard and heavy — they do best when taken every waking hour or two. Also consider fresh ginger, which you can add to your recipes. Once you recuperate, look to immune modulators (page 162) to strengthen your immune system so that you can better fend off future infections. Other immune herbs include oregano, thyme, elecampane, rose hips, berberines, and alder.

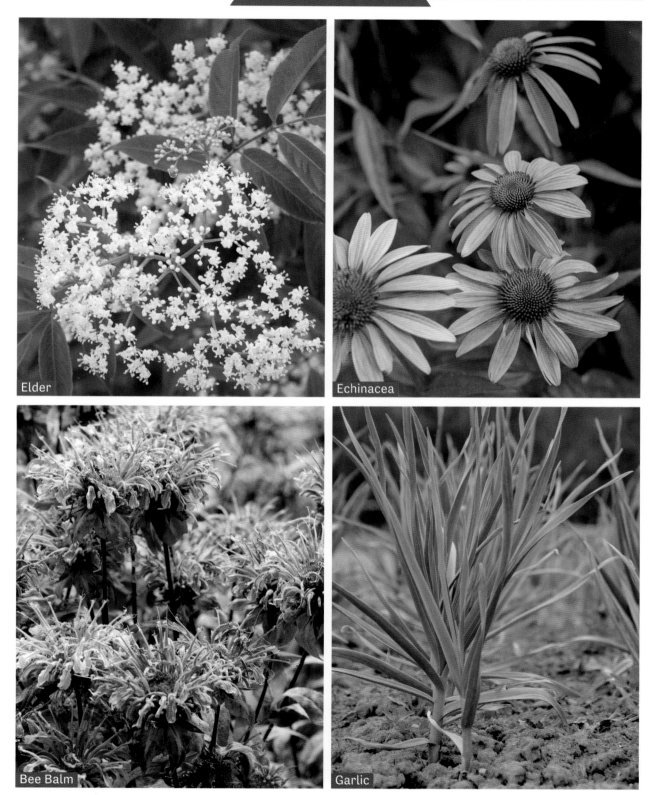

Elder

Echinacea

Bee Balm

Garlic

Elder

Elder provides two medicines. The summer flowers ease allergies and cold symptoms with gentle antihistamine activity and break a fever via diaphoretic effects. The berries prevent viral infections by keeping the virus out of cells, inhibiting its ability to hijack your cells, reprogram them to make more viruses, and spread more virulently. Think of the plant's properties as a force field. Elder is my go-to cold and flu remedy. It works well and tastes great. This wild shrub of damp places can be pruned into an arching small tree on the edge of or in back of the garden. It prefers partial to full sun and moist, rich soil. Use the berries and flowers dry or cooked, not fresh. The fresh berries and to some extent the flowers can be incredibly nauseating and mildly toxic. Don't consume the leaves, stem, or root, which is violently nauseating and more toxic. See page 265 for more.

Best in: tea, syrup, oxymel

Bee Balm

Oregano gets all the press, but consider bee balm instead. It combines antimicrobial compounds found in oregano (carvacrol) *and* those contained in thyme (thymol). It's gorgeous and much more robust than oregano — easily gathered in large quantities. Bee balm, oregano, savory, and friends warm, move, and dry up mucus and have direct antimicrobial activity on contact (throat and gut from tea, nasal passages in a steam) and also target the lungs. Seek bee balm species with a strong bite, like *Monarda fistulosa*. Plant this aggressive spreader in its own bed or along the edge of your property in moist, rich soil and full to partial sun. See page 249 for more.

Best in: tea, fresh or dried herb tincture, honey, oxymel, glycerite, steam

Echinacea

All parts of echinacea stimulate the immune system, boost white blood cells, and increase lymph detoxification to eliminate "dead bodies" and "debris" of the infection battle. Though popular now for viral infections, it was traditionally used for bacterial infections, early stages of sepsis and "bad blood," as well as a topical and internal antivenom remedy for snake and other potentially dangerous bites (these days it's prudent to head to the ER instead). Use all parts, but the fresh root is the most potent part of this prairie wildflower. See page 264 for more.

Best in: fresh plant tincture, tea, flower essence

Garlic

Garlic fends off vampires and infections of various sorts. It stimulates immune function and makes you less hospitable to germs. If tolerated, eat as many raw chopped garlic cloves as you can — with honey, in hummus, as a purée, in fire cider (page 236), and in broth, soup, salads, and other dishes. This works particularly well for throat and lung infections. You'll reek, and garlic is just too irritating to the gut and mucous membranes for some people. Plant the bulbs in nutrient-rich, well-worked soil in late fall to harvest the next season. See page 268 for more.

Best in: food (pesto, hummus, soup), fresh tincture, broth, vinegar, honey

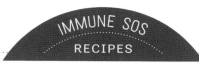
DARCEY BLUE'S ELDERBERRY SYRUP

MOST PEOPLE SIMMER THEIR ELDER SYRUP, but I love this technique from herbalist Darcey Blue of Shamana Flora. Of all the elder syrups I've tried, this one works the best for me and keeps well.

¼ cup dried elderberries

2 tablespoons dried elderflowers

Optional additions: 2 teaspoons each gingerroot and cinnamon chips, or whatever inspires you (cloves, elecampane, rose hips)

4 ounces boiling water

2 ounces 151- or 100-proof vodka

¼–½ lemon, juiced

About 4 ounces raw honey

Suggested tools: 16-ounce jar with lid, strainer and large spoon or cloth, medium to large glass measuring cup, 8-ounce bottle

Combine the herbs in a jar, cover with boiling water and vodka, stir, cover, and let sit for a day (longer is fine — pop it in the fridge or freezer). Strain and squeeze out as much liquid from the herbs as possible. Add lemon juice. Measure and add an equal amount of honey (approximately 4 ounces), whisk or stir vigorously to dissolve the honey. Though this is relatively shelf stable, I prefer to keep my main bottle in the fridge or freezer — it stays liquid. Take ½–1 teaspoon (3–5 squirts off a dropper bottle) daily as a preventive or every few hours during an acute or impending infection.

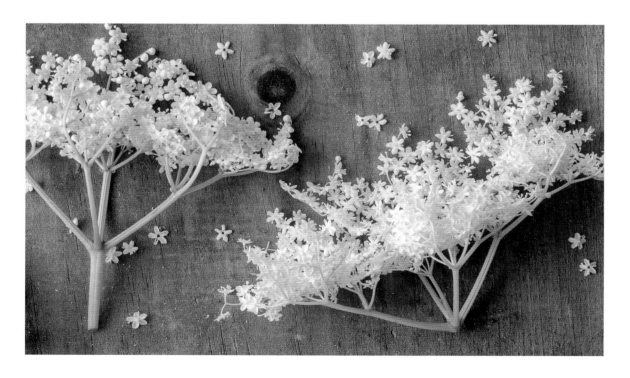

ELDER-ROSE HIP OXYMEL

THIS SWEET-TART VINEGAR-HONEY EXTRACT is perfect for people who want a relatively shelf-stable elderberry syrup without any alcohol or refined sugars. It's supereasy to make. If you have them, schizandra berries and hibiscus flowers are nice additions, and these ingredients also blend well with elderberries and honey as a tea.

¼ cup dried elderberries

¼ cup dried rose hips

½ cup apple cider vinegar (preferably raw)

½ cup honey (preferably raw)

Suggested tools: 12-ounce or larger jar with lid

Combine the herbs in the jar, cover with vinegar, then add honey. Shake or stir well to combine. Let macerate (steep) for 2–4 weeks, shaking every day or two. Strain and press out as much liquid from the herbs as you can. Dose it the same as elderberry syrup: ½–1 teaspoon daily as a preventive or every couple of hours for an acute or oncoming infection.

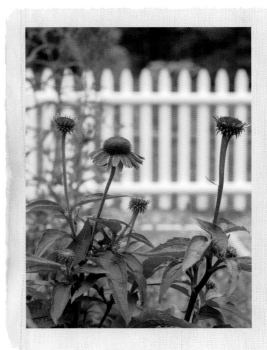

Echinacea Tincture

Echinacea is most potent and palatable (though it's not yummy, so let's get it over with fast) as a fresh plant tincture. Most of us simply make the basic fresh tincture (page 38) using any part of the plant — roots being most potent. Then take ½–1 teaspoon as often as you can think of it (every 1–2 waking hours or so) starting with the first tickle of an infection until it has cleared. Good-quality echinacea numbs the tongue, tastes weird, and makes you salivate.

Bee Balm Honey

The first herb-infused honey I ever made was of bee balm on one of our Southwest School of Botanical Medicine field trips with Michael Moore. Honey does a nice job mellowing the sharp, spicy, oregano punch of bee balm. You can use the raw method, but I prefer the cooked technique on page 48 to evaporate the moisture so the honey doesn't go bad. Try a spoonful for sore throats or stir it into hot water for an instant tea. You can use any species of *Monarda* that tastes good. *M. didyma* (shown) tastes good, but *M. fistulosa* remains my fave.

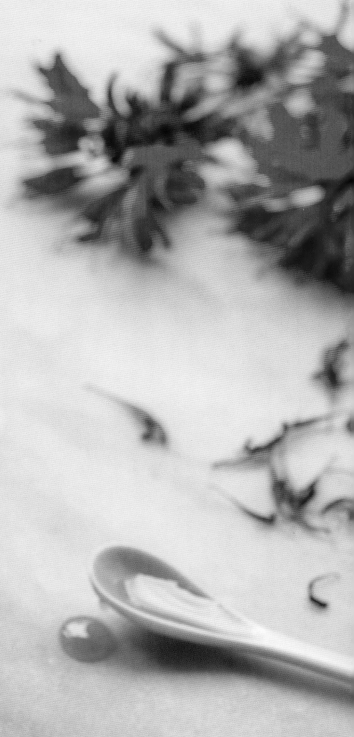

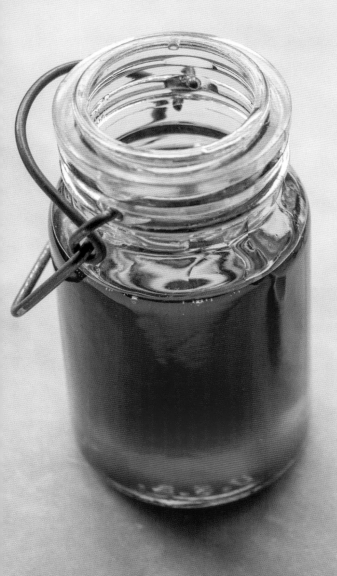

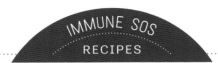
BEE BALM-MINT TEA

THIS WARMING SPICY-SWEET TEA soothes the soul on a cold, dreary day. It's also great at the onset of a cold or flu. Bee balm offers the same antimicrobial essential oil compounds as oregano and thyme. Mint and honey buffer its bite and help soothe the throat and coughs.

1 tablespoon dried bee balm (or oregano and/or thyme)

1 tablespoon dried apple mint (or spearmint)

1 tablespoon honey (optional)

Suggested tools: 12- to 16-ounce mug or teapot with infuser

Combine your herbs in a container or infuser, cover with 12–16 ounces of boiling water, and let steep for 20 minutes. Strain (optional) and stir in honey, if desired.

More Ways to Support Your Immune System

Fire cider: Take it by the spoonful or shot glass to prevent and during acute infections to help kill germs and warm the body. See page 236.

Cough relief: Horehound or wild cherry bark cough syrup, tincture, or infused honey for wet or dry coughs (respectively). See page 177.

Ginger tea: A go-to in our house! Steep 1 inch of fresh gingerroot, sliced thin or grated, in a thermos with two wedges of lemon and honey to taste for 30 minutes.

Immune support broth: Simmer mushrooms and astragalus regularly to prevent infection. Calendula, ashwagandha, and nettle — as well as garlic and onions — add extra medicine, if desired. See the Nutri-Broth with Mushrooms on page 81 for inspiration.

Holy basil green tea: This is great for general immune support and at the first sign of a cold or flu. Steep 1 teaspoon holy basil (tulsi) and ½ teaspoon quality green tea (I prefer jasmine pearls) in 16 ounces of water for 2–5 minutes.

Antimicrobial tincture blend: This can be used topically, as a gargle or sore throat spray, mouth rinse, ingested for a wide range of bacterial and fungal infections including respiratory, urinary tract, and intestinal/dysbiosis. Equal parts Oregon grape root (or other berberine-rich herb such as goldenseal or barberry), bee balm, alder bark, and myrrh, plus 1 percent clove tincture (optional).

Deep immune chai: Add two slices of chaga, a handful of astragalus, 1 teaspoon of ashwagandha, and/or 1 teaspoon of chaga to the Chai Base (page 78) for general immune support and as a preventive.

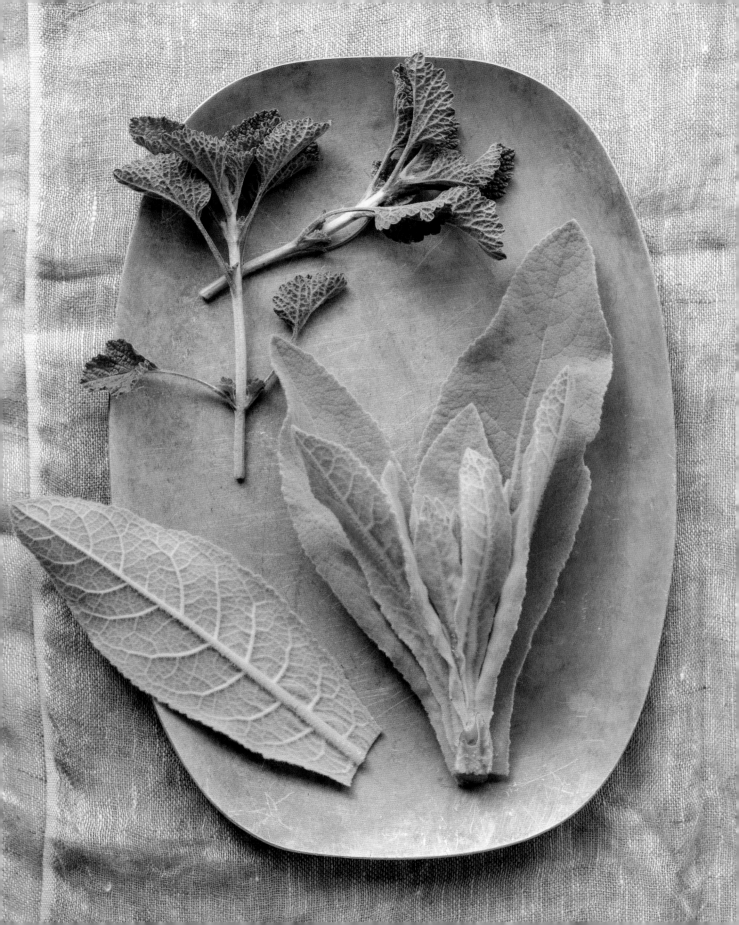

LUNG TONICS

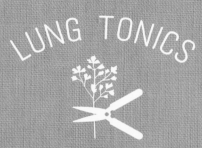

If you suffer from chronic respiratory issues like asthma, chest congestion, chronic bronchitis, and allergies, take comfort in the wonderful lung tonic herbs you can grow in your backyard: mullein, horehound, wild cherry, marshmallow, and plantain. Consider each plant's actions to choose the best ones for you. These are not one-size-fits-all. Each has a different role to play in respiratory health: thinning mucus to clear phlegmy coughs; relaxing irritated, dry, spastic coughs; soothing and opening the lungs. Remember that some respiratory conditions warrant immediate medical attention, including serious infections, difficulty breathing, and pressure that feels like an elephant is sitting on your chest. Certainly use herbs concomitantly, but medications remain best for acute asthma attacks and pneumonia. Other lung herbs include elecampane, thyme, peppermint, Korean mint, bee balm, and New England aster.

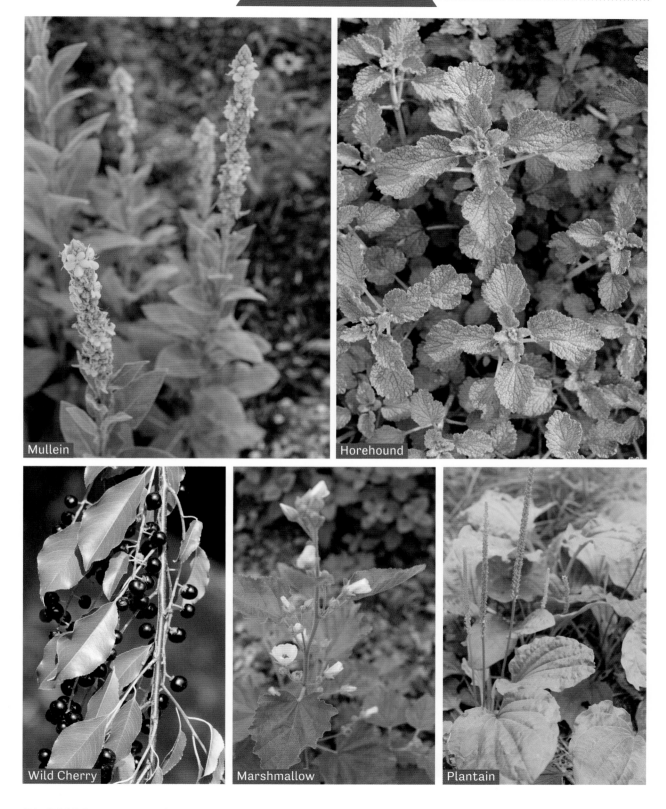

Mullein

Horehound

Wild Cherry

Marshmallow

Plantain

Mullein

Mullein's soft, flannel-like leaves help you remember it's a soothing herb. Mullein opens constricted airways, moistens the lungs, and eases and cools inflammation and irritation. It can be used solo but makes a lovely supportive herb in almost any lung blend. Let this attractive biennial weed seed itself throughout the garden. Harvest the leaves anytime they look happy, preferably before the plant blooms. Strain out the hairs with a cloth or coffee filter. See page 288 for more.

Best in: tea, tincture, syrup, glycerite

Horehound

This wrinkly, silvery herb tastes *intensely* bitter with an oily texture. It's rich in essential oils even though it doesn't taste or smell aromatic. Horehound thins and moves mucus, and is a classic for wet coughs, making them more productive. Think of it for any respiratory issue with thick mucus congestion, including allergies and postnasal drip. It's too bitter for tea but excels as a fresh plant tincture. It thrives in dry, sunny spots near Mediterranean herbs like lavender and thyme. See page 275 for more.

Best in: tincture, syrup, glycerite, cough drop, honey, capsule

Wild Cherry

The bark of this common wild tree (and its scrappy cousin chokecherry) has an excellent, longstanding reputation for easing dry, irritated, spastic coughs. That's why many commercial cough drops and syrups are cherry flavored (albeit now artificially). Turn to cherry bark whenever the lungs are dry, irritated, and tight — for example, from wood smoke or chronic asthma. Cherry bark is safe and most effective used dried without too much heat exposure. See page 306 for more.

Best in: tincture, tea, honey, syrup, glycerite

Marshmallow

Best known for its slimy, soothing properties for the gut, marshmallow similarly soothes the respiratory system, supporting stronger herbs in formulas when dryness, inflammation, and irritation are present. Consider marshmallow syrup as a base for a cough elixir, mixing it with horehound, mullein, and/or wild cherry bark tinctures. This tall flowering herb brings subtle beauty to the garden. See page 283 for more.

Best in: tea, syrup, broth, lozenge

Plantain

This soothing gut herb also crosses over nicely to the respiratory tract. Although not as overtly slimy as marshmallow, it soothes and heals inflamed tissue and gently tones mucous membranes. As with marshmallow, plantain's not a key lung herb but plays a supportive role in blends. See page 293 for more.

Best in: tea, syrup, glycerite, broth

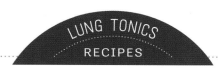
SOOTHING LUNG TEA

THIS BLEND TASTES PLEASANT and helps open and soothe irritated lungs and respiratory tissue — be it a chronic respiratory condition like asthma, an angry red sore throat, or irritation in the lungs. (Note that some conditions may warrant medical attention and diagnosis. This blend is not particularly antimicrobial.) Fennel seed and peppermint both help break up mucus and ease spasms — choose whichever flavor you like best. Choose fennel seed if you'd like a gentler approach. You'll want to strain this through fine woven cloth or paper to keep all of the mullein's hairs out of your tea.

1 teaspoon mullein leaf

1 teaspoon marshmallow leaf and/or root

1 teaspoon plantain leaf (optional)

1 teaspoon fennel seed or peppermint

Optional additions: nettle leaf, wild cherry bark, yerba santa, thyme, goldenrod, licorice, passionflower, evergreen

Suggested tools: 16- to 32-ounce mug or teapot, cloth or paper tea bag or coffee filter

Steep your herbs (in a tea bag or loose) in 16–32 ounces of hot water for 15 minutes. If your herbs were loose, strain it through a piece of cloth or coffee filter before drinking. Drink 1–3 cups daily as needed.

More Ways to Use Respiratory-Supporting Herbs

Nettle-peppermint-marshmallow tea: See page 183. Feel free to swap out the peppermint for Korean mint or fennel seeds. Violet leaf is a soothing addition, too.

Respiratory broth: Reishi, chaga, nettle, plantain, marshmallow leaf or root, and/or ashwagandha, with optional oregano, thyme, garlic, and/or bee balm added at the end.

Bee balm honey: See page 170.

Fire cider: See page 236. When things need to be kicked up and out.

Herbal steam: See page 57. This can feature any combination of mint, oregano, bee balm, thyme, rosemary, and/or Korean mint.

Allergy tincture blend: See page 182. This blend and its variations also help soothe and open the lungs.

Lung support tea: Great herbs include peppermint, fennel seed, Korean mint, anise hyssop, marshmallow, plantain, nettle, mullein (strain hairs well through cloth or coffee filter), thyme, bee balm, oregano, and wild cherry bark.

HOREHOUND COUGH SYRUP

ALTHOUGH MANY PEOPLE make syrups by simmering herbs in water, straining, then adding an equal amount of sugar to preserve it, this "syrup" is more like a cross between a raw honey and fresh plant tincture. You get honey's additional cough-relieving properties, and the alcohol better extracts the horehound while also preserving your syrup. This makes a potent and long-lasting shelf-stable remedy.

2⅔ ounces chopped fresh horehound

3 ounces 100-proof vodka

2 ounces local raw honey

Suggested tools: 8-ounce jar, jelly bag or metal mesh strainer with spoon

Chop your herbs and shove them in the jar (it's okay to leave the stems on). Add the vodka. Top off with honey and cap it. Shake vigorously to combine, then shake it every day or two. Strain after 1 month, squeezing as much liquid out of the herbs as you can. Take ½ teaspoon as needed for coughs (especially wet coughs) and thick mucus congestion.

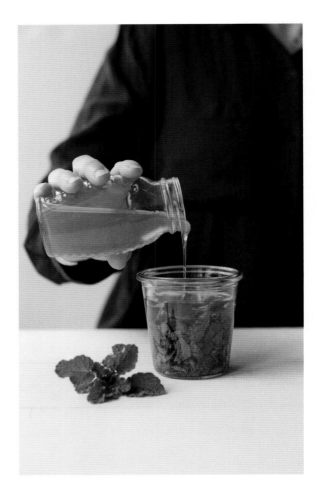

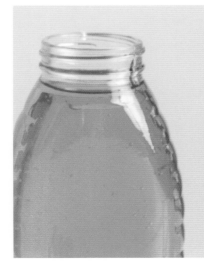

Raw Wild Cherry Honey

Use dried wild cherry or chokecherry bark, twigs, or strips to make this yummy, super-soothing, fast-acting cough remedy. Loosely fill your jar with the cherry bark and twigs, following the instructions for a raw honey on page 49. I particularly like this infused honey once it's crystallized. Slowly licking it off of a teaspoon prolongs the soothing effect, giving it more contact on the throat and a better opportunity to act. Store-bought cherry bark tends to be poor quality, but bark that you process yourself (even if it's been hanging out in the pantry for a few years) works fantastically and has a lovely amaretto-like flavor.

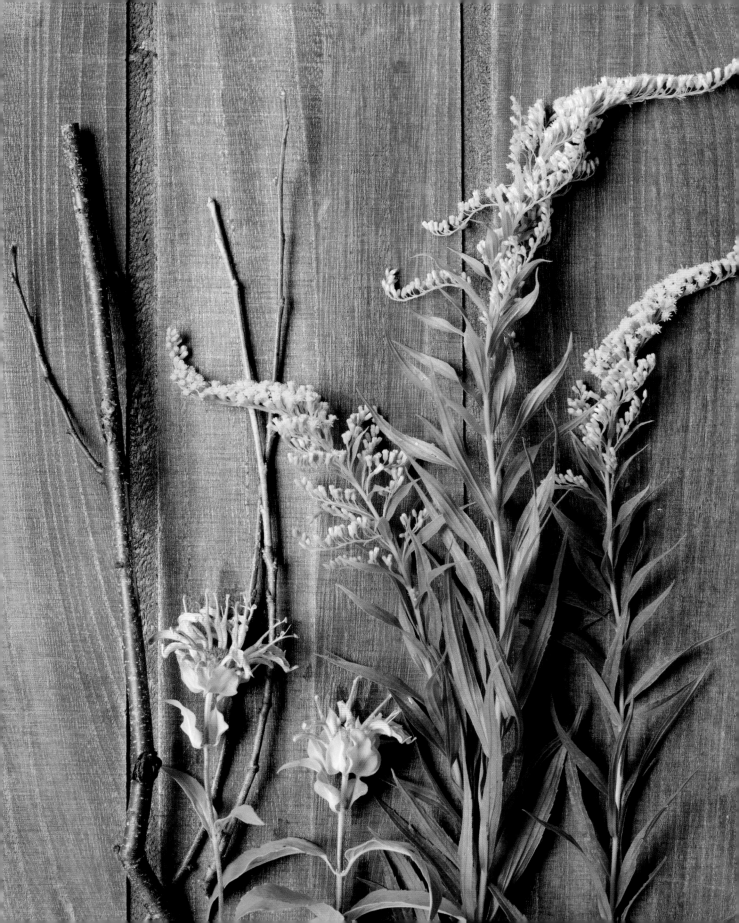

ALLERGY AND SINUS

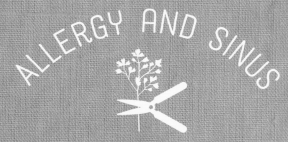

Most of our allergy relief herbs are common weeds, though you can certainly incorporate them into the unkempt edges of your landscape. Turn to nettle, goldenrod, horehound, bee balm, and berberine-rich herbs like goldenseal to dry or move out mucus, ease up on histamine, and fight sinus infections. Also employ them in respiratory infections, congestion, asthma, and chronic lung conditions. Match the individual situation to the actions of each herb for the best results. For example, horehound helps move and thin excess mucus, and berberine-rich herbs quickly dry things up while bee balm fights infections. Other allergy and sinus herbs include marshmallow, thyme, mullein, New England aster, fennel, peppermint, reishi, chaga, cherry bark, and peach twig.

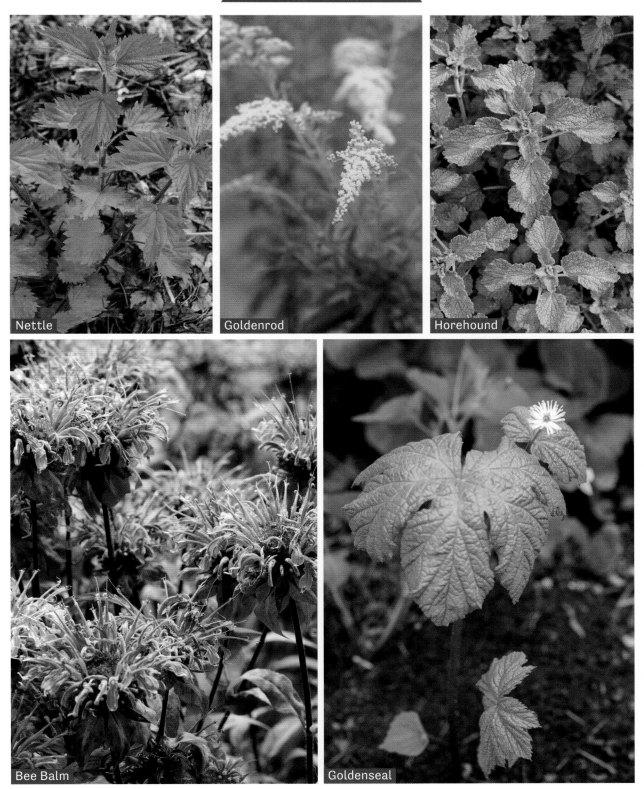

Nettle

Goldenrod

Horehound

Bee Balm

Goldenseal

Nettle

Fresh nettle tincture provides safe, fast-acting relief for environmental allergens like ragweed and animal dander. The more the fresh plant stings (and I mean *stings* — this plant bites back), the better an antihistamine it is. Just a few drops of the fresh plant tincture brings allergies down a notch, and it combines well with goldenrod. Dried nettle tea has subtle but useful benefits long term for allergies and respiratory issues. Wear gloves and long sleeves while harvesting and processing. See page 289 for more.

Best in: tincture or juiced (strongest), tea, broth, food (cooked, juiced, or dried)

Goldenrod

This late-summer field wildflower gets unduly blamed for hay fever because it blooms and grows alongside the more inconspicuous culprit, ragweed. Goldenrod offers fantastic antihistamine and mucus-thinning and -moving properties for allergies, sinus congestion, and sinus infections. Welcome it along unkempt edges of your yard alongside other garden brutes. Harvest the tops just as they're beginning to bloom. See page 269 for more.

Best in: tincture, tea, vinegar, oxymel

Horehound

Horehound gets a solid mention in the Lung Tonics garden on page 175, but it bears repeating because these same properties make it a favorite for allergy and sinus blends. It's my go-to herb for thick mucus and phlegm, common in sinus and allergy issues. Postnasal drip, nasal congestion, and chest congestion all respond well to horehound, which blends well with goldenrod to thin and move crud out. This plant prefers arid environments, growing wild throughout the country. This *bitter* silvery herbaceous plant thrives in dry spots of the garden near lavender and thyme. See page 275 for more.

Best in: tincture, syrup, glycerite, cough drop, honey, capsule

Bee Balm

Pockets of bee balm grow wild throughout the country, but it's better known as an ornamental perennial. Medicinally, it bridges oregano and thyme — potently antimicrobial, warming, drying, opening, mucus moving, expectorant, with an affinity for the lungs. Unlike its culinary cousins, bee balm's a tall, robust plant with gorgeous flowers, easy for ample harvests. Try it with honey for sore throats, in tinctures with goldenrod for sinus infections, and as a steam for chest congestion. See page 249 for more.

Best in: tea, tincture, oxymel, glycerite, honey, steam

Goldenseal

Cultivated goldenseal root and leaf work systemically and quickly to dry up excess secretions (called catarrh) and tighten and tone mucous membranes. It also fights bacterial and fungal infections, but only on *contact*. Add it to sinus rinses and combine with echinacea in throat spray. Other berberine-rich herbs, including barberry and Oregon grape root, can be used similarly. See page 270 for more.

Best in: tincture, glycerite, vinegar, topical tea/wash/nasal rinse

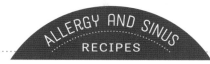
ALLERGY TINCTURE BLEND

THIS BLEND CAN BE HELPFUL IN CHRONIC ALLERGIES, hay fever, and chronic asthma. While some people may only need to take it as needed when allergies kick in (preferably starting 2 to 6 months before allergy season begins), people with chronic allergic or asthmatic conditions can take it daily. New England aster would work well here, too, especially for someone with allergy-induced asthma and congestion. Consider adding peach twig for people with lots of hypersensitivities that cause hives.

3 parts nettle tincture

3 parts goldenrod tincture

2 parts horehound tincture

1 part mullein tincture

1 part fennel seed or thyme tincture

Suggested tools: 2-ounce dropper bottle

If you already have the individual tinctures prepared, simply measure them by volume and pour them into the same bottle (for example, 5 ml per "part," which will not quite fill a 2-ounce bottle). If you need to make a combo tincture from scratch, measure the fresh herbs by weight (it's okay if the fennel is dried) — each part can be ½ ounce so you'll have 5 ounces total — chop and shove them into a 16-ounce jar. See fresh plant tincture instructions on page 38. Take 1–2 ml (¼–½ teaspoon) of the blend, diluted in water, as needed or 2–3 times per day

VARIATIONS

Simple Nettle: basic but often effective

Nettle-Goldenrod: seasonal and animal allergies, histamine overload

Nettle-Goldenrod-Horehound: thick mucus conditions, to drain

Goldenrod-Bee Balm: sinus infection, to drain

Goldenrod-Bee Balm-Berberine: sinus infection, to dry

Horehound-New England Aster-Goldenrod: congestion, mucus, asthma

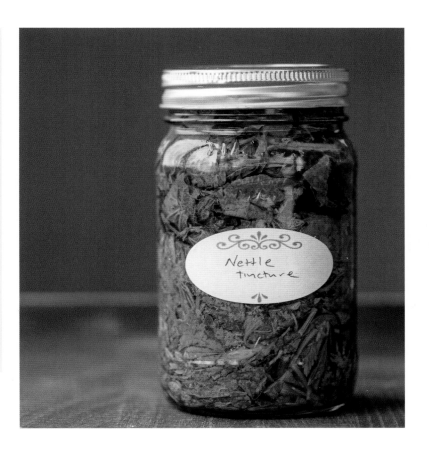

NETTLE-PEPPERMINT-MARSHMALLOW TEA

IF YOU'RE A PEPPERMINT TEA FAN, you'll enjoy this delicious blend. The primary flavor of mint mellows nicely with the other ingredients, including a velvety mouthfeel from the gentle mucilage of marshmallow. It's hard to categorize this tea blend and fit it into one of this book's garden themes even though it's one of my favorites. These multifaceted herbs soothe the lungs and have mild antihistamine properties yet are also rich in nutrition, stimulate digestion, soothe and heal the gut, and have mild detoxifying properties. (My favorite version of this tea also has a teaspoon of violet leaves, and I powder up a peppermint-free version — with all the additional ingredients — to add to my dog's food for general health.)

1 teaspoon nettle leaf

1 teaspoon marshmallow leaf

1 teaspoon peppermint leaf

Sprinkle of calendula petals (optional)

Optional additions: violet leaf, plantain leaf, gotu kola, evergreens

Suggested tools: mug with infuser

Steep the herbs in 12–16 ounces of hot water for 15 minutes or longer, strain, and enjoy. Drink 1–3 cups daily, as desired as a tonic beverage tea.

Bitter Berberines

"Berberines" is my collective term for herbs rich in the terribly bitter bright yellow alkaloid called berberine. These herbs include goldenseal, Oregon grape root, and barberry (the three most commonly available), as well as coptis, goldthread, and yellow root. The roots contain more berberine, but the leaves also contain some, as well as other compounds that make the berberine more effective. These herbs dry excessive mucus secretions quickly, tone mucous membranes, and soothe bacterial and fungal infections on contact. Although goldenseal is one of the stronger and most well-known berberine-rich herbs, it's also unethically wildcrafted and slow growing. Only use organically cultivated goldenseal, and feel free to substitute Oregon grape root (cultivated or sustainably wildcrafted only where abundant) or barberry (an easy-to-find invasive shrub). Learn more on page 271.

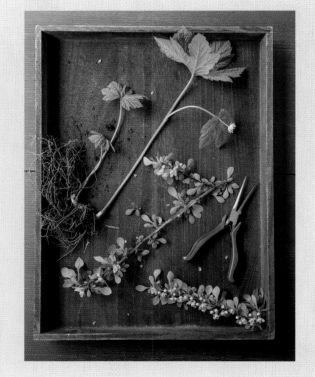

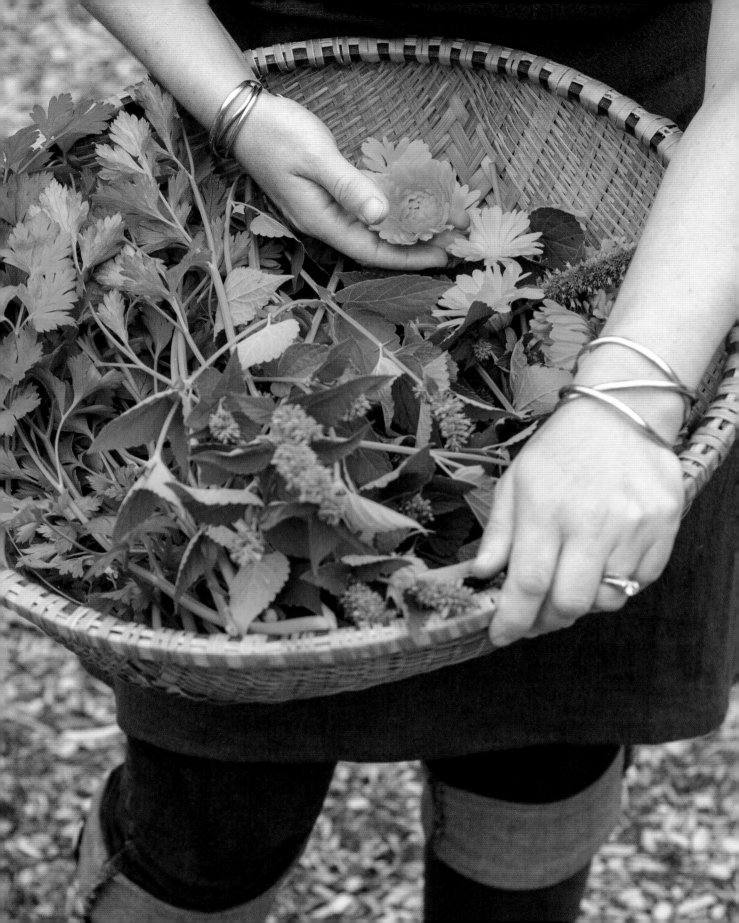

Skin Care and First Aid

THESE GARDENS focus on the topical use of plants. We start with general skin care, then move on to first aid treatments and preparations for repelling and managing insect bites and poison ivy.

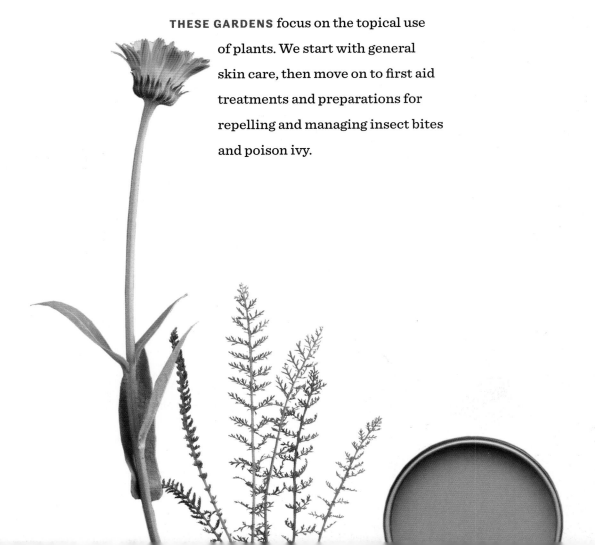

TYPES OF HERBS FOR SKIN CARE

When it comes to general skin care and first aid, we turn to a variety of categories of herbs depending on what is needed for the situation. Often, we bring two or more categories together in one formula or protocol. For example, rose hydrosol toner (astringent) plus calendula-comfrey cream (vulnerary, moisturizer) for aging skin, or honey (vulnerary) plus lavender (antimicrobial) for a wound or burn.

Vulnerary Wound Healers

Vulnerary herbs promote wound healing and connective tissue integrity. They often increase the speed or improve the quality of the healing process. These properties make them useful for cuts and scrapes, as well as in general skin care, especially if the skin is aging, sensitive, irritated, or otherwise less than ideal. We use this same category of herbs to heal the gut lining, but here we apply them topically. Vulneraries include St. John's wort, gotu kola, lavender, calendula, plantain, and comfrey, as well as honey. If moisture is needed, oil-based remedies and demulcents like marshmallow or aloe may be employed.

Astringent Toners

These herbs contain tannins, a category of constituents that bind to protein in tissue, tightening, toning, and strengthening its surface. They also tend to be antimicrobial to varying degrees. Strong tannins are used to tan leather — transforming it from flaccid skin into tight, waterproof material. We want far gentler tannins for health purposes. We use them internally for gut healing, bleeding, and diarrhea. Topically, we use them to tighten and tone the skin. Gentle astringents include rose petals and plantain while stronger ones include witch hazel, oak, and alder.

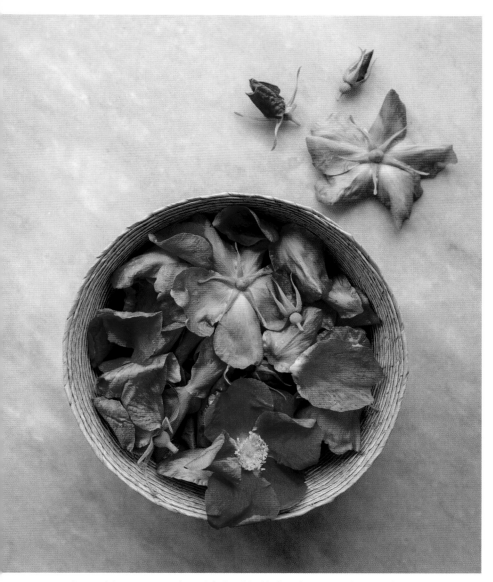

Roses tighten, tone, and nourish the skin. Hydrosols, water infusions, glycerites, and diluted essential oil all work wonderfully.

Antimicrobials

Antimicrobials disinfect wounds and address fungal, bacterial, or viral (wart) skin issues. If a wound appears infected, it's important to deal with that infection first before speeding up the healing process. Otherwise you might seal the infection in. For serious wounds, irrigation with saline solution and charcoal plasters, honey, and fresh leaf poultices (yarrow, chaparral) work best. Freshly made herbal teas, soaks, compresses, tinctures/liniments, and vinegars also work well. In general, oils, salves, and creams are less preferred and can make some infections worse. Antimicrobial herbs include thuja, yarrow, milder calendula, and lavender. Though not featured in this book, the southwestern herb chaparral is also fantastic.

Itch Relief

These herbs help with rashes, bug bites, and poison ivy, soothing the skin and relieving inflammation. Calendula, plantain, and lavender are prime examples.

Bug Repellent

These herbs help keep mosquitoes, ticks, and other nasties a little farther away. Most of these plants are highly aromatic, including lavender, rosemary, and catnip. Yarrow also works well.

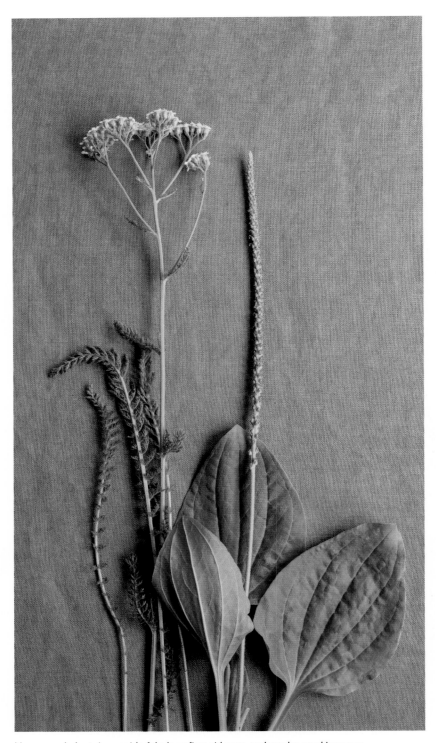

Yarrow and plantain provide fabulous first aid care, and can be used in many ways. Notably, yarrow poultice or liniment helps disinfect and stop bleeding wounds. Plantain poultice, oil, or salve helps draw out bug bite venom, poison ivy, and splinters. Together, they make a great anti-itch bug bite rub.

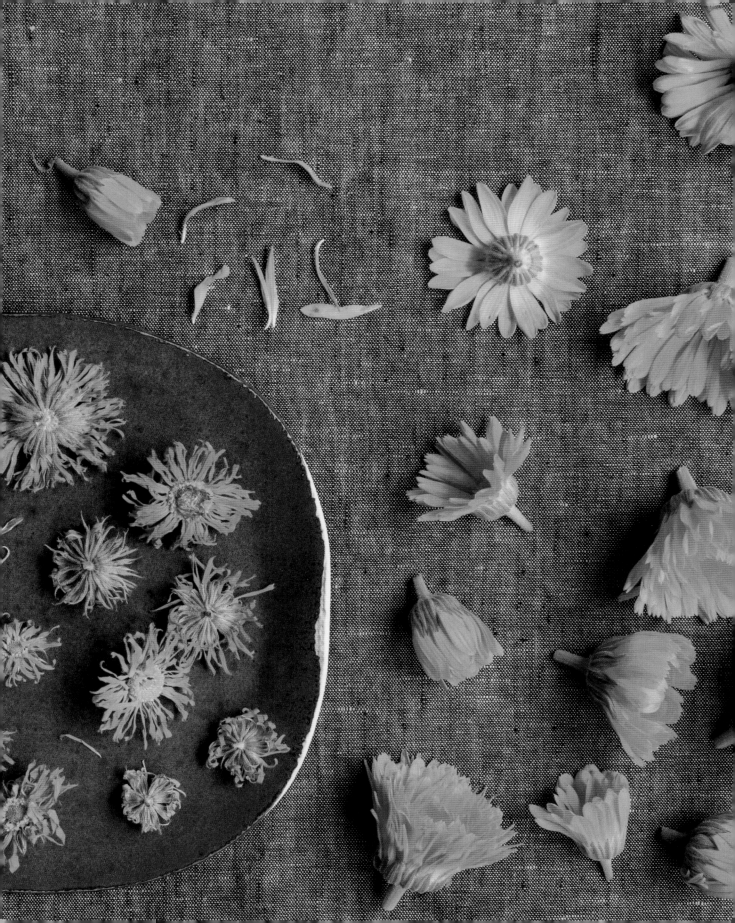

SUPER SKIN

This garden features some of our best herbs for daily skin care as well as everyday skin conditions including rashes and wrinkles. Vulneraries like calendula, gotu kola, comfrey, and lavender increase the speed and improve the quality of wound healing and promote the integrity of connective tissue. Gentle astringents like rose tighten and tone the skin, while anti-inflammatory and soothing herbs relieve skin irritation. When dealing with skin issues, also address the root causes, such as topical irritants, food allergies or sensitivities, nutrient deficiencies, sluggish detoxification, and/or stress. If you were to keep just two herb-infused oils on your shelf, whip up calendula and St. John's wort infusions. Other skin care herbs include plantain and lemon balm.

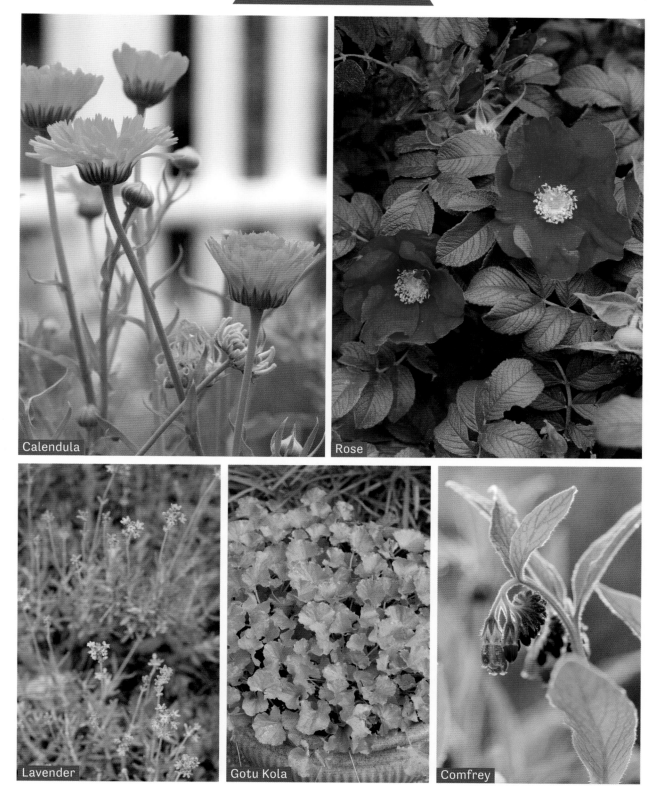

Calendula

Rose

Lavender

Gotu Kola

Comfrey

Calendula

Calendula soothes itchy, irritated, and inflamed skin — including most rashes from infections, heat, and various forms of dermatitis such as eczema – offers mild antimicrobial activity, and even soothes hemorrhoids. Look no further than these gorgeous flowers for baby's skin issues like diaper rash, cradle cap, and dryness. Calendula's quite safe and easily tolerated, but it sometimes *causes* itchiness in people with daisy-family flower allergies. Plant these cheery flowers in full sun and good soil with regular moisture. See page 255 for more.

Best in: oil (preferably alcohol-intermediary plus heat), salve, cream, bath/soak, compress

Rose

As a mild astringent, rose petals gently tighten and tone the skin while their presence in aromatic essential oils nourish and soothe it. Use rose hydrosol or tea as a lovely toner, and add the hydrosol or glycerite to creams. Though divine, 1 ounce of pure rose essential oil requires *1 ton* of rose petals and sells for $600 to $1,000. If you decide to splurge, purchase it in miniscule quantities and dilute one drop in a carrier oil like coconut to stretch it out. Or simply use roses in homemade remedies. See page 296 for more.

Best in: glycerite, hydrosol (with 10 percent rose liniment), bath, topical tea rinse or spritz, essential oil

Lavender

Lavender functions in almost every way your skin might need: it serves as a mild antimicrobial as well as a potent and soothing anti-inflammatory, anti-itch, and vulnerary remedy. It even repels insects! Lavender works well for almost any skin type for both acute care and daily use. The essential oil is, thankfully, far less expensive than rose, requiring "only" 16 pillow-sized pounds of buds to make 1 ounce. Mild recipes like hydrosols, liniments, topical teas, and herb-infused oils are also lovely. See page 279 for more.

Best in: hydrosol (combine with lavender liniment), liniment, topical tea, bath, soak/compress, oil, essential oil

Gotu Kola

Gotu kola offers many beneficial properties, appearing in several gardens in this book. For skin care, it's one of our best vulneraries — not only speeding healing but working on a deeper level to ensure the tissue remodels well with minimal scarring. Studies support its use for skin, gums, gut, and other tissues. Gotu kola also boosts circulation and the integrity of blood vessel lining so that it's more flexible and less prone to breakage, used topically and internally for varicose veins, hemorrhoids, spider veins, and bruises. Consider it, alongside roses, green tea, and lavender, for aging skin. See page 272 for more.

Best in: oil, bath, liniment, internal applications

Comfrey

Comfrey soothes with mucilaginous compounds as well as allantoin, which improves skin integrity. Comfrey *rapidly* heals wounds, sometimes too fast and not as well as calendula, St. John's wort, and gotu kola. I prefer to use comfrey on old scars, for aches, pains, bumps, bruises, and general skin health. Add it to rash and fungal formulas to promote skin healing and integrity. Use the fresh poultice on small burns and nettle stings for fast, soothing, cooling relief. See page 260 for more.

Best in: oil, salve, cream, double-extraction liniment (low alcohol), poultice

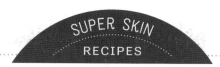

Healing Herbal Skin Care Simples

Calendula Oil

Calendula tops my list for herb-infused oils to keep on hand. It shines for irritated, itchy conditions ranging from dry skin to eczema, diaper rash, and other forms of dermatitis and even hemorrhoids. You can make this via any oil infusion method, with fresh or dried plants, but the most potent oils are made using the alcohol-intermediary method followed up with heat. See directions on pages 62 and 64. Instead of straining right away, pour the "slop" from the blender into a mason jar to heat for a few days, *then* strain it out. Recently dried flowers make the most amazing deep yellow-orange oil. I love it as is, but it also makes a fabulous salve and cream solo or alongside St. John's wort or gotu kola.

Rose Hydrosol

Rose essential oil has profound nourishing, soothing, and healing properties for the skin, but it's incredibly expensive and often adulterated. It takes 1 ton of rose petal to make 1 ounce of rose essential oil, which can easily cost $600 to $1,000. In contrast, you can make a rose hydrosol in the kitchen with a basket full of rose petals. Harvest them first thing in the morning for the best aroma. I use rugosa rose, but any unsprayed, strongly aromatic rose will work. See page 58 for directions and take note of shelf stability issues addressed there. A hydrosol extracts some essential oil diluted in distilled water. Use your rose hydrosol straight as a toner and aromatherapy mist or as an ingredient in formulas such as creams. Rose Glycerite (page 119) is quite nice, too.

Comfrey Root Liniment

Even though we often make comfrey leaves into comfrey oil, its wound-healing constituent allantoin is more soluble in hot water. Follow the directions for a decoction tincture on page 42 using fresh or dried comfrey roots with a final 20 to 25 percent alcohol (comfrey's mucilage repels high-proof alcohol) — just an hour or two of simmering will do, no need to concentrate it down unless you want to. We call topical tinctures "liniments," and this should *only* be used topically because of comfrey root's potential liver toxicity when taken internally. Comfrey promotes rapid wound healing, helps with old scars, and eases aches and pains. I *don't* use it in deep wounds because it can trap in infection (it's not antimicrobial) and increase the scarring in new wounds (it's fast, not sophisticated). The liniment makes a great ingredient in calendula-comfrey cream (to heal rashes from eczema and other conditions) and in antifungal blends (to promote healing alongside herbs with direct antifungal activity like thuja and chaparral).

CALENDULA-COMFREY CREAM

THIS RECIPE uses my base "perfect cream" formula outlined on page 66. Follow those directions using these ingredients for a rich, healing face and body cream that is particularly soothing for eczema and dry skin. If you don't have enough calendula oil on hand, you can replace up to 4 ounces of it with grapeseed oil — this will also make it a lighter, less greasy cream. This recipe makes about 14 ounces of cream. Feel free to halve or double the batch.

VARIATION

Gotu Kola–Calendula Cream: Great for aging skin, use a mix of calendula- and gotu kola–infused olive oils. Replace the comfrey liniment with more distilled water or rose hydrosol.

Oils

6 ounces calendula-infused olive oil (page 62)

1½ ounces coconut oil

1 ounce cocoa or shea butter

¾ ounce beeswax

Waters

2 ounces comfrey root decoction liniment (page 192)

2 ounces vanilla extract

1½ ounces distilled water

A few drops of lavender essential oil (optional)

See page 66 for supplies and directions.

Adding Sunscreen, Three Ways

DIY sunscreen is a bit of a gamble since each ingredient could increase or decrease the effects of sun exposure on your skin. Greasy products tend to make you more likely to burn, yet some ingredients offer variable sun protection. DIY sun creams work well for day-to-day sun exposure but will probably not be strong enough for, say, fair skin on a full day of kayaking.

Add Unscented SPF 30 Sunscreen: Mix organic store-bought cream 1:1 with whatever home-made cream you've already made.

Add Zinc: Buy zinc oxide powder. Wear a mask to ensure you don't accidentally inhale it. Use 20 percent zinc in your recipe to get 20+ SPF — about 3 ounces of zinc for the above recipe. Stir it into your oils after you remove them from heat. Play around with small quantities first to find an amount that works for your skin and isn't too pasty white when applied.

Use Sun-Protective Ingredients: Various herb-infused oils and skin care ingredients have modest sunscreen properties (perhaps 4–10 SPF) and/or help protect the skin from sun damage. These include coconut oil, unrefined sesame oil, hemp oil, shea butter, and infused oils made with St. John's wort, chaparral, comfrey leaf, and/or green tea.

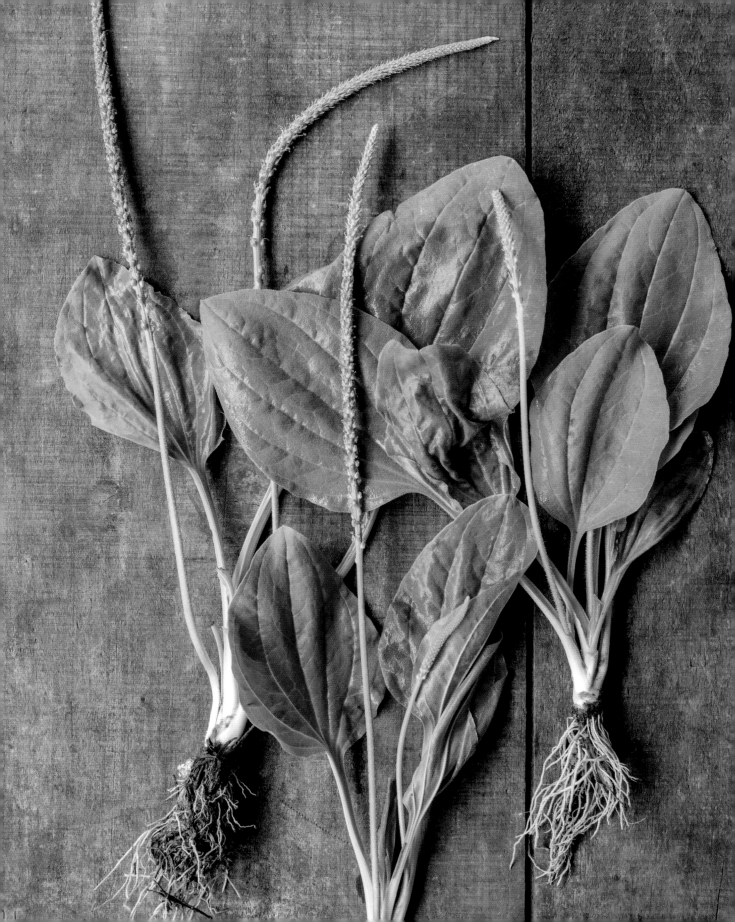

FIRST AID

In this garden, we explore herbs for cuts, scrapes, burns, bruises, boo-boos, skin infections, and minor bleeding. The array of herbs here won't necessarily fit neatly into one garden bed but are easy to incorporate into the yard. Calendula's a proper garden herb for a sunny location. Weedy yarrow, plantain, and St. John's wort can be invited into your garden, but they often prefer the spot they chose. Plant trees like thuja and witch hazel in partial- or full-shade edges of the yard if they don't already grow wild near you. Expand your first aid repertoire with the skin care, topical pain, and bite/poison ivy care herbs featured throughout this section. Other first aid herbs include gotu kola, lavender, goldenseal, alder, aloe, comfrey, bee balm, and oregano.

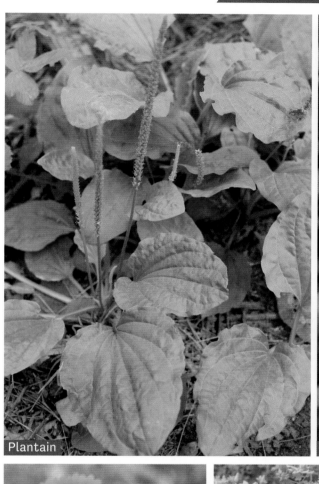

Plantain

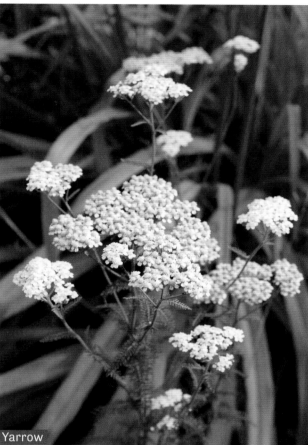

Yarrow

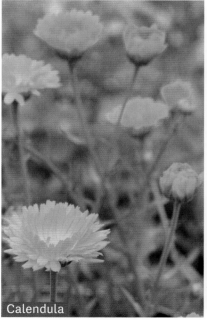

Calendula

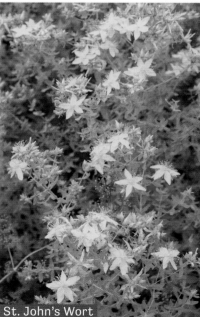

St. John's Wort

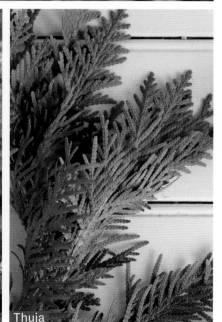

Thuja

Plantain

"White man's footprint" pops up where we step — pavement cracks, footpaths, lawns. Colonists brought this hitchhiker for food and medicine, but America already had its own native species. The fresh chewed leaf poultice draws out bee sting and bug bite venom, poison ivy's itch, and even splinters — it's better than calendula. The sooner applied, the better. Other preparations work, but not quite as well. Plantain soothes, tones, and heals both topically and internally. Easily wildcrafted or introduced to the garden. See page 293 for more.

Best in: fresh leaf poultice, oil (alcohol-intermediary), salve, liniment, topical vinegar, bath/compress/soak, sitz bath

Yarrow

Yarrow heals wounds like nothing else. Named *Achillea* after the Greek war hero Achilles, it was traditionally used for soldiers' battlefield wounds. The fresh leaf poultice stops bleeding, allays infection, eases pain and itches, and promotes healing with minimal scarring. Yarrow offers more powerful antimicrobial and anti-infection properties than most vulneraries, and a whole lot more. Topically, it repels insects, astringes hemorrhoids, and tones varicose veins and other varicosities. See page 307 for more, including additional *internal* uses.

Best in: poultice, liniment, topical vinegar, bath/compress/soak, sitz bath, oil

Calendula

Calendula's the go-to for itchy, irritated, rashy skin conditions (though plantain's superior for bug bites and poison ivy) including eczema, allergic skin reactions, and other forms of dermatitis and conjunctivitis (when combined with berberines). It begins working almost instantly and can be used long term in chronic and dry skin situations, even for babies. Add lavender essential oil to bump up the anti-itch action. If you have daisy-family flower allergies, spot test first — it *makes* a few people itchy. See page 255 for more.

Best in: oil (alcohol-intermediary plus heat), salve, cream, tea/bath, compress, sitz bath

St. John's Wort

This multipurpose first aid herb heals wounds (minor and after the remodeling phase), rashes, and bedsores. Specific for burns including sunburns, it also acts as a light sunscreen. It relieves pain, especially nerve pain, and may heal nerve damage long term. Alongside its antiviral properties, St. John's wort excels for all forms of herpes outbreaks including shingles. Use fresh buds and flowers. See page 299 for more, including how to harvest and prepare this plant for maximum potency.

Best in: oil, liniment, salve, cream

Thuja

Also called arborvitae, this potent antimicrobial evergreen fights fungal infections, warts/HPV, and other "icky critter" skin issues. Use the evergreen needles topically. Thuja grows wild in various areas throughout the country and also makes a fine landscape plant with tall, dense growth that can be shaped into a hedge. Just be sure it gets enough water. The southwestern herb chaparral is somewhat similar and also invaluable for first aid wound care. For warts, celandine works even better. See page 302 for more.

Best in: oil, salve, cream, liniment, vinegar, soak

SUPER SKIN SALVE

USE THIS ALL-PURPOSE HEALING SALVE on scrapes, rashes, cracked skin, hemorrhoids, minor wounds — you name it! Safe for kids and pets, too.

1 ounce beeswax

1 ounce St. John's wort oil (page 215)

1 ounce calendula oil

1 ounce plantain oil

1 ounce gotu kola oil

20 drops lavender essential oil (optional)

Check out the suggested tools and directions for making a salve on page 64. Keep a couple in roll-on tubes for easy first aid on the go.

VARIATIONS

Calendula: Favorite for babies, rashes, and sensitive skin. Use 4 ounces of calendula in place of the various herb oils. Skip the lavender essential oil for babies.

Calendula and St. John's Wort: Rev up your calendula salve by using 25 to 50 percent St. John's wort oil with or without the lavender.

Plantain: If poison ivy or bug bites are your enemy, then turn to 100 percent plantain salve with lavender and perhaps a few drops of peppermint essential oil.

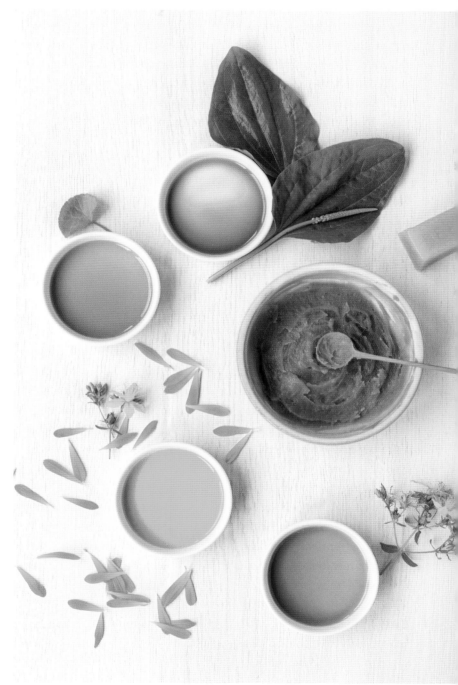

ICK STICK THUJA SALVE

ALTHOUGH IT'S USUALLY BETTER TO FIGHT FUNGUS WITH REMEDIES based on alcohol, vinegar (both antimicrobial), or hot water soaks, thuja's so potent that it holds up well as an oil or salve. This broad-spectrum antimicrobial helps eliminate various fungi including *Tinea* species like ringworm, foot fungus, and jock itch, as well as viral infections like warts. Stick with it until the infection is well cleared, and address the root cause. Root causes may include microbe exposure, weak immune system, reduced vitality, or too much sugar. (For warts, fresh mashed aerial parts of greater celandine applied overnight often work even better, clearing infections in just one or two applications.)

1 ounce thuja oil

¼ ounce beeswax

Optional additions: 15 drops tea tree essential oil, 10 drops oregano essential oil, 3 drops black pansy flower essence

Suggested Tools: salve jars or tubes (for 2½ ounces total volume)

Check out the suggested tools and directions on page 64. If you prefer more of an ointment consistency, use ⅛ ounce beeswax instead.

First Aid Simples

For more intense herbal first aid training, check out Sam Coffman's *The Herbal Medic Book*.

Lavender Essential Oil or Hydrosol/Liniment: rashes, bites, repellent, disinfect, heal wounds, burns

Plantain Poultice: bug bites, bee stings, poison ivy, splinters

Plantain Oil: itchy bites, poison ivy (or Plantain-Yarrow Bite Rub, page 205)

Comfrey Oil: bumps, bruises, aches, sprains

St. John's Wort Oil: rashes, burns, sores, cuts, scrapes, nerve pain, herpes (page 215)

Calendula Oil or Salve: eczema, diaper rash, hemorrhoids

Thuja Salve: antifungal, antiwart

Yarrow Poultice: stop bleeding, heal wounds, manage infection

Yarrow Liniment: clean wounds, repel insects, antimicrobial

Aloe or Prickly Pear: burns, minor wounds, sunburns

Witch Hazel Hydrosol/Liniment: infections, bites, hemorrhoids

Honey: burns, wounds

Peach Twig Tincture/Liniment: allergies, hives, bug bites, bee stings

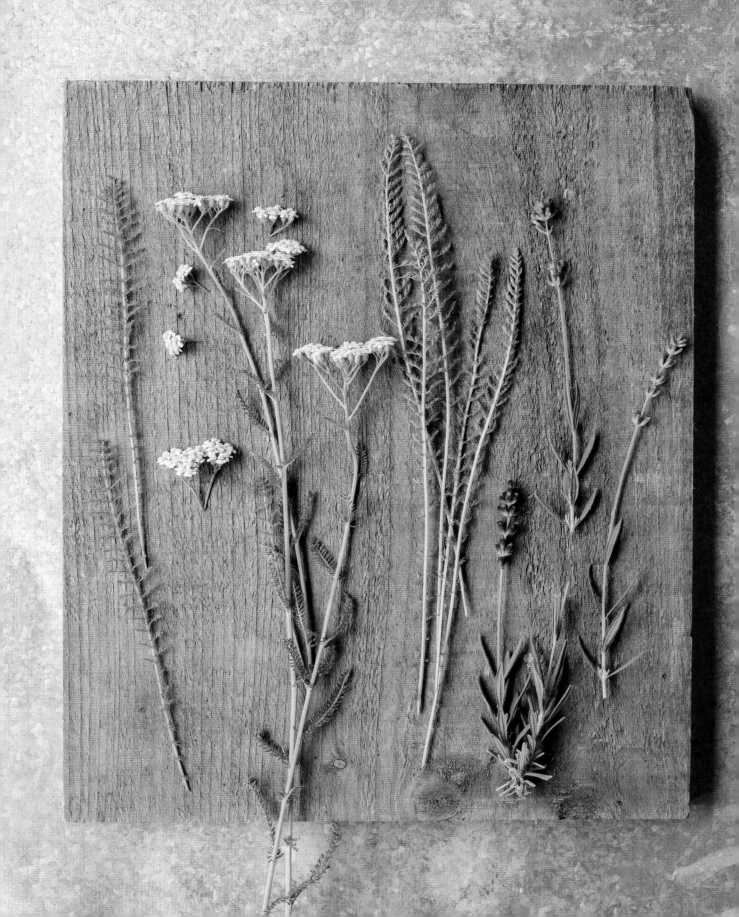

INSECT REPELLENT
AND BITE CARE

If you're a gardener, biting insects and ticks come with the territory. Fortunately, lavender, yarrow, plantain, and catnip — all of which also offer other healing virtues — repel those nasty buggers and ease the itch if and when you do get bit. Welcome all these herbs into your formal garden, though you may prefer English plantain over broad leaf for aesthetics. For insect repellents, a blend based on about 20 percent essential oils, applied frequently, works *best,* but try homemade liniments and other preparations as a base. Other insect-repellent herbs include rosemary, alder, witch hazel, and peach twig and leaf.

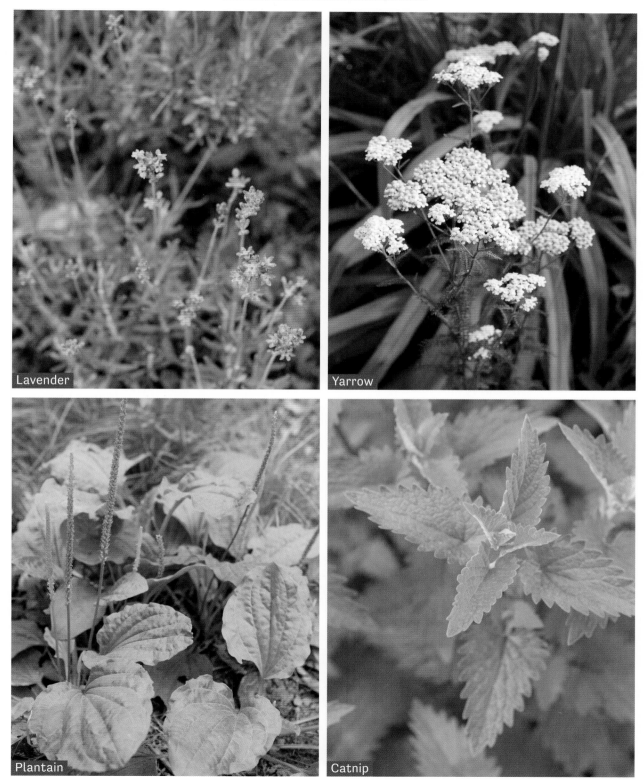

Lavender

Yarrow

Plantain

Catnip

Lavender

Most people think of citronella as the first-line herbal insect repellent, but lavender does a stellar job and may be superior for ticks. Also dab it on bites and dilute the essential oil in remedies to disinfect and ease the itch. The essential oil will be far stronger, but milder homemade preparations also help. Lavender blends particularly well with rose geranium as a tick repellent and for general skin care. Lavender sanitizer wipes work in a pinch as a repellent and for postbite care, too. See page 279 for more.

Best in: essential oil, liniment, oil (alcohol-intermediary), hydrosol

Yarrow

Yarrow's one of the few insect repellent herbs that is *not used* as an essential oil but rather a tincture that you spray topically. Sensitive folks who can't handle strong smells from essential oils or simply want a gentler, safer option appreciate this. Studies support yarrow extract's ability to ward off mosquitoes and ticks. It offers disinfectant and skin-healing properties, too. Combine the tincture with plantain oil to rub onto itchy bites. Yarrow offers a host of additional skin benefits, including disinfecting wounds, speeding wound healing, and stopping bleeding, not to mention more internal uses. See page 307 for more on this multipurpose herb.

Best in: liniment, vinegar, poultice

Plantain

Nothing squelches the itch or sting of a bug bite quite like fresh plantain leaf poultice. Other preparations work in a pinch. This common weed draws, heals, soothes, and cools inflammation, making it broadly useful for many skin conditions including bug bites, stings, and poison ivy — it is superior to calendula for these kinds of itchy rashes. You may not need to plant this common weed, just search around the lawn and yard edges. English plantain's pretty enough for the garden. See page 293 for more.

Best in: poultice, oil, liniment, vinegar, compress, bath

Catnip

Studies have found that catnip essential oil repels mosquitoes, and you can use catnip liniment as a base for your homemade bug sprays. Catnip's simultaneously easy yet finicky in terms of growing conditions. It might not come back the next year, then take over a whole stretch of yard elsewhere. Don't take it personally if it doesn't take to a new location. It'll show up again somewhere. It prefers warm spots and good soil, tolerating a range of moisture and light conditions. See page 257 for more.

Best in: liniment, vinegar, hydrosol

HERBAL INSECT REPELLENT

REACH FOR THIS BEFORE YOU HEAD OUTSIDE, and reapply frequently. Feel free to tinker with the recipe based on personal tastes, what works best with your individual body chemistry, and what you have on hand. And remember, you can use just plain old yarrow tincture in a pinch! Feel free to try a blend of yarrow and catnip tinctures, too.

1½ ounces yarrow tincture

¼ ounce rosemary tincture

¼ ounce lavender essential oil

20 drops geranium essential oil (optional)

Suggested tools: 2-ounce spray bottle

Combine your ingredients, shake vigorously, and spray every 15–30 minutes when you're outside.

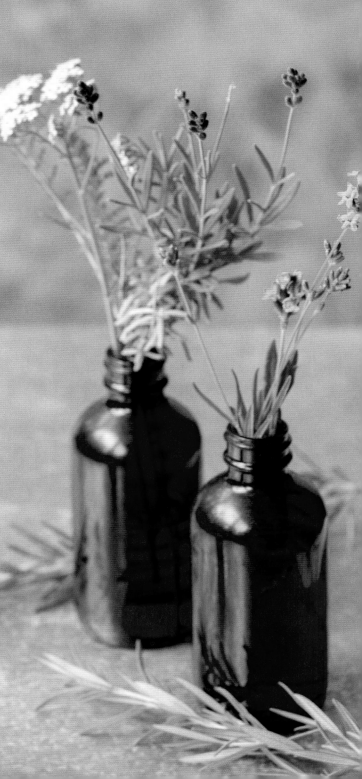
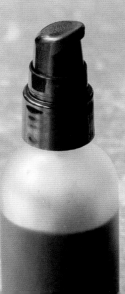

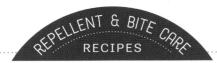

Bite and Rash Relief

Plantain Poultice

Nothing impresses quite like fresh, crushed plantain leaves on a bug bite, bee sting, or poison ivy. It immediately draws out the itch and inflammation. Even people with bee allergies will find it useful (but still get that EpiPen to be safe), and it may help avert cellulitis. The sooner it's applied, the better. Essential first aid for picnics and herb walks — teach the kids!

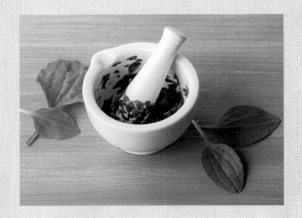

Plantain-Yarrow Bite Rub

Simply combine plantain-infused oil and yarrow tincture 1:1 to dab or rub onto bites to disinfect, heal, and stop the itch. The ingredients will separate, so shake vigorously before applying. I like keeping them in a small roll-on tube. Feel free to add a few drops of lavender essential oil and perhaps a little bit of peppermint, but it works well without essential oils, too.

Poison Ivy Relief

Bugs aren't the only thing that make us itch in summertime. Fortunately, several herbs lend a hand for the maddening itch of poison ivy, oak, and sumac rashes.

Plantain: poultice, compress, oil, or salve

Lavender: essential oil (diluted), compress, liniment

Oatmeal: bath, compress

Grindelia*: fresh flowering parts of this West Coast plant work better than possibly anything else; apply as a liniment

Jewelweed*: Crush and rub the fresh aerial parts of this plant on the area, preferably as soon as you're exposed, then rinse it off. You can also simmer the whole fresh plant and freeze in ice cube trays to apply as needed.

*These herbs are not otherwise covered in this book but are so effective they're worth mentioning.

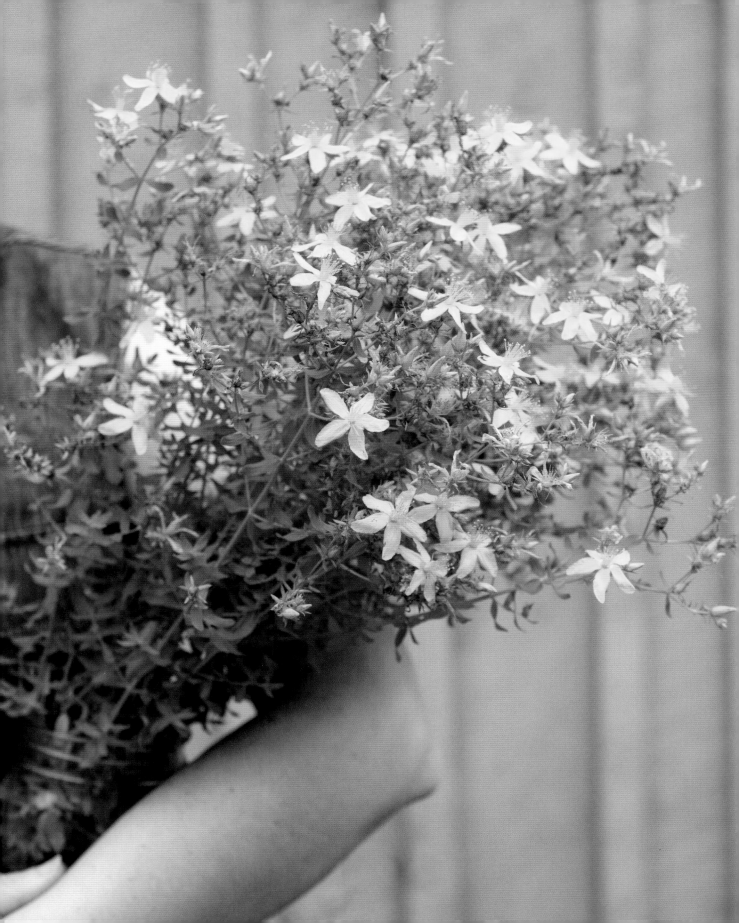

CHAPTER

EIGHT

Pain Relief

CHRONIC PAIN AFFLICTS more Americans than diabetes, heart disease, and cancer combined, and the most common medications come with a slew of side effects including liver toxicity, gastric inflammation, and addiction. In contrast, the herbs we use to manage both acute and chronic pain boast a higher degree of safety with fewer side effects; however, they're not a simple "this for that" substitution. In herbal medicine, we do our best to get to the root cause of symptoms — this can include diet and lifestyle changes. When it comes to herbs, they're specific for certain people and types of pain, and they often work better over the long haul. Our most famous anti-inflammatory and pain herbs include turmeric and ginger (from the tropics) and boswellia (from the Middle East), but several other great pain herbs grow well in North American gardens.

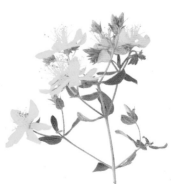

TYPES OF HERBS FOR PAIN

To manage pain, match yourself up with the best herb for your situation or combine herbs with different modes of actions for a multifaceted approach.

Anti-inflammatories

These herbs may work on the same principle as cyclooxygenase (COX) and lipoxygenase (LOX) inhibitors, two classes of drugs that help regulate the levels of the inflammation-promoting prostaglandins and leukotrienes produced respectively by the COX and LOX enzymes, or they may possess some other mechanism that controls inflammation.

COX inhibitors include non-steroidal anti-inflammatory drugs (NSAIDs) like aspirin and ibuprofen. That said, herbal anti-inflammatories provide gentler, more well-rounded benefits. They may not be as strong or work as quickly, but they have few side effects and often promote better health over time than their drug counterparts. Natural alternatives to these drugs range from meadowsweet, birch, willow bark, rosemary, ashwagandha, and holy basil to more exotic herbs like turmeric, ginger, and boswellia.

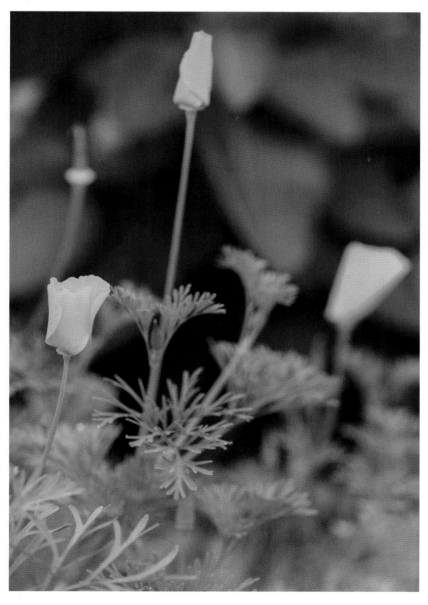

California poppy acts as a mild analgesic and nociceptive pain reliever. I prefer to use the whole plant rather than just aerial parts, because the roots are stronger.

Crossover Herbs

Several herbs can be used both topically and internally for pain management.

Birch: general anti-inflammatory

California Poppy: general analgesic

Cramp Bark: muscle cramps

Horsetail: bone breaks, joints, wounds, arthritis

Meadowsweet: general anti-inflammatory

Solomon's Seal: joint pain, sprains

St. John's Wort: nerve pain/damage

Analgesics and Nociceptives

These pain relievers work more directly on the nerves, preventing them from transmitting the message of pain to the brain and body. Tylenol is analgesic. Poppy-family herbs — in this book, the supersafe and nonaddictive California poppy — fall into this category. Cayenne and, to a lesser extent peppermint, works by depleting the pain neurotransmitter substance P. St. John's wort helps relieve pain while improving nerve healing and function.

Antispasmodics and Muscle Relaxers

These herbs tend to relax tense muscles, ease spasms, and reduce muscle pain. Herbs in the previous two categories also work, but others like blue vervain, cramp bark, black cohosh, betony, and peppermint are more specific.

Connective Tissue and Joint Support

These herbs help relieve pain while aiding the repair of connective tissue, joints, broken bones, tendons, and ligaments. Different herbs tend to target specific types of tissues. These herbs include Solomon's seal, mullein root, and horsetail. Comfrey, arnica, and elder leaves work well for bruises and aches when applied topically.

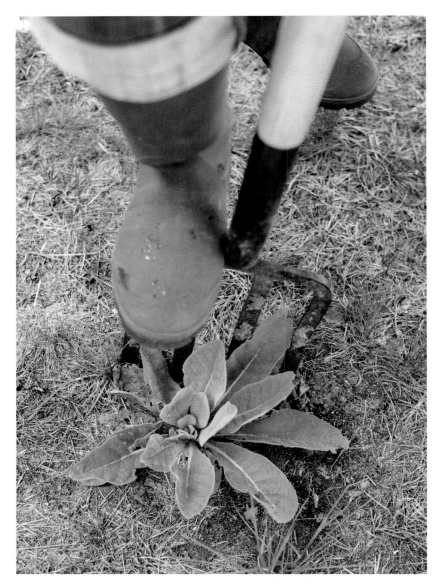

Dig mullein root before it flowers in spring or in the fall to support tendons, ligaments, and joints.

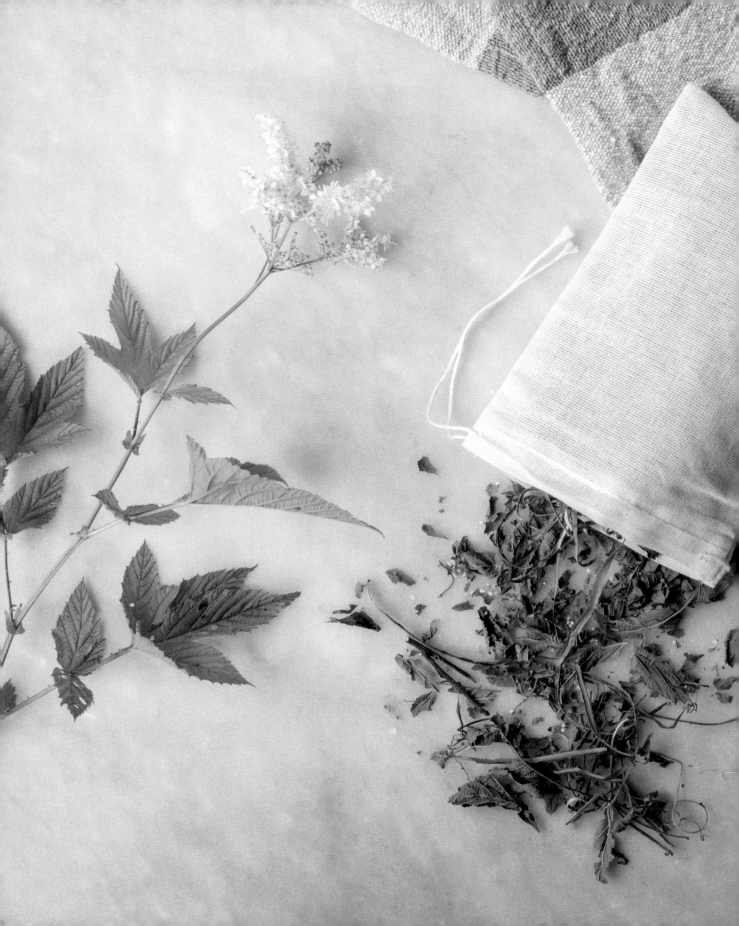

TOPICAL PAIN RELIEF

When dealing with pain, try a two-pronged approach: apply something externally and take something internally. Topical pain remedies like meadowsweet, birch, cayenne, and cramp bark tend to work quickly but are often more superficial in terms of long-term pain management. Nonetheless, their support for acute pain can be invaluable, and some topicals — like St. John's wort and comfrey — do indeed support long-term healing of the underlying condition. Also see the Aches and Pains garden (page 217); many of these herbs can also be used topically, and vice versa. Other topical pain-relief herbs include peppermint, Solomon's seal, horsetail, and ginger.

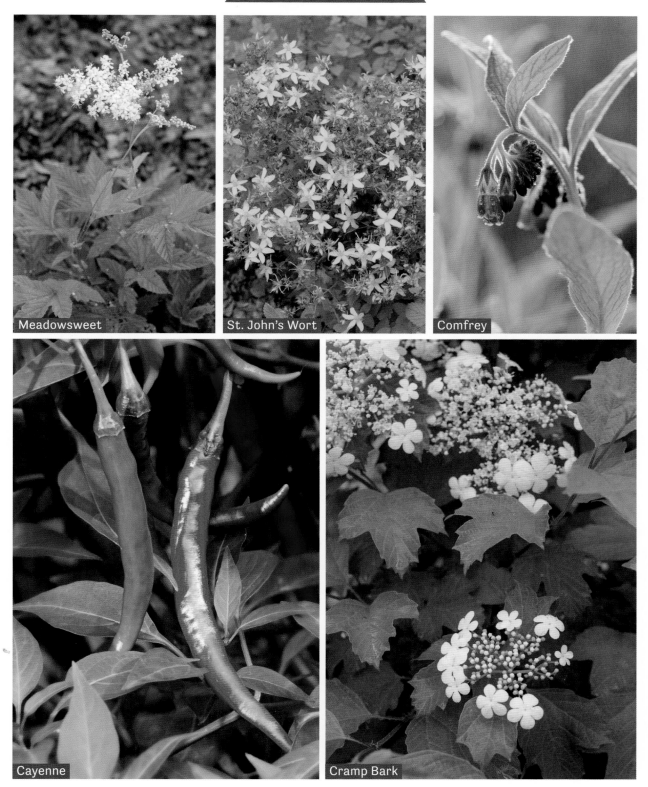

Meadowsweet

St. John's Wort

Comfrey

Cayenne

Cramp Bark

Meadowsweet and Birch

Meadowsweet thrives in either a tidy Victorian garden or a sprawling meadow, preferring good soil, adequate moisture, and full sun. As an inspiration for the creation of aspirin, it's rich in pain-relieving salicin and methyl salicylate. Black birch bark emphasizes the wintergreeny methyl salicylate. Use both "herbal aspirins" topically or internally for acute pain issues. Though weaker than its conventional counterparts, meadowsweet is much safer for higher doses and for long-term use. See pages 284 and 251 for more.

Best in: bath, liniment, oil (internally: tea, tincture)

St. John's Wort

This invaluable wound-healing first aid herb also soothes and heals nerves when they're inflamed, irritated, or damaged. It may instantly relieve pain and, with long-term use, delivers deeper healing. Its nerve-healing and antiviral properties make it useful for treating all types of herpes outbreaks. You'll make a vastly more potent oil if you use fresh buds and flowers from a sunny, dry spot after a hot-as-Hades week. The redder the oil gets, the better. You don't need to worry about drug interactions or sunburns with topical use. See page 299 for more.

Best in: oil, liniment, salve, cream (internally: tincture)

Comfrey

This speedy wound and bone healer is even more valuable topically for pain. A review of 26 human studies confirmed its efficacy and safety for ankle distortion, back pain, abrasion wounds, and osteoarthritis. Think of it as a local arnica alternative for sprains, tendon and ligament issues, aches and pains, and bruises. Use the oil plain or with liniments to improve their glide. Comfrey's almost too easy to grow. Due to its potential liver toxicity, only use it topically or internally as a flower essence. See page 260 for more.

Best in: oil, cream, liniment, poultice, compress, flower essence

Cayenne

Capsaicin cream's probably the best-researched, strongest topical herbal remedy for pain. This spicy constituent of cayenne depletes substance P, a neurotransmitter that sends pain signals to the brain. Cayenne burns a bit when you first apply it, but eventually that sensation diminishes. Consider it for osteoarthritis, shingles, and nerve pain. Not everyone tolerates the burning, irritating properties of this herb, and keep it away from sensitive spots (eyes, nose, genitals). See page 258 for more.

Best in: oil, liniment, cream

Cramp Bark

Gorgeous white flower clusters and red berries make this tall shrub a lovely landscape addition. Prune it to maintain a nice shape and ensure plenty of bark medicine for muscle cramps. This antispasmodic, muscle-relaxing herb targets menstrual cramps when taken internally. Use it externally for general muscle tension and spasms, including backaches. It combines well with cinnamon and ginger. Recent homegrown harvests work much better than store-bought material. See page 261 for more information.

Best in: bath, compress, liniment (internally: tincture, tea)

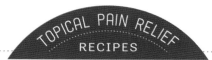
SORE MUSCLE BATH

MEADOWSWEET IS THE STAR in this bath blend, and you could use that as a single ingredient in a pinch. Herbalists Henriette Kress and Rosalee de la Forêt gave me the inspiration for this recipe — it's perfect after a long day of gardening or for a sprain or a pulled muscle.

1½ ounces meadowsweet

½ ounce cramp bark

Suggested tools: half-gallon mason jar and hand strainer or a large tea bag (nylon stockings work well)

Combine the herbs in a half-gallon jar, cover with boiling water, let steep 30 minutes, then strain into a full bathtub. Or place the herbs in a large tea bag or stocking, place in the tub with extremely hot water, and wait until the bathwater reaches a comfortable temperature. Some practitioners prefer ice water for the bath to reduce inflammation, but more recent research suggests that heat helps the body heal more effectively (and it relaxes muscles) — choose whichever feels best to you.

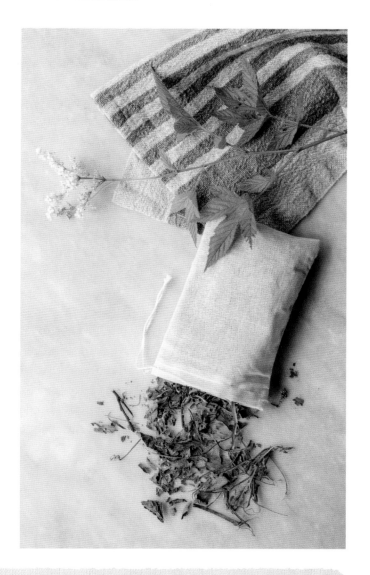

Cramp Bark Tincture with Glycerine

If you have issues with menstrual cramps, you'll want to dig deeper to address the root cause (excessive inflammation and estrogen? magnesium deficiency? undiagnosed endometriosis?), but in the meantime, cramp bark tincture provides excellent pain relief for many women within minutes. Follow the instructions on pages 38 and 40 for a fresh or dried herb tincture, but add 10 percent glycerine to your solvent — it helps discourage the tendency of the tincture to get clumpy from tannins precipitating out. Freshly made tinctures and homegrown cramp bark provide the most effective remedy. It loses potency dramatically after 1 to 3 years. Take 2 squirts (2 to 4 ml, or ½ teaspoon) diluted in water every 15 minutes until the cramps subside.

St. John's Wort Oil

The most versatile oil you can stock in your medicine cabinet, St. John's wort oil offers all-purpose healing properties as well as pain relief, nerve healing for deeper injuries and herpes outbreaks (including shingles), a light sunscreen, a burn remedy, and more. It's safe for babies, too, and the drug interactions are not a concern with topical use. It should be made with fresh buds and flowers (more harvesting tips on page 299). Unfortunately, these materials make the oil less shelf stable, which means that you need to find a fresh stand every year. Oils made with dried flowers or with leaves are far less effective. The redder the finished oil, the better. See directions for a fresh oil infusion on page 62. You can blend the finished product 1:1 with St. John's wort tincture for a nice oil/liniment.

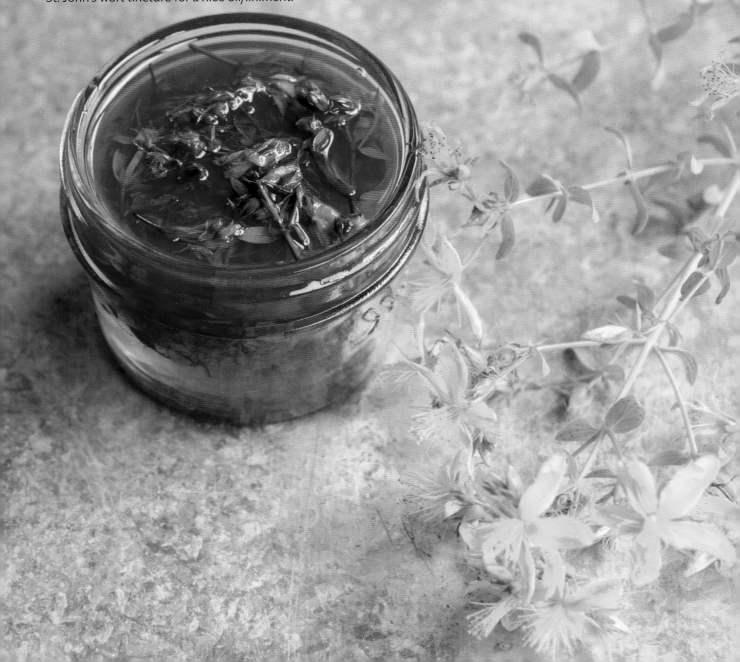

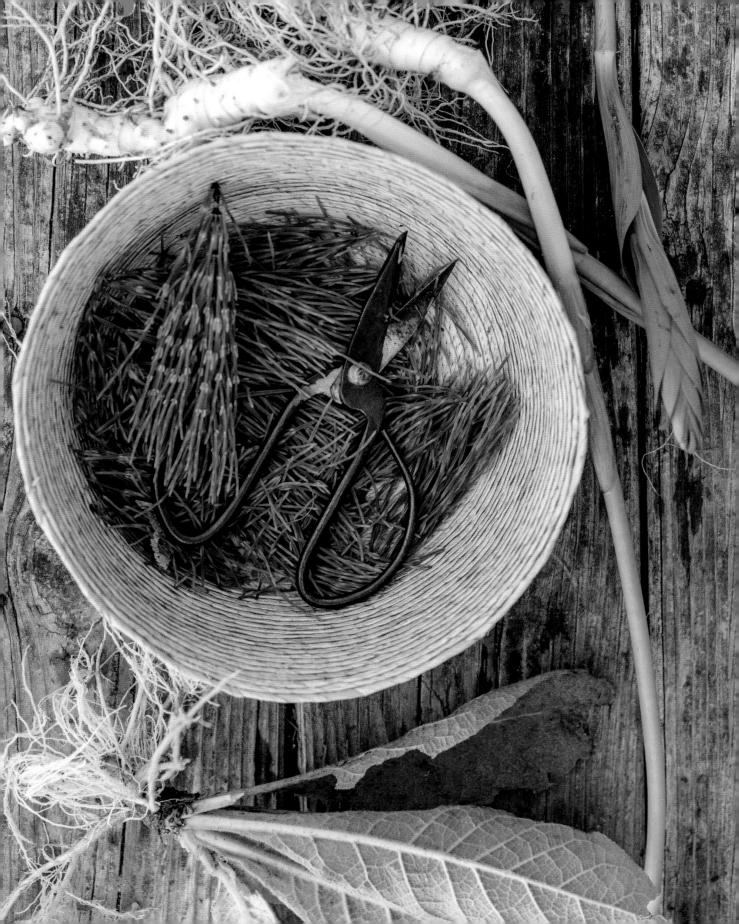

ACHES AND PAINS

None of these herbs acts like an NSAID for quick, all-purpose pain relief. Yet blue vervain, black cohosh, Solomon's seal, horsetail, and mullein root are invaluable for specific types of pain. Some work quickly, others take time, but they work best when well matched to the person and situation. All grow easily in the garden, though horsetail can be a bit of a weed. North American wildflowers black cohosh, Solomon's seal, and blue vervain bring subtle beauty to a part-shade garden. Also look to the topical pain herbs on page 213, many of which can also be used internally. Other pain-relief herbs include betony, pleurisy root, meadowsweet, birch, cramp bark, St. John's wort, ashwagandha, holy basil, and rosemary.

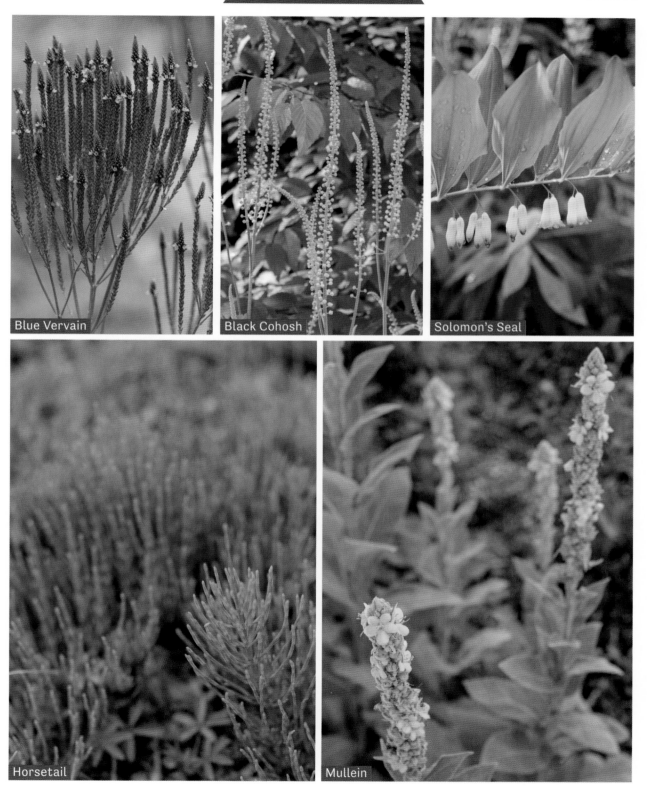

Blue Vervain

Black Cohosh

Solomon's Seal

Horsetail

Mullein

Blue Vervain

Blue vervain grows wild on riverbanks, preferring partial shade and moist, rich soil. It's tall and erect with pretty purple flowering spikes. The bitter flowering tops relax both physical and emotional tension, especially for type A control freak list-makers with a susceptibility to neck and shoulder tension and headaches. Just a few drops of the tincture will ground and relax most people. It has a long history of use for many health issues and deserves an herbal renaissance of recognition. See page 253 for more.

Best in: tincture, flower essence, possibly vinegar, oxymel, tea — so bitter!

Black Cohosh

Black cohosh favors the same woodland ecosystems as Solomon's seal, and one plant reaches 2 to 3 feet wide and 6 to 7 feet tall. Harvest the roots after 3 to 5 years, at which point the plant will be large enough to offer *plenty* of medicine; be sure to leave or replant some roots for future harvests. Black cohosh has many uses. It balances estrogen levels and lifts the dark cloud of depression. As an analgesic, it eases the aches and pains of arthritis and rheumatism and relaxes and relieves uterine cramps. See page 252 for more.

Best in: tincture (preferably fresh)

Solomon's Seal

This attractive woodland perennial thrives in rich soil, and just one plant quickly multiplies for good root harvests within just a few years. Solomon's seal's white, knobby rootlike rhizomes look like the joints of the spine. Jim McDonald teaches us to use it both topically and internally for chronic joint pain as well as problems with tendons and ligaments, including osteoarthritis, sprains, and strains. See page 301 for more.

Best in: tincture, tea, food, topically: liniment, mixed into cream, oil

Horsetail

Gardeners usually hate horsetail, which thrives in rich, moist, and soggy soil near waterways, because it's almost impossible to eradicate. However, the medicinal species stays a manageable height and doesn't outcompete other plants. Horsetail is rich in silica, a mineral that supports healthy connective tissue. Try this underrated herb both internally and externally for healing wounds and bone breaks, maintaining joint health, and relieving arthritis. Studies support its benefit for rheumatoid arthritis and wound repair. See page 276 for more.

Best in: tea, broth, tincture, topically: oil, liniment, cream

Mullein

We don't really know how mullein works, but herbalists Matthew Wood and Jim McDonald teach us to use it to cushion to joints, promote spinal alignment, and heal tendons and ligaments. It blends well with Solomon's seal and horsetail. In the garden, mullein prefers dry, sunny locations. Sprinkle its seeds and let it move around your garden year to year. This biennial weed's silvery soft foliage and tall flower stalks are a welcome sight. Harvest the roots before the flower stalk appears. See page 288 for more.

Best in: tincture

ACHES AND PAINS, STRAINS AND SPRAINS TINCTURE/LINIMENT

THIS MULTIPURPOSE MIX can be used topically and internally for joint, bone, tendon, and ligament pain, for both acute and chronic issues. You can make separate tinctures to combine as needed or make one combination blend in spring from scratch. Tinker with the herb proportions based on how much you can harvest.

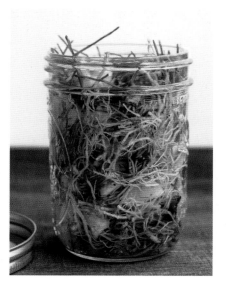

1 ounce fresh Solomon's seal root

1 ounce fresh horsetail

⅔ ounce fresh mullein root

5⅓ ounces high-proof alcohol

Suggested tools: harvesting and processing equipment (garden fork to dig up the roots, scissors for the horsetail, pruners to chop roots), 8-ounce jar with lid, scale

Follow the instructions on page 38 for making a fresh plant tincture. Once strained, take 0.5–1 ml (15–30 drops, diluted in water) as needed, 1–4 times daily. You can also rub a bit directly on the affected area. Topically, you can use the tincture straight, shake it vigorously with oil (comfrey-infused oil would work well), stir it into premade cream, or use it for the "waters" in the cream recipe on page 66.

More Ways to Use Pain-Relieving Herbs

Ashwagandha and holy basil tinctures: This is a great combo for when pain, inflammation, mood, and stress issues overlap. See pages 247 and 274 for more on these herbs.

Solomon's seal, mullein root, and horsetail: In formula or as simple tinctures or teas, they are excellent for joint, bone, tendon, and ligament issues. Horsetail and/or Solomon's seal can also be added to bone broth for joint support.

Blue vervain tincture: You can use just a few drops of this nice simple tincture for muscle spasms, neck tension, and stress tension headaches. Betony (page 250) works similarly.

Black cohosh tincture: Just 5–15 drops of tincture can help relieve rheumatic aches and pains as well as dark cloud depression and uterine pain.

Ashwagandha-turmeric golden milk: A great regular tonic for mood, inflammation, and pain support. Recipe inspiration on page 247.

Ginger, turmeric, boswellia, and rosemary: While not all of these are garden-friendly, they can be profoundly useful solo or in formula for pain and inflammation as tinctures, food, or pills.

Flower Essences for Pain

Don't forget about flower essences when working with pain. They can be used solo or added to any kind of formula including tinctures, glycerites, and topical preparations. Blue vervain is among my favorite remedies for a stiff neck or headache caused by physical or emotional tension. Others include comfrey (deep healing), dandelion (another one for tension release), lowbush blueberry (resilience), and echinacea (healing after trauma). For restoring physical vitality on various levels, try essences derived from nasturtium, forsythia, red maple, lilac, and chili pepper blooms. Get directions on how to make and use flower essences on page 68.

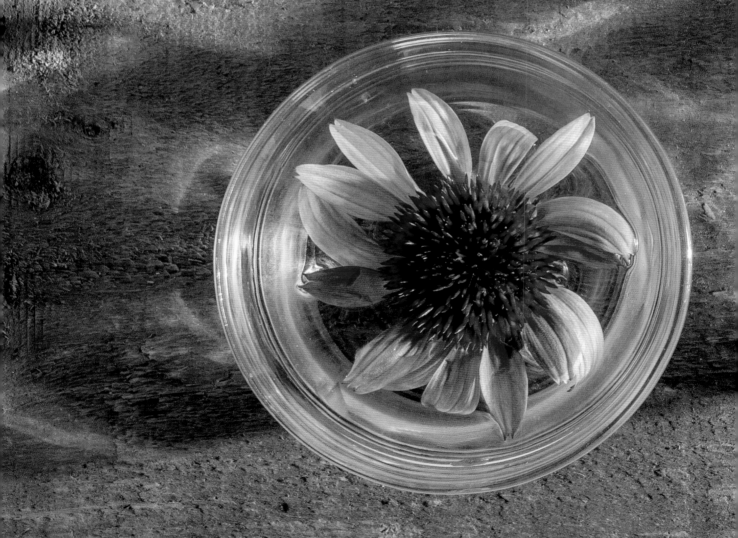

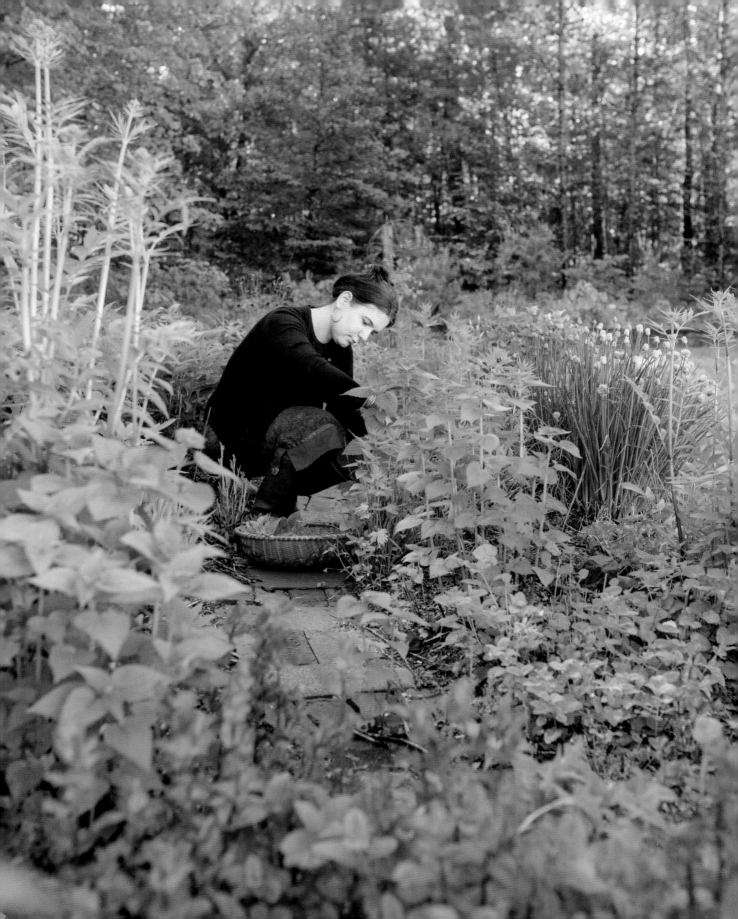

Heart and Love

IN THESE GARDENS, we turn our attention to the cardiovascular system and the female reproductive system. (Sorry guys, most "men's herbs" don't grow that easily in the garden, but check out nettle root, mullein root, ashwagandha, and autumn olive berries.) These gardens incorporate many lovely herbs — from stately linden trees, robust black cohosh, and thorny roses to pungent garlic.

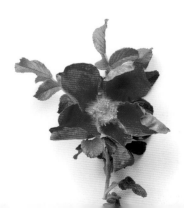

SPECIFIC TYPES OF HEALING HERBS

When working with the heart and reproductive organs, here are some herbal categories to consider.

Heart Tonics

These tonics have broad-based benefits for the cardiovascular system. While many of them do improve circulation (our upcoming category), they offer additional benefits. They may modestly reduce cholesterol or hypertension, strengthen the heart muscle, improve pumping ability, increase the integrity and flexibility of blood vessel lining, and ease emotional stress that manifests as heart symptoms. Common commercially available heart tonics include hibiscus flowers, dark purple grapes/red wine, and cacao, as well as hawthorn, garlic, and linden.

Circulation Enhancers

These herbs promote healthy circulation by improving blood vessel lining integrity, increasing blood flow, and making the blood less thick, sticky, and likely to clot. In combination, these properties help optimize the delivery of nutrients and removal of waste throughout the body and take pressure off the heart. This category of plants can be useful as a source of heart tonics, in cases of poor circulation, and for both the prevention of varicose veins and alleviation of their symptoms. Pungent herbs and vegetables are also circulation enhancers. Heart herbs may interact with heart medications — double-check with your pharmacist. Garden-variety circulation enhancers include gotu kola, garlic, and rosemary.

Herbs That Gladden the Heart

These herbs lift the spirits and ease stress and anxiety that's felt in the heart. Consider them for grief and trauma as well. They also help heal the heart when stress is an underlying factor in heart disease — for example, stress-induced hypertension — although you'll want to combine them with more overt cardiac herbs. They include roses, linden, lemon balm, holy basil, and motherwort.

Hawthorn can be harvested in spring and then again as a fall berry. It gently benefits the heart in almost every way possible!

Hormone Balancers

These herbs address reproductive hormone imbalance directly by increasing, decreasing, or modulating the production, binding, or excretion of reproductive hormones. Often we don't know exactly how they work. Many other commercially available herbs fit into this category, including dong quai, vitex, saw palmetto, maca, soy, and flax. Garden-variety herbs that increase or modulate estrogen production include black cohosh and red clover.

Tissue Toners

These herbs tighten and tone tissue, particularly the uterine lining. They may help prepare for a swift birth, promote healing after labor, ease excessive discharge or heavy menstrual bleeding, or address prolapse. They're generally gentle astringents safe for regular use and don't have a substantial hormonal effect. They include lady's mantle, raspberry leaf, and roses.

Uterine Antispasmodics

Although these gardens do not directly address menstrual cramps and uterine tension, several herbs in this book do indeed help here, relaxing the uterine muscles, relieving menstrual pain, and easing labor contractions. They include black cohosh, cramp bark, and valerian, as well as culinary spices ginger and cinnamon.

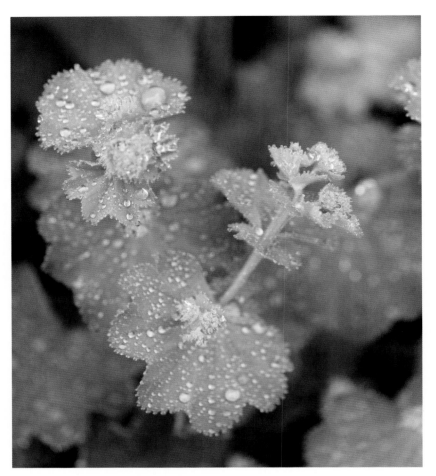

Lady's mantle makes a nice addition to shady, moist gardens. The attractive foliage catches the dew — reported in Ireland to have various magical properties — and can also be made into a pleasant tea for uterine health.

Safety Tip

Please seek professional guidance if you take medication, have a serious heart condition, or are experiencing heart symptoms that have not been properly diagnosed by a medical professional. These herbs might still be useful, but life-threatening conditions are beyond the scope of safe self-treatment and may require immediate medical attention. Once you have a diagnosis, a professional herbalist or naturopathic doctor can guide you in which herbs are most appropriate and safe to use long term. Some of these herbs may interact with medications.

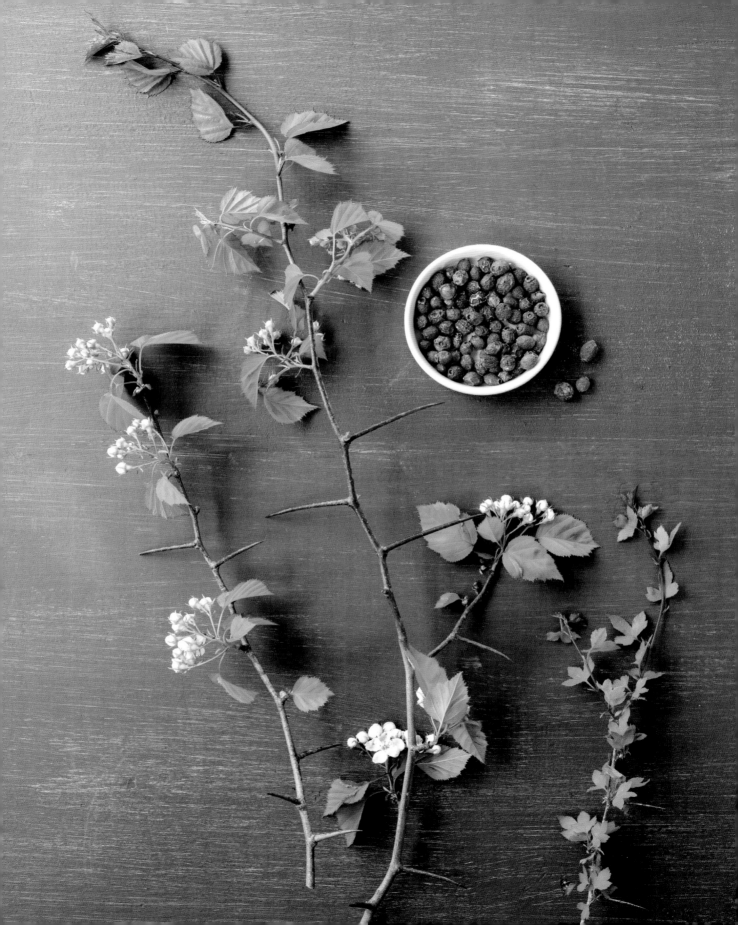

GLADDEN THE HEART

Hawthorn, linden, rose, and motherwort cross the mood-heart divide and could just as easily be used as nervines for stress and anxiety and to support the nervous system (page 103). Your heart serves as a major center of emotion for the body, and these herbs have an affinity for stress or mood dysfunction that manifests as heart issues. Think of these herbs when grief breaks your heart, trauma causes pain and tightness in your chest, and panic attacks feel like heart attacks. In overt heart conditions, don't rely solely on these herbs — it's a good idea to seek professional guidance — but these herbs can still play a supportive role in a treatment protocol. Other gladdening herbs include holy basil, lemon balm, and passionflower.

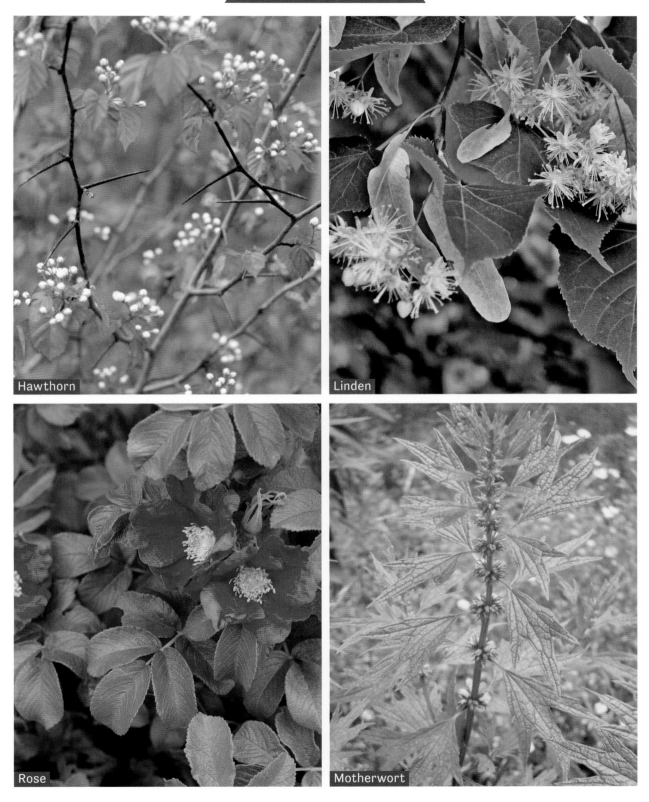

Hawthorn

Linden

Rose

Motherwort

Hawthorn

Of all the herbs in this garden, hawthorn has the most profound, direct cardiovascular effects, yet it also works on an emotional level. As a heart tonic, it's best taken in large daily doses for months to begin seeing its beneficial effects, then continued over the long term for supportive treatment and prevention of chronic and acute cardiovascular problems including congestive heart failure, heart attack, hypertension, and angina. Use the fall berries and/or spring leaves, flowers, and thorns. Hawthorn grows as a shrub to small tree, scrappy or shapely depending on the species and how you prune it. It takes *several* years to produce flowers and fruit, and the shrub can be planted as a hedge or as a specimen plant in the back or center of your garden. See page 273 for more.

Best in: tincture, tea, jam, oxymel, honey, powder, cordial, food, flower essence

Linden

Linden's heart-shaped leaves immediately bring cardiovascular health to mind. Use the intoxicatingly aromatic flowers with the attached leaflike bract. Linden offers a delightful honeylike aromatic, sweet flavor and light astringency on the tongue. The French and other Europeans love to sip linden (also called *tilleul*) tea after dinner to lift and calm the spirits. Consider it for stress-induced hypertension and as a general heart tonic. City landscapers plant linden along streets and parks. It can get quite tall (read: unreachable), so seek out a small to medium-sized species, prune carefully, and employ a ladder and a spotter. See page 282 for more.

Best in: tea, cordial, fresh or dried herb tincture, honey, glycerite, oxymel

Rose

The beauty and aroma of roses immediately lift the spirits and foster love and healing. Use rose to bring a heart blend together or solo for a pick-me-up. Sprinkle the petals into tea blends, infuse the fresh flowers in water (you benefit from seeing, smelling, and tasting them), and make sweet preparations. Time and cool temps best extract rose's aroma without too much bitter astringency. See page 296 for more.

Best in: glycerite, water, seltzer, tea, honey, cordial, elixir, flower essence, hydrosol

Motherwort

Motherwort tastes *terribly* bitter. This bitter flavor grounds people who fly off the handle easily. Motherwort gives love to those who use it. It helps take the edge off people who feel underappreciated and on the edge of rampage, particularly mothers of young children and perimenopausal and PMS-ing women, though men can certainly use this plant, too. It fosters warm boundaries, so you can take better care of yourself and get off the emotional roller coaster while still remaining friendly to others. It's specific for stress, anxiety, and panic attacks that manifest as tachycardia, arrhythmias, chest tightness, and possibly even atrial fibrillation (of course see a doctor to rule out serious cardiovascular events first). See page 287 for more.

Best in: fresh tincture, flower essence, vinegar

Hawthorn Tincture

No herb cares as deeply for the human heart as hawthorn. It makes a lovely tincture fresh or dried. We most commonly use the fall-harvested berry, but you can add in the spring-harvested leaves, buds, flowers, and even a twig or thorn or two. If you're working with fresh herbs, tincture them separately, then combine the finished extracts, using 30 to 50 percent leaf/flower to 70 to 50 percent berry. See pages 38 to 45 for tincture instructions. Feel free to add 10 to 20 percent honey for flavor. This will keep for at least 5 years. Take ½ to 1 teaspoon 2–3 times per day.

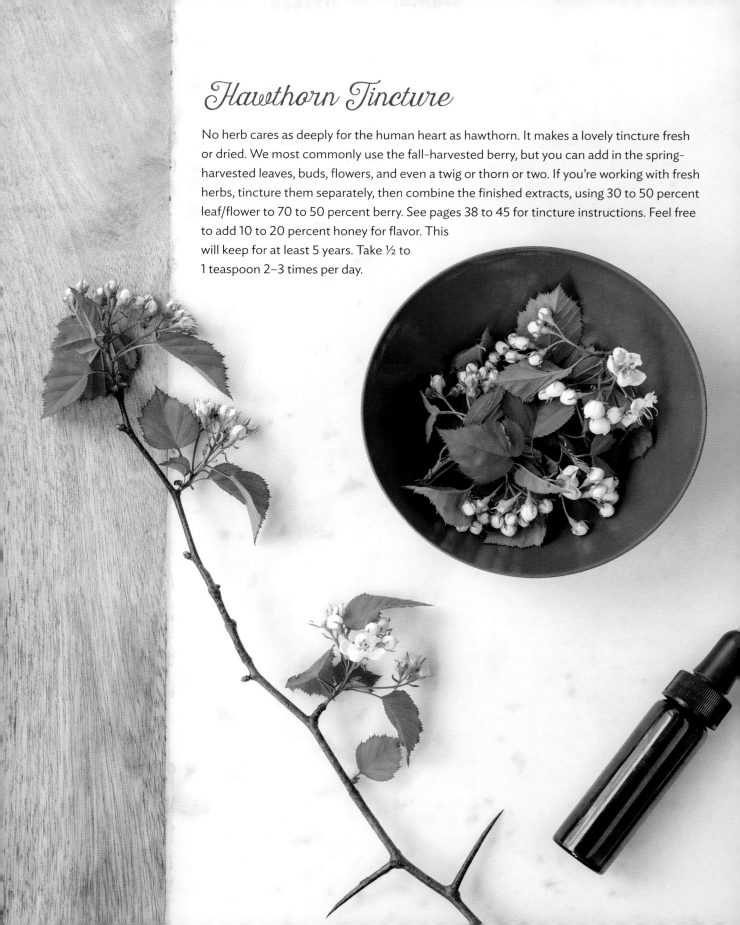

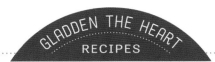

PEACEFUL HEART TEA

ENJOY THIS TASTY, HEART-CALMING TEA as a daily tonic or whenever you feel like your heart needs a lift.

2 heaping teaspoons linden

1 teaspoon holy basil

1 teaspoon lemon balm

½ teaspoon hawthorn berry and/or leaf and flower

½ teaspoon passionflower (optional, calming)

Suggested tools: infuser teapot or mug

Steep the herbs in 12–16 ounces of hot water for 15 minutes, strain. Sweeten with honey, if desired. Enjoy once or twice daily.

Linden-Honey Cordial

The honeylike aromatic flavor of linden marries so well with actual honey, you can enjoy them together in this delightful after-dinner cordial. Simply follow the instructions on page 54 using fresh or dried linden flowers and good-quality honey as your sweetener. Sip it straight from a dainty cordial glass or mix it into seltzer. If you'd like, garnish it with citrus zest or a sprig of lemon verbena.

More Ways to Use Heart-Gladdening Herbs

Motherwort tincture: Fantastic for interrelated heart-stress/anxiety conditions as a daily tonic, as well as in acute anxiety-induced states. For an alcohol-free option, try vinegar.

Rose glycerite: Heals and lifts the heart on an emotional level, for immediate and daily use. Also consider honey, tea, hydrosol, and elixir forms.

Linden tea, cordial, or tincture: Excellent solo or in blends to gently calm and uplift the spirits and the heart.

Passionflower tea or tincture: Use solo or in blends when stress, anger, or agitation trigger heart conditions, such as hypertension and tachycardia.

Holy basil and lemon balm: These herbs can be used solo or in formula for additional, happy-calm, heart-tonic support. They also have overt, cumulative benefits for cardiometabolic disease, reducing blood sugar, bad cholesterol, and inflammation.

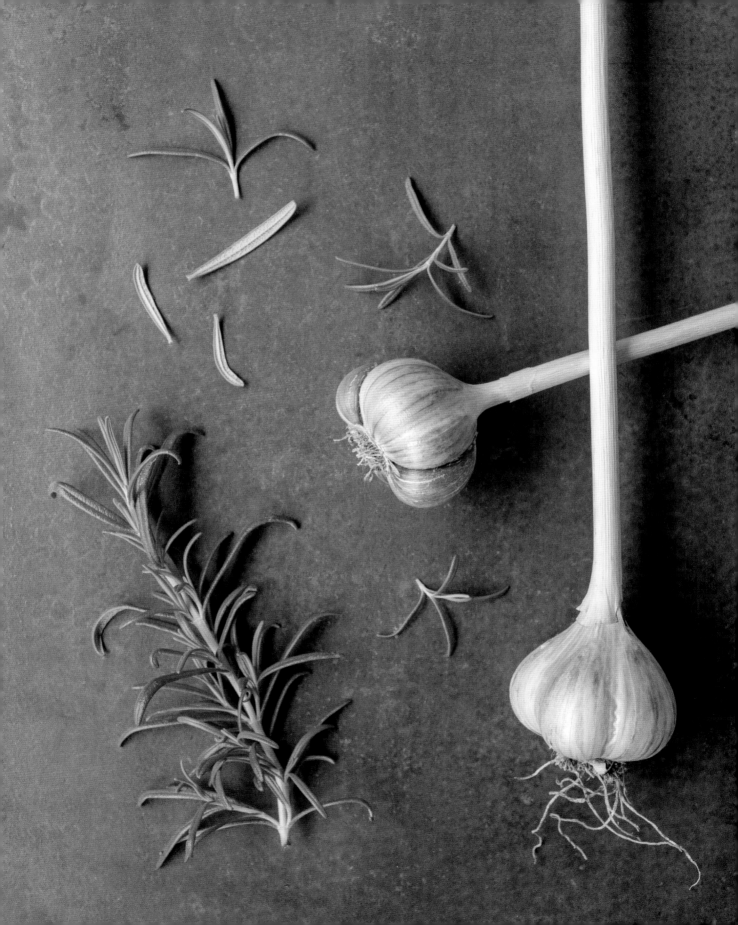

GET THE BLOOD MOVING

In contrast to the herbs in the Gladden the Heart garden, plants such as garlic, cayenne, rosemary, and artichoke are more specifically cardiovascular, well suited for improving blood circulation and increasing blood vessel lining integrity as well as encouraging other heart-healthy actions. All do well in a garden bed with good soil but have different water needs. Hawthorn remains the heart star. When laying out your garden plan, keep in mind that the hawthorn tree takes several years to bear fruit, and artichoke plants could exceed 4 feet in height and width in one season. Other cardiotonic herbs include yarrow and holy basil.

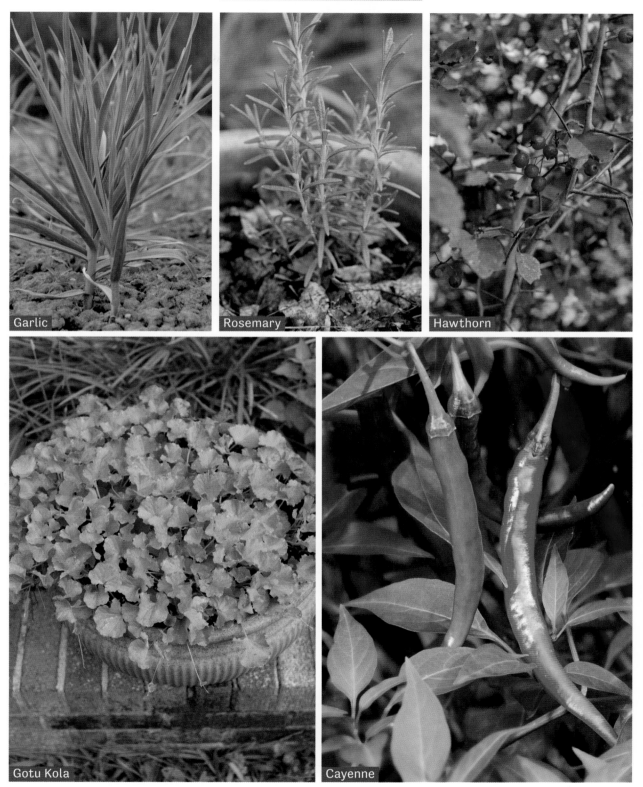

Garlic

Rosemary

Hawthorn

Gotu Kola

Cayenne

Garlic

This cardiotonic *modestly* reduces blood pressure and cholesterol; its effects are more widespread. Garlic reduces inflammation and thins the blood by reducing platelet aggregation (clumpy stickiness), atherosclerosis, and fibrin (clots and coagulation). The raw, minced cloves work best, but it makes breath — and your whole body — *stink*. Garlic's contraindicated alongside blood-thinning medications, with bleeding disorders, and prior to surgery. Plant the bulbs in nutrient-rich, well-worked soil in late fall to harvest the next season. See page 268 for more.

Best in: food (pesto, hummus, soup), tincture, broth, honey, vinegar, oxymel

Rosemary

Most people don't think beyond chicken and oven-roasted potatoes when they grow this culinary herb. Yet rosemary provides potent antioxidant, anti-inflammatory, and circulation-enhancing properties. Enjoy the fresh needles in food and use it as a synergist in medicinal blends. It's an excellent blood-moving, warming herb for formulas. It has *many* other medicinal benefits as well. Best fresh, serviceable dried. See page 297 for more.

Best in: food, tea, tincture, vinegar, oxymel

Hawthorn

This tree's berries, leaves, and flowers slowly and gently improve cardiovascular health from many angles, with tonic effects and foodlike safety. Hawthorn modulates blood pressure; strengthens the heart muscles; protects against and heals damage; fights oxidative stress and inflammation; improves heart rhythm, circulation, and the tone of blood vessels; modestly lowers bad cholesterol; and even gladdens the heart. It's extremely safe, but double-check herb-drug interactions. See page 273 for more.

Best in: tincture, jam, tea, oxymel, honey, powder, cordial, food, flower essence

Gotu Kola

Don't overlook this multifaceted herb for cardiovascular health. Gotu kola strengthens the integrity of blood vessel lining while improving circulation, particularly useful for poor vascular tone and blood stagnation. Consider it for varicose veins, hemorrhoids, and even more serious conditions like chronic vascular insufficiency and prevention and postacute care of deep vein thrombosis (acute cases *demand* medical oversight). Apply gotu kola topically for superficial conditions and take internally to support collagen integrity and wound-healing from the inside out. See page 272 for more.

Best in: tea, tincture, food, powder, juiced

Cayenne

Historically, Samuel Thompson and Dr. Christopher made cayenne famous for heart health and to increase overall vigor. Slowly incorporating modest foodlike doses into your health care regimen works best to get the blood moving and improve circulation. Add just a pinch to increase the effects of other herbs in your blend. Too much may actually trigger a fatal response. Cayenne loves dry heat without much competition, such as a minimally watered terra-cotta pot next to a brick or stone wall. See page 258 for more.

Best in: low dose in tea, food, vinegar, oxymel, tincture

FIRE CIDER

THE NAME OF THIS TRADITIONAL herbal recipe was coined by my teacher Rosemary Gladstar, who shared it freely with students and her community. This blend of spicy, pungent herbs preserved in apple cider vinegar (and, if desired, additional honey) is a delicious addition to the kitchen that can be taken by the spoonful or shot glass as a daily heart tonic. It also happens to be great for the immune system and fending off pathogens. Turmeric isn't a standard ingredient, but I love the color and healing properties it imparts.

Suggested tools: Knife and cutting board, food processor, large jar with plastic lid, strainer

Coarsely chop and mince your herbs. You can toss it all into the food processor or do it by hand. Let sit for 10 minutes before putting it in the jar and covering everything with vinegar and your desired amount of honey (perhaps 25 percent). Shake regularly and strain after about a month. I particularly love to use fire cider to make salad dressing (see page 237).

1 onion or shallot

1 head of garlic bulbs, peeled

1 inch gingerroot

½ inch horseradish root

1 or more hot peppers, to taste

1 teaspoon turmeric powder

Raw apple cider vinegar

Raw, local honey (optional)

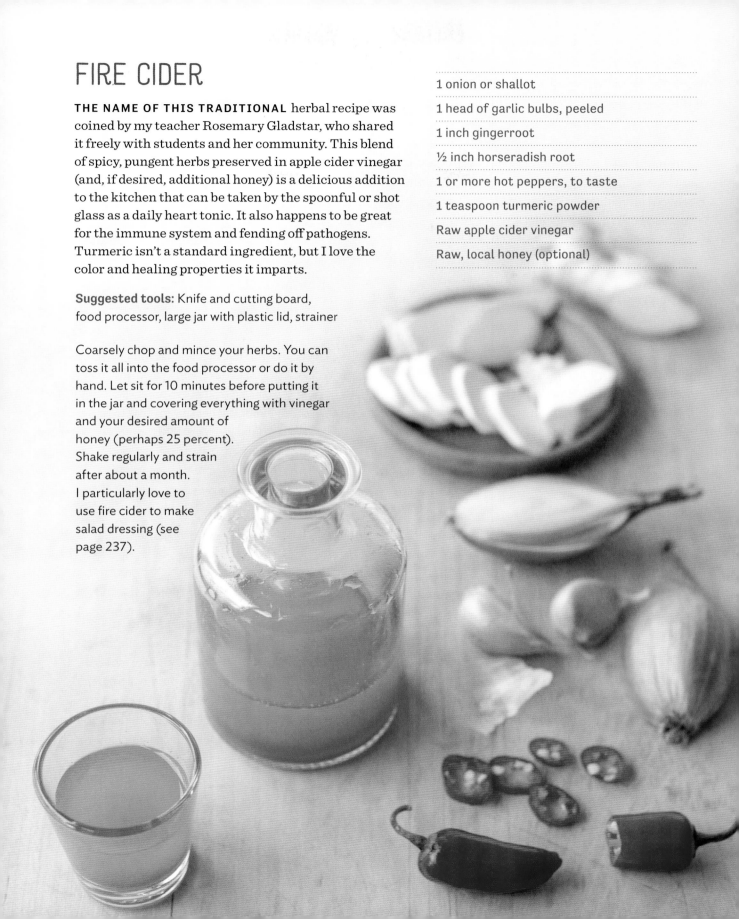

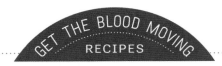
Fire Cider Recipes and Variations

Fire Cider–Maple-Mustard Dressing: This sweet-spicy dressing tastes delicious for fall salads with some crisp bitter greens, sliced apples, dried cranberries, cheddar, and/or pepita pumpkin seeds. Whisk vigorously or zip up in a compact blender 2 parts fire cider, 1 part maple syrup, 1 part stone-ground mustard, and 1 part olive or vegetable oil. This dressing will keep in the fridge for months (the olive oil will solidify).

Thai Curry Fire Cider: To the basic fire cider recipe (including the turmeric), add 2–4 chopped lemongrass stalks and 2 cinnamon sticks. This gives the recipe a little something special.

Thai Curry Paste: Purée shallot, ginger, garlic, hot peppers, chopped lemongrass stalks, and fresh or powdered turmeric (no vinegar, honey, cinnamon, or horseradish) to make Thai curry paste to use immediately or freeze in ziplock bags. Just break a chunk off to use as needed. Sauté in coconut oil, add coconut milk, a little fish sauce, and a squeeze of lime — so good with veggies, chickpeas, or chicken!

HEART TONIC TINCTURE BLEND

YOU CAN EASILY ADAPT this basic recipe for your individual needs. This combination offers broad cardiovascular benefits. Note that garlic and rosemary are best fresh whereas the other plants can be used fresh or dried. It's easier to make these tinctures as separate plant extracts to blend as needed. See tincture directions on page 38.

3 parts gotu kola tincture

2 parts hawthorn berry tincture

2 parts hawthorn leaf and flower tincture

1 part rosemary tincture

1 part artichoke leaf tincture (optional)

1 part garlic tincture (optional)

5 drops hawthorn flower essence (optional)

Suggested tools: measuring shot glass, 4-ounce dropper bottle, small funnel

To make a 4-ounce bottle, use 12 ml per "part," pour into the bottle. Shake to combine. The daily dose would be 2–5 ml (½–1 teaspoon) twice daily with meals.

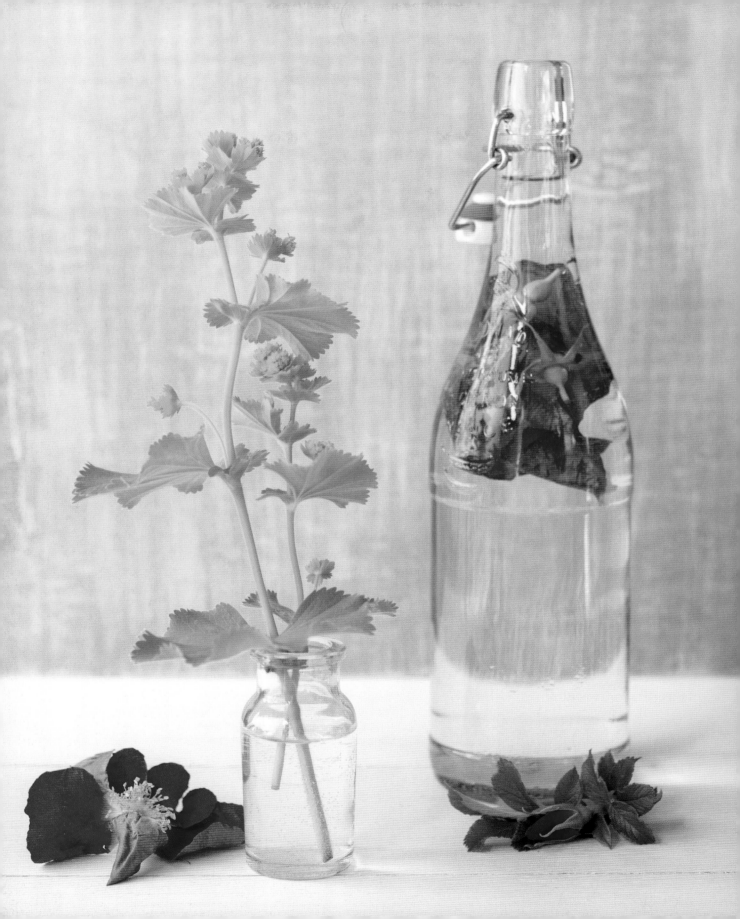

THE WOMAN'S GARDEN

Enjoy the subtle beauty of these womanly herbs. Lady's mantle, rose, raspberry leaf, and red clover make delightful tonic teas for the uterus and reproductive system. Depending on your own personal health needs and gardening interests, you can easily expand your selection. The woodland wildflower black cohosh (not so tasty and best as a tincture) is easy to grow in part shade and acidic soil but requires several years to reach harvest. Other women's herbs include cramp bark, blue vervain, motherwort, and sage.

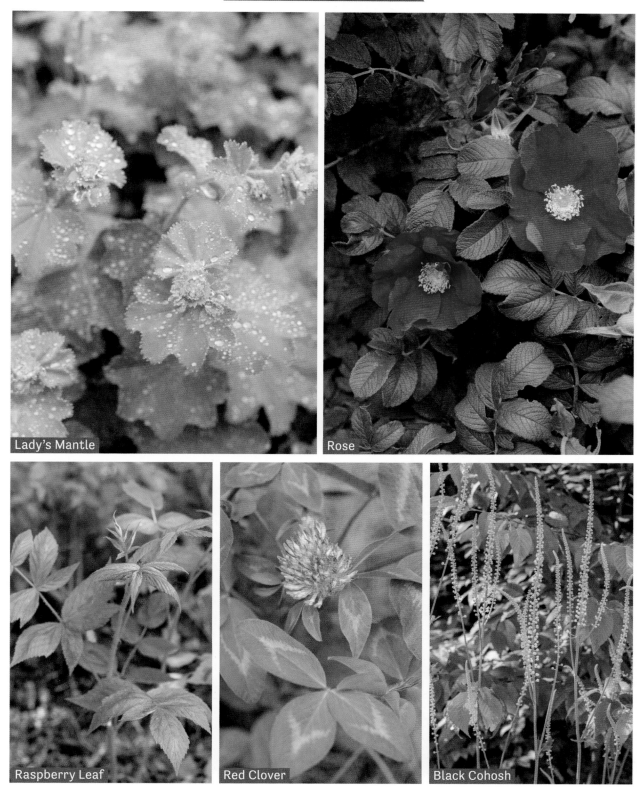

Lady's Mantle

Rose

Raspberry Leaf

Red Clover

Black Cohosh

Lady's Mantle

The subtle beauty of lady's mantle graces many formal gardens. The ornamental dew-catching leaves outshine summer's chartreuse blooms. It's gorgeous for edging beds and providing mounds of silvery-green contrast. Popular in Ireland and surrounded by lore, it thrives in dreary climates and moist, slightly shady pockets of the garden. True to its lineage, lady's mantle offers classic gentle rose-family astringent properties. It tightens and tones the uterus and may help relieve prolapse and excessive nonpathogenic leukorrhea (discharge). It tastes similar to green tea. See page 278 for more information.

Best in: tea

Rose

Roses bring in feminine energy with red-pink color and floral aroma, then tighten and tone with gentle astringency, complementing lady's mantle and raspberry leaf. Add the blossoms to tea to gladden the heart, promote healing after trauma, and support self-love and self-care. Let this thorny shrub sprawl as a hedge along a border or wall, or seek better-behaved heirloom specimens for the garden. See page 296 for more information and additional uses.

Best in: tea, glycerite, hydrosol, infused water, seltzer, elixir, cordial, honey

Raspberry Leaf

Scraggly wild raspberry really takes over with its persistent underground root runners, so wildcraft it or plant it *outside* your garden on the edge of the forest or a building. Yet another rose-family astringent ("YARFA"), raspberry leaf claims fame as the *most* popular, safe women's tea herb. Science supports its ability to strengthen the uterine muscles, and it provides calcium, iron, and vitamin C — important nutrients for women. Low doses are safe and recommended during the last trimesters of pregnancy to prepare for a swift birth. Harvest leaves from the first-year canes. See page 294 for more.

Best in: tea

Red Clover

This pretty cover crop wildflower earns a spot on the edges of your garden or lawn. Harvest the purple flower heads (including the attached leaves), and process fresh or dry promptly in the dehydrator for a pleasant tea. Rich in minerals and a source of plant estrogens, turn to red clover to nourish the body, modulate estrogen function, ease perimenopausal symptoms, and strengthen the bones. Its effects on breast cancer are mixed. See page 295 for more, including additional uses.

Best in: tea, tincture, vinegar

Black Cohosh

Black cohosh modulates estrogen levels and pituitary-gonad communication, and also relaxes tension and inflammation in the uterus. It relieves hot flashes and night sweats, eases menstrual cramps and contractions, and alleviates cycle-related depression. Although many other less garden-friendly herbs support women's hormones (particularly vitex, shatavari, fenugreek, and dong quai), this woodland wildflower lends itself well to the temperate garden. It prefers decent soil in partial shade to full sun. Dig 3- to 5-year-old roots. See page 252 for more.

Best in: tincture

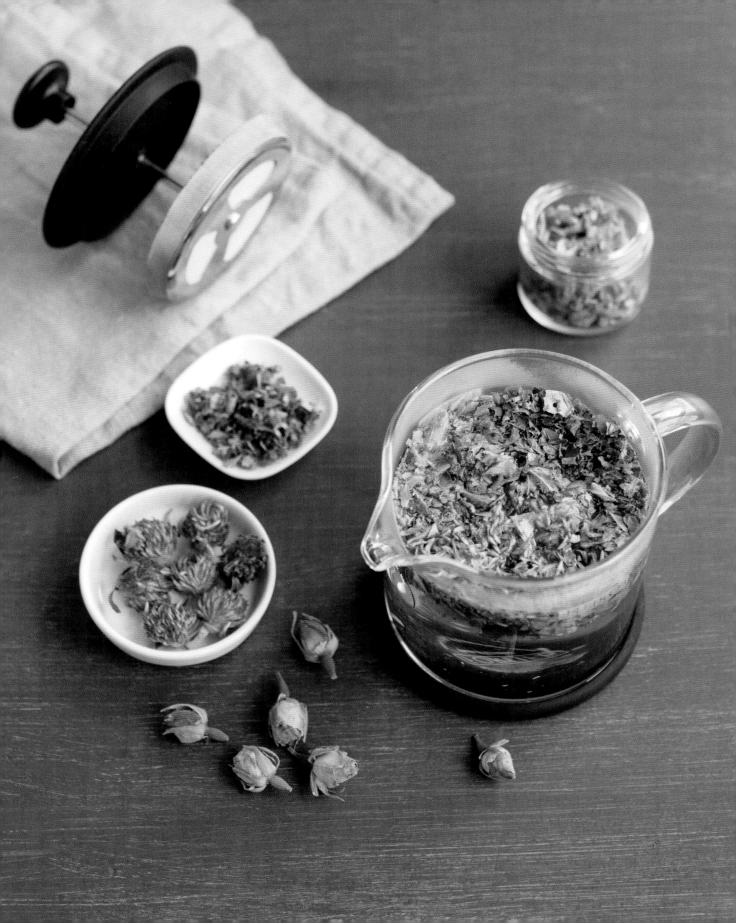

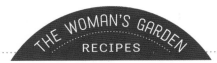
LADY TEA

THIS SUBTLE AND DELICIOUS TEA leaves a puckery-astringent feel on the tongue (similar to green tea) and has a delicate rose aroma. Enjoy it daily as a tonic or as desired as a beverage tea. The studies are mixed on whether red clover increases or decreases breast cancer risk. Feel free to omit it. The other herbs tone reproductive tissues (in women and men) and cause no hormonal effects at all. It makes an elegant iced tea.

2 parts raspberry leaves

2 parts lady's mantle leaves

1 part red clover blossoms

½ part rosebuds or petals

Honey to taste (optional)

Optional additions: fennel or linden

Suggested tools: French press, infuser teapot, or mug with infuser

Steep 2 tablespoons of the blend (or approximately 1 heaping teaspoon per part of herb) in 16 ounces of not-quite-boiling water for 15 minutes or longer. Strain, sweeten, and enjoy 1–2 cups daily hot or iced.

More Recipe Ideas for Women's Health

Cramp bark: Excellent as a tincture or tea for symptomatic relief of menstrual cramps. Page 261

Nutri-lady tea: Combine nettle, oatstraw, red clover blossoms, and/or raspberry leaf — all nutritives with an affinity for women's health — with flavorful herbs like mint, holy basil, or lemongrass as a daily beverage tonic tea or super infusion (page 35) for uterine health, bone strength, and overall well-being.

Black cohosh: You'll want to let it grow for 3 to 5 years before you dig up the roots. But what you get will be vastly superior to what's available on the market. Fresh roots offer twice the strength of dried, so you can get away with half the dose. Also, much of the black cohosh on the market is unethically wildcrafted and/or adulterated with liver-toxic Chinese cohosh species. You know it's great quality when you make your own, and black cohosh is easy to grow. This is a versatile herb. Use 5–10 drops a few times a day for a range of hormonal and nonhormonal uses. See page 38 for fresh plant tincture instructions and page 252 for more about black cohosh's uses.

Other herbs to try: Many more women's herbs help balance hormones, but most are difficult to grow or process in their usable parts. That said, Southwest-loving vitex berries grow easily as a shrubby tree in warmer climates; fenugreek seeds act as a phytoestrogen and blood sugar balancer but may be difficult to harvest in abundance; Indian shatavari root survives in Zones 8 and warmer. Angelica roots are easy to grow and help relax uterine cramps, but its relative Chinese dong quai requires special processing to make it active. White peony root decreases inflammation and balances progesterone and testosterone levels. The Mexican herb damiana can be grown in a container in full sun, brought in during winter.

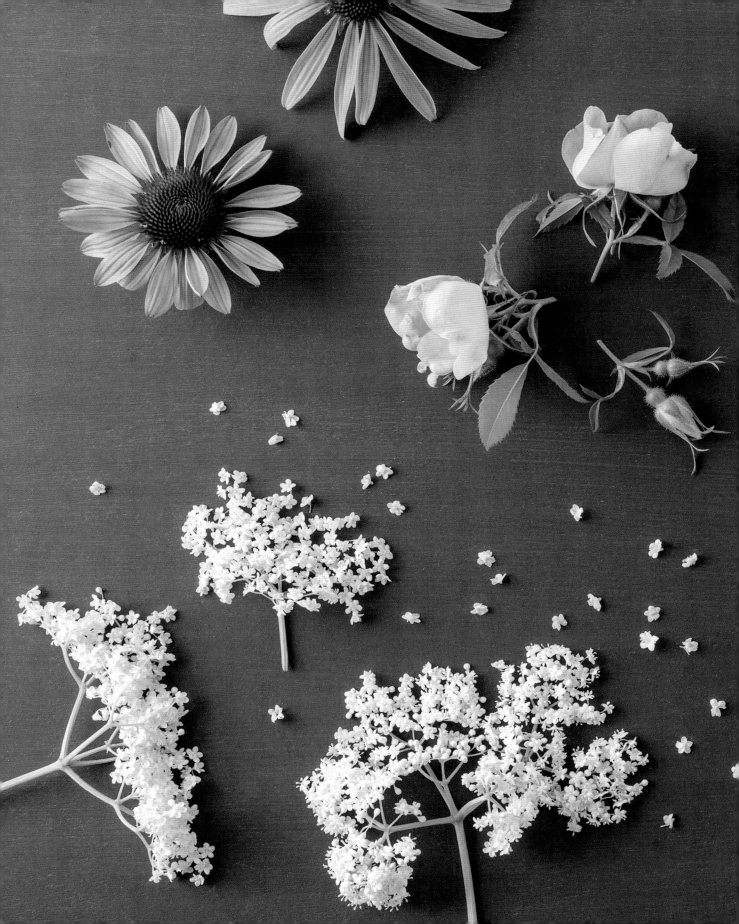

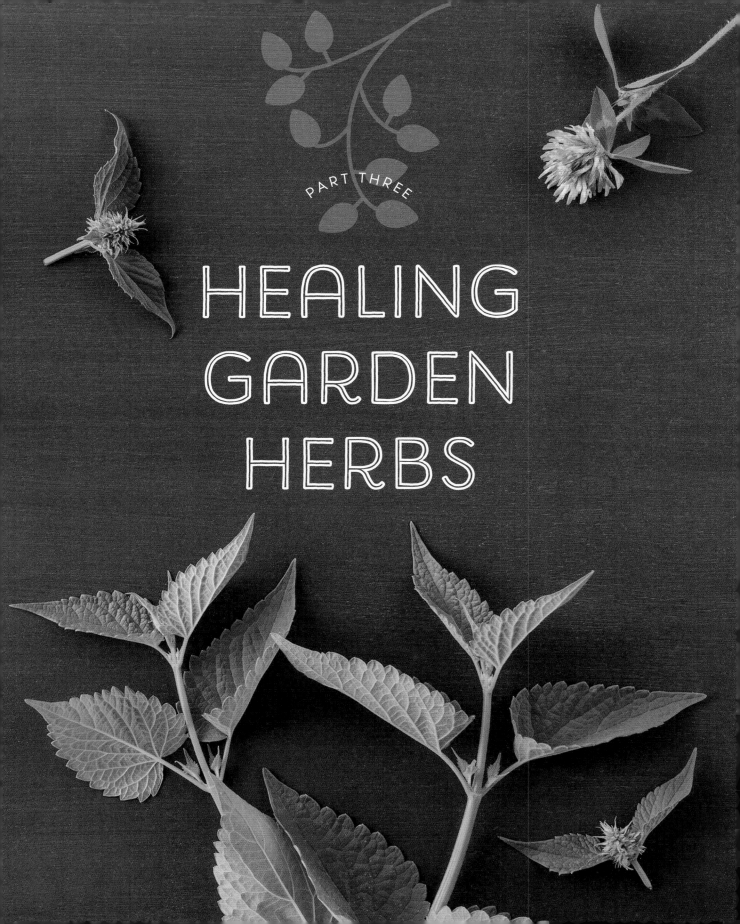

HEALING GARDEN HERBS

See pages 17–18 for sun and water icon keys

ARTICHOKE

Cynara scolymus

Daisy Family (Asteraceae)

Body Systems: Digestive, Detoxification, Metabolic, Cardiovascular

  annual Zones 4–7, perennial Zones 8–11

A MEDITERRANEAN FOCAL POINT

This formidable Mediterranean native thrives in well-prepared heavily mulched, compost-rich, mildly acidic soil with *plenty* of room to grow. One plant can reach 4 to 6 feet in height *and* width! It can be challenging in cooler climates; start it indoors. In subtropical climates, it will produce for several years. Cardoon (*C. cardunculus*) has similar properties.

SIMPLE BITTER FOR YOUR AILS

The Arabs, Greeks, and Romans cultivated artichoke and cardoon for food and medicine for millennia, and from those populations it spread to the world. The leaves act as a simple bitter (see page 134) to promote digestion and liver detoxification, much like the more famous gentian root, yet far easier and more sustainable to grow and harvest in abundance. We use bitters to increase gastric juice and enzyme production, ease many cases of reflux and heartburn, improve peristalsis (the muscle action that moves food through the GI tract), encourage the liver to detoxify more efficiently, improve bile production and excretion, increase our ability to digest fats, indirectly move the bowels, reduce blood sugar, regulate appetite, control sugar cravings, and more. Human studies support its benefits in dyspepsia, gastric motility, cholesterol, hypertension, and appetite control. As a flower essence (page 68), artichoke increases your understanding of and empathy for individual humans and humanity as a whole.

FLOWER VEGETABLE

Enjoy globe artichoke flower buds as a vegetable. Cut them before they bloom, and steam for approximately an hour. I love them with a sprinkle of salt, but most people dip them in butter or lemon butter. Both globe artichoke and cardoon leaves can be used medicinally, but globe artichoke is preferred as a vegetable. Well-cooked stems are delicious. Inulin fiber in the bud and stem feed beneficial gut bacteria.

SAFE FOR MOST PEOPLE

Known for its safety, artichoke is among our better-tolerated bitters. As with other bitters, it may aggravate a hyperacidic gut and hypoglycemia, and should not be used in an acute ulcer or bowel obstruction. Large doses may cause nausea. Watch for the sharp spines on the bud bracts — trim them off with scissors if you like — and remove the hairy "choke" from the center of the bud before you eat it.

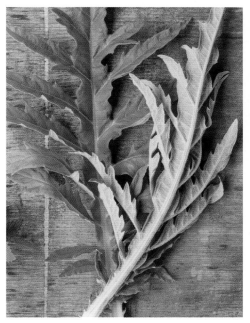

Harvesting, Preparing, and Using Artichoke

Harvest the leaves at any time. Use fresh or dried. The bitterness — and potency — mellows with cooking. Take it with meals in a small dose — sip, spray — it works better if you taste it. It's too bitter as tea, but enjoy a splash of a bitter blend (with aromatic carminatives and a hint of sweetness) in seltzer.

Parts Used: leaves

Tincture or Vinegar: ½–2 ml, 1–3 times daily, solo or in formula with meals
• Fresh 1:2 in 95 percent alcohol or dried 1:5 in 50–60 percent alcohol

Cordial, Oxymel, Elixir, or Glycerite: 1 teaspoon to 1 ounce

Recipes: Bitters Spray, page 141; Heart Tonic Tincture Blend, page 237

Enjoy unopened artichoke buds as a vegetable, but turn to the bitter leaves for stronger medicine. Give it *space* in the garden.

ASHWAGANDHA

Withania somnifera

Nightshade Family (Solanaceae)

Body Systems: Nervous/Adrenal, Mood, Inflammation/Pain, Immune, Reproductive, Thyroid, Cognition/Brain

  tender perennial, Zones 8–11

AN AYURVEDIC PANACEA

Ayurvedic practitioners revere ashwagandha as one of the most effective, multipurpose, safe medicinal plants for vitality. Start seeds indoors (easy to germinate) and/or plant seedlings outdoors after the threat of frost. Treat it like an annual in cool climates and grow it like tomatoes: ashwagandha loves heat, sun, and well-drained soil (rich to sandy) without competition from nearby plants.

THE STRENGTH OF A STALLION

According to ancient wisdom, taking ashwagandha regularly for a year will give you the strength of a stallion for the next 10 years. This includes deep energy, physical strength, calm mind, better sleep, perky and stable mood, cognitive prowess, more muscle, nourished nerves, less pain, reduced cancer risk, healthy immune and respiratory systems, stronger thyroid function, improved libido, enhanced hormones and fertility, and more. Ashwagandha is one of my favorite herbs for myself and clients. You often see results within a few days, with further improvement over time.

FANCY, FATTY FORMULATION

Ayurvedic practitioners often stir the powder into hot milk (cow, coconut, or almond), ghee, or other warm, fatty substance based on the belief that this would better send ashwagandha to the fat-lined nervous system. It's a great addition to "golden milk," which is traditionally made with turmeric, honey, hot milk, and a pinch of black pepper. I add a pinch each cardamom and nutmeg and sometimes blend in egg and vanilla extract (eggnog!).

A VERY SAFE NIGHTSHADE

Ashwagandha is extremely safe, but avoid it if you react to other nightshade-family plants like tomatoes and potatoes. To avoid overstimulating the thyroid, seek an herbalist's or naturopathic doctor's guidance if you have hyperthyroid disease or are on thyroid medications and want to use herbs (always keep your medical doctor in the loop, too).

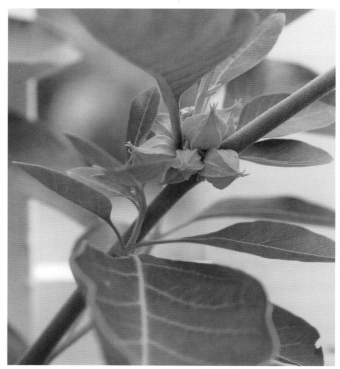

Ashwagandha's name means "smells like horse" because of the strong scent of the roots. Don't dry ashwagandha near other herbs as it can flavor them.

Harvesting, Preparing, and Using Ashwagandha

Dig up the root in the fall before frost in its first year in cool climates or, in warmer zones, the second fall when the berries are ripe red-orange. Clean and dry. (Some herbalists tincture it fresh, but I prefer dried.)

Parts Used: roots

Tea: ¼–1 heaping teaspoon powdered or 1 tablespoon cut/sifted roots per cup, simmered 10+ minutes, 1–3 times daily

Tincture: 2–5 ml, 1–3 times daily, solo or in formula
• Dried 1:5 in 50–60 percent alcohol

Powder/Capsules: 1–6 g per day in capsules or mixed into hot milk, ghee, honey, spices

Recipes: with Chai Base, page 78; Stress Support Tincture Blend, page 107, Mellow Me Glycerite, page 125. Also feel free to add it to Aches and Pains Tincture, page 220

BACOPA

Bacopa monnieri

Plantain Family (Plantaginaceae)

Body Systems: Cognition/Brain, Nervous

   annual (perennial, Zones 8–11)

A CREEPING WATER PLANT

Aquarium supply stores commonly sell *Bacopa* genus plants, but only this species has the reputation as a supreme brain, memory, and nerve tonic in the Indian healing system of Ayurveda. Bacopa likes it wet and warm and can be grown in the water or in soil that stays consistently damp. It's a native wildflower growing in sludgy, sometimes questionable-quality sites in California and the Gulf Coast. Mine thrives in a medium pot in a moist, partly shade spot with timed irrigation twice a day. You can let it sit in a dish of water. If you have a marshy area or water feature, plant it on the edge, but be aware that it may spread and become invasive. It has a succulent appearance similar to purslane with small white flowers and a hanging vinelike growth pattern. It's sometimes categorized within the figwort (Scrophulariaceae) plant family.

ANCIENT AYURVEDIC CALMING BRAIN TONIC

Ayurvedic texts primarily refer to bacopa as brahmi, a name sometimes applied to gotu kola, which shares some attributes and works well alongside bacopa. Bacopa is among our most esteemed memory and cognition tonics and also acts as a calming (but not sedating) nervine. Therefore, it helps provide calm focus and is useful in stress, anxiety, and mood issues as well as in cognitive formulas as a nerve tonic and protective, healing remedy. Several preliminary human studies support the ancient uses of this plant, particularly for memory and cognitive issues such as speed of free recall and shifts of attention, and for improving performance and learning in school-aged children with attention deficit hyperactivity disorder (ADHD). Consider it in blends for brain trauma. It may mildly boost thyroid function as well; studies show it increases levels of the thyroid hormone T4 but not T3. As a flower essence bacopa ignites joie de vivre — pleasure and joy in your life!

SAFE FOR CHILDREN AND ADULTS

Extremely safe for children and adults, though it is extremely bitter and may be better balanced with warming carminative herbs like ginger, cardamom, nutmeg, or holy basil. Take with food if it upsets the stomach. Though it is not likely to interact with medications, use cautiously alongside calcium channel blockers, anticonvulsants, thyroid, and mood medications.

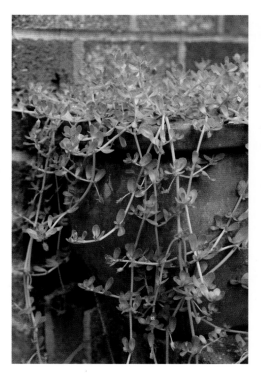

This water-loving creeper can be added to water features and aquariums or grown in a well-hydrated pot.

Harvesting, Preparing, and Using Bacopa

Harvest happy aerial parts regardless of flowering. Use fresh or dried. Its bitter flavor makes it unpalatable in tea and cordials, though you could try a small amount with tastier herbs.

Parts Used: leaves/aerial parts

Tincture: 1–5 ml, 1–3 times daily, solo or in formula
- Fresh 1:2 in 95 percent alcohol (best) or dried 1:5 in 50–60 percent alcohol
- Add 10 percent glycerine to stabilize tannins and improve shelf life

Capsules/Powder: 500–1,000 mg crude herb daily

Juice: 2–3 teaspoons per day

Recipes: Stress Support Tincture Blend, page 107; Brain-Boosting Tincture Blend, page 112

BEE BALM

Monarda spp.

Mint Family (Lamiaceaė)

Body Systems: Immune, Respiratory, Digestive, Nervous/Adrenal, Skin, Antimicrobial

   perennial, Zones 4–9

A POLLINATOR PLANT WITH POWER

Most gardeners plant bee balm — also called wild bergamont and Oswego tea — in their gardens unaware of its culinary and medicinal uses. They love the gorgeous red, magenta, and purple blooms and its ability to attract bees, butterflies, hummingbirds, and hummingbird moths. Yet *Monarda* makes a fine substitute for oregano and thyme, and it's easier to harvest in abundance. It prefers full to dappled sunlight in rich, semimoist soil. It can be a "garden brute," spreading vigorously via underground root runners and by seed. Plant in its own bed, on the less-maintained edges of your property, or let it duke it out with other garden brutes. Don't stress about powdery mildew — it's part of growing bee balm. Use any bee balm species with strong oregano-thyme flavor. I prefer the potent *M. fistulosa* (lavender blooms) and *M. punctata* (spotted), though *M. didyma* (scarlet, magenta varieties) sure is pretty.

ANTIMICROBIAL PUNCH

Rich in carvacrol (which gives oregano its bite) and thymol (that distinctive Listerine/thyme flavor), bee balm hits two home runs for antimicrobial, carminative, and expectorant activity. Honey mellows its bite, making bee balm tea a delightful, warming treat on dreary days and at the first sign of infection. Use it for thick and stuck mucus. It helps fight germs and promote expulsion of mucus and dry congestion. As you consume bee balm, oregano, and/or thyme, your body excretes the essential oils via the lungs, which targets and disinfects the area. *Monarda* also addresses sore throat pain and infection, makes a superb infused honey (also nice for coughs!), and can be used as a steam.

WARMING DIGESTIVE AND MORE

Carminative bee balm increases digestive function and helps fight pathogens in the digestive tract as well as vaginal yeast infections (skip the honey). Use it as a soak or compress for fungus and mildly infected wounds. In rare cases, people experience a profound calming nervine effect. Try it as an herbal Earl Grey bergamot tea stand-in. As a flower essence (page 68), *M. fistulosa* helps cool down people who tend to get hotheaded easily, saying and doing things they might regret later. *M. didyma* brings joy to life, helping you let go of inhibitions that prevent you from having fun.

AS SAFE AS OREGANO

Bee balm is incredibly safe and can be used as an oregano/thyme-like seasoning. Its warming, drying activity (so perfect for cold-damp respiratory states) makes it less appropriate for people who are already in hot-dry states. It acts as an emmenagogue, so avoid it during pregnancy.

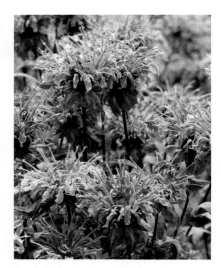

Bee balm brings stunning beauty to the garden along with its oregano/thyme-like medicinal action.

Harvesting, Preparing, and Using Bee Balm

Harvest bee balm before or just as it flowers, before the powdery mildew sets in (which happens quickly postflower). Excellent fresh or dried.

Parts Used: aerial parts, leaves, flowers

Tea: 1 heaping teaspoon dried herb/cup, infusion, 1–3 cups daily

Tincture: 1–3 ml, 1–3 times daily, solo or in formula
• Fresh 1:2 in 95 percent alcohol or dried 1:5 in 50–60 percent alcohol

Honey, Vinegar, Oxymel, Glycerite: 1 teaspoon as needed

Food: leaves (quite a punch!) and individual flowers (sweet) fresh or dried for thyme/oregano flavor and color

Topical: soak, bath, compress, oil, liniment , vinegar

Recipes: Floral Ice Cubes, page 96; Bee Balm Honey, page 170; Bee Balm–Mint Tea, page 171

BETONY

Stachys officinalis

Mint Family (Lamiaceae)

Body Systems: Digestive, Nervous, Pain, Musculoskeletal, Respiratory, Liver Detoxification

  perennial, Zones 4–8

PRETTY MEDICINAL HERB

Betony catches the eye in the garden with its robust mound of oval, scalloped leaves and tall purple flowering spikes that attract winged pollinators. It gets bigger each year, divides easily, and occasionally self-seeds. Be aware that another plant is also called "betony" and "wood betony," *Pedicularis* spp. Totally unrelated, both look somewhat similar and are used for pain, *Pedicularis* being more impressive but also less easily cultivated and only abundant wild in pockets of the country.

ALWAYS THE BRIDESMAID

Betony is a virtual panacea in the garden, yet with so much competition from other herbs that do similar things, it's easily overlooked. It shares many of the benefits of fellow mint-family herbs: digestive aid, calming nervine, focus enhancer, respiratory tonic, and antidepressant. Perhaps it's best known as an antispasmodic anti-inflammatory with an affinity for headaches and muscle tension. It tastes predominantly bitter (and is indeed a mild digestive bitter, page 134) but is not so terrible tasting. Blending it with mint, holy basil, or other tasty herbs will brighten its flavor in tea.

LORE AND HISTORY

This is a plant full of lore, planted and carried for protection against evil, negative spirits, and posttraumatic stress disorder. These uses date back to ancient Greek healers, the medieval saint Hildegard von Bingen, and other precursors of modern herbalists. As a flower essence (page 68) and a medicinal herb, betony helps ground and center energy, ease anxiety, and restore the body.

SAFE FOR MOST PEOPLE

Little modern safety data exists, but betony has a long history in Europe with a reputation for a high degree of safety.

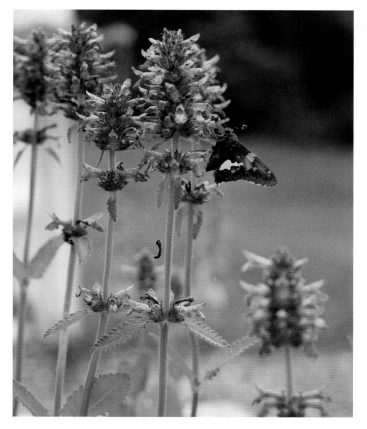

Harvesting, Preparing, and Using Betony

Harvest the leaves anytime; flowers when they're newly open and happy — mixing the two is preferred. Use fresh or dried.

Parts Used: aerial/leaves and flowers

Tea: 1 heaping teaspoon dried herb/cup, infusion, 1–3 cups daily

Tincture: 1–3 ml, 1–3 times daily, solo or in formula
• Fresh 1:2 in 95 percent alcohol (best) or dried 1:5 in 50–60 percent alcohol

Glycerite, Oxymel, Syrup: 1 teaspoon as needed

Recipes: consider adding it to Stress Support Tincture Blend, page 107; Good Mood Tincture, page 119; sleep tinctures, page 131; Bitters Spray, page 141

The Italian phrase "Sell your coat and buy betony" refers to the panacea-like benefits of this beautiful, easy-to-grow herb.

BLACK BIRCH

Betula lenta

Birch Family (Betulaceae)

Body Systems: Musculoskeletal, Pain, Inflammation, Detoxification

   perennial, Zones 3–7

FAST-GROWING TREE

Birches grow quickly in recently logged or cleared land. Black birch and its close relative yellow birch (*B. alleghaniensis*) are unique among the birches for their wintergreeny aroma (scratch and sniff a branch) and pain-relieving properties. Young trees work well; for older trees, you'll need to remove the outer bark. They're easy to forage in their range and can be cultivated. They eventually grow into very large trees. Black birch has attractive dark bark and catkins and is among the first trees whose leaves turn yellow in fall. Older yellow birch has metallic gold, shiny, peeling bark. The two species are nearly indistinguishable when young.

HERBAL ASPIRIN

Sweet black and yellow birch bark contain an aspirin-like methyl salicylate. Unlike bitter salicin (the plant constituent from which aspirin is synthesized), methyl salicylate tastes and smells sweet, wintergreeny. Use it solo or in formula for acute pain of varying types including headaches and muscle aches. Try it internally and/or topically. I prefer to use it alongside other pain herbs with varying mechanisms for the greatest relief and, due to the potential toxicity, I keep the birch dose low (about 5 percent of the formula) for occasional use only. Use wintergreen leaf (*Gaultheria procumbens*) identically.

A TASTY BEVERAGE

Birch beer soda and twig tea both taste quite nice. I take some twigs, break them up into pieces, and shove them into a thermos with white pine or hemlock tree needles — a delicious tea to sip while trekking in the snow! Tap older trees for sap as you would maple. Use the spring leaves of most birch species as a tea for mild detoxification via the kidneys. As a flower essence (page 68), birch helps us be more flexible.

OCCASIONAL USE ONLY

While the birch leaf tea is relatively safe, the methyl salicylate in the birch bark and wintergreen leaves can be liver toxic in high or long-term doses. These essential oils are highly concentrated and potentially toxic (1 drop equals approximately 81 mg of aspirin, and less than a teaspoon can kill a child). Use birch bark and wintergreen remedies cautiously, taking occasional low doses.

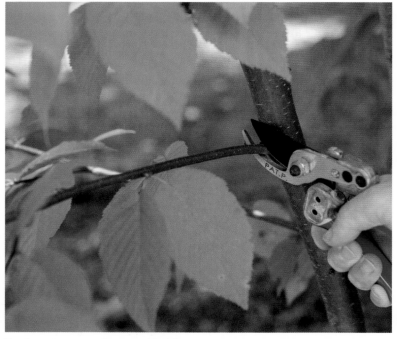

Break a twig or scratch a young black birch branch to release the sweet medicinal wintergreeny aroma.

Harvesting, Preparing, and Using Birch

Harvest young branches with a diameter of up to 1 inch, shaving off the bark and chopping up twigs. Best fresh; serviceable dried. Harvest and dry leaves in spring shortly after they unfurl while still bright green.

Parts Used: bark, twigs, (different uses) leaves

Tea: 1 teaspoon dried herb/cup, infusion, 1–3 cups daily

Tincture or Glycerite: 5–20 drops, as needed
- Fresh bark 1:2 in 95 percent alcohol (best) or dried 1:5 in 50–60 percent alcohol

Topical: oil (alcohol-intermediary), salve, cream, liniment, soak/bath

BLACK COHOSH

Actaea racemosa

Baneberry Family (Actaea)

Body Systems: Endocrine, Reproductive, Inflammation, Mood

   perennial, Zones 3–8

AT-RISK WOODLAND FLOWER

Black cohosh (formerly called *Cimicifuga racemosa*) is easy to grow. Due to overharvesting — it's on the United Plant Savers' "at risk" list — and adulteration issues in commercial preparations, this plant deserves a spot in your garden. Just be patient because you'll need to wait at least 3 years to harvest the roots. This is not a dainty wildflower. Black cohosh is not picky about sunlight or watering, but it does like rich soil and commands both vertical and horizontal space, surpassing 5 feet in height when in bloom and widening each year. Grow it along with fellow woodland wildflowers goldenseal, bloodroot, trillium, Solomon's seal, and wild ginger.

ESTROGEN BALANCE

Black cohosh's reputation as a "women's herb" that offers the estrogen support needed to allay hot flashes and night sweats during perimenopause is well deserved. While no herb works all the time, this one works well for most women. It doesn't work as a phytoestrogen but instead seems to improve brain-ovary hormone communication to regulate estrogen, follicle stimulating hormone (FSH), and luteinizing hormone (LH). It eases uterine tension, contractions, and inflammation, making it useful for shrinking fibroids (70 percent decrease in fibroid size in 3 months, better than medications) and in polycystic ovary syndrome (PCOS; increasing fertility and improving hormone levels), endometriosis, and menstrual cramps. Studies also support its ability to protect bones after menopause and act as an antiproliferative in breast cancer. Hormonal shifts can take at least 3 months to kick in.

LIFT DARK MOODS AND EASE PAIN

Black cohosh lifts the black cloud of depression. Consider it for hormonal mood issues. In combination with St. John's wort, it's been shown to relieve menopausal depression in studies, and it works well for women with PMS depression who get worse with the herb vitex. Black cohosh also reduces systemic inflammation and rheumatism, making it useful in rheumatoid and osteoarthritis. As a flower essence (page 68), black cohosh helps you stand up for yourself, confront abusive relationships, break bad cycles, and lift the dark moods associated with emotionally toxic environments.

ENSURE QUALITY

True black cohosh and the standardized extract Remifemin are safe; however, commercial black cohosh is associated in several cases of liver toxicity around the world — relatively rare considering its widespread use and likely related to intentional adulteration with liver-toxic Chinese species. Due to its complex effects on hormones, I would avoid using it for men, children, during pregnancy, or while nursing unless you're taking it under professional guidance. Even though studies suggest it decreases breast cancer risk, most people avoid it as its estrogenic effects are not well understood.

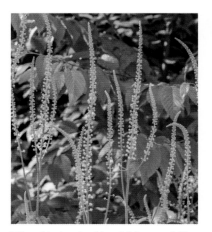

When black cohosh's tall fairy wand-like flowers appear, you might be surprised by their mothball fragrance!

Harvesting, Preparing, and Using Black Cohosh

After 3 to 5 years of growth, use a sharp-pointed shovel and a lot of jumping to lop off one-third of the root crown and/or dig it all up and replant a few leftover rhizomes. Fresh roots have double the strength of dried. Not so tasty — a good candidate for tinctures and capsules. Use low doses.

Parts Used: roots

Tincture: 5–20 drops, 1–3 times daily, solo or in formula
• Fresh 1:2 in 95 percent alcohol (double-strength) or dried 1:5 in 50–60 percent alcohol

Capsules/Powder: 50–100 mg crude herb daily

Topical: Feel free to add the tincture to liniment-oil rubs and creams for pain

BLUE VERVAIN

Verbena hastata

Verbena Family (Verbenaceae)

Body Systems: Mood, Musculoskeletal, Nervous, Endocrine, Metabolic, Immune, Detoxification

   perennial, Zones 3–7

PRAIRIES AND WATERWAYS

This wildflower adapts well in the garden, the clusters of electric purple-blue flowers catch your eye throughout its bloom cycle. It prefers slightly moist spots and rich soil. Water regularly in dry, sunny spots or the stress can welcome pests and disease. When happy, it reaches 5 feet high and self-seeds readily.

TENSION RELEASE

Early American herb doctors relied on this New World native regularly for a wide range of conditions.

Eventually it was forgotten and is now experiencing a resurgence of appreciation, particularly for its ability to quickly release both emotional and physical tension. Matthew Wood talks about it for type A control freak, workaholic list-makers who get a stiff neck and headaches easily, and I can attest to this both personally and clinically. The bitter flavor helps ground people with "wind" or "vata" energetic patterns, who exhibit tension and quivering and are prone to extremes and ever-changing symptoms including emotional lability. Blue vervain helps create balance. As a flower essence (page 68), blue vervain also helps release emotional and physical tension.

METABOLIC, LIVER, IMMUNE

If you read about blue vervain in herbals, you might wonder if everyone's talking about the same plant — its uses vary so widely! Blue vervain is a bitter liver and digestive tonic, eases metabolic wobbles (i.e., emotional lability associated with being "hangry" or having low blood sugar), and helps support the immune system during oncoming or acute infections, primarily as a fever-thwarting diaphoretic. This makes it useful in a variety of formulas for mood issues and chronic infections like Lyme disease and Epstein-Barr virus, as well as for maintaining blood sugar stability, providing endocrine support via liver and mood activity, and alleviating PMS, sugar cravings, and sluggish digestion. According to Michael Moore, other *Verbena* and *Glandularia* species can be used relatively interchangeably — some of which are quite showy and thrive in hot, arid climates.

SAFE BUT BITTER

Blue vervain is safe for most people, including children; however, it's incredibly bitter, which makes it unpalatable in tea and nauseating in large doses. Often, just a few drops of the tincture will work its magic. If you want larger doses and are prone to low blood sugar, take it with food.

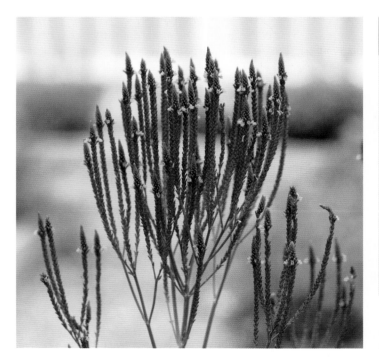

Harvesting, Preparing, and Using Blue Vervain

Harvest the top one-third to two-thirds of blue vervain when it's in bloom and happy. Use fresh or dried. It blends well with a range of herbs depending on what you're using it for. Other forms can be used if you don't mind its bitterness.

Parts Used: aerial parts, preferably in flower

Tincture: 3–60 drops (2 ml), 1–3 times daily, as needed, solo or in formula
• Fresh 1:2 in 95 percent alcohol or dried 1:5 in 50–60 percent alcohol

Recipes: Flower Essences for Pain, page 221

Blue vervain's erect growth pattern reminds us of the tense type A person it helps the most.

BURDOCK

Arctium lappa

Daisy Family (Asteraceae)

Body Systems: Lymph, Liver, Detoxification, Nutritive, Digestion, Gut, Colon

   biennial, Zones 3–7

BIG LEAVES, SWEET ROOT

Even if you're not familiar with burdock, you've likely pulled its round, hooked seed heads (literally the inspiration for Velcro) from your clothes. This biennial produces large leaves, sometimes confused with rhubarb. In the second year, it puts forth tall flowering stalks with purple flowers that look like those of the thistle plant (yet the burdock plant itself isn't prickly like a thistle). It prefers moist, rich soil in full sun or partial shade, often on the edge of a forest, meadow, woodland path, or field. The interchangeable *A. minus* looks similar, just smaller.

LIVER AND LYMPH TONIC

Burdock makes friends with other weedy, bitter root medicines like dandelion, yellow dock, and chicory. It has similar benefits for the liver, mildly improving detoxification as well as digestion and elimination. Burdock tastes milder, slightly sweet, though. It's one of our safest, gentlest, yet still quite effective bitter detoxifying herbs for a wide range of people. Burdock also supports lymph detoxification and, to a lesser extent, kidney detoxification, which makes it a really nice well-rounded alterative for whole body detoxification support. It is particularly useful in skin issues and as a supportive remedy for allergies. Seeds have somewhat similar properties but are too tedious to harvest and process. As a flower essence (page 68), burdock helps cleanse the body to clear the consciousness.

SPECIAL INULIN FIBER

Burdock contains ample amounts of inulin, common in daisy-family roots. This complex fiber helps feed beneficial bacteria to boost the microbiome. Burdock also offers sodium-leaching diuretic properties, which may help manage hypertension (though hypertension can be difficult to address solely with herbs, and it's deadly if left uncontrolled).

SAFE FOR MOST PEOPLE

Of all the bitter, detox herbs, burdock tends to be the most well tolerated by the broadest range of people. That said, inulin falls into the category of a "FODMAP," a group of plants with complex starches that ferment in the guts of people with small intestinal bacterial overgrowth (SIBO) and certain forms of dysbiosis — for them, inulin may cause horrendous gas, pain, bloating, diarrhea, and worsening of symptoms. If this is you, get your gut in gear before reintroducing burdock.

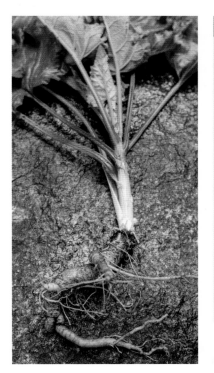

Harvesting, Preparing, and Using Burdock

Dig up roots (not easy!) in fall of the first year or spring of the second. That is, *before* the plant puts up a flower stalk. Use fresh or dried. Tastes pleasant.

Parts Used: roots

Tea: 1 heaping teaspoon dried herb/cup, decoction, 1–3 cups daily

Tincture: 1–5 ml, 1–3 times daily, solo or in formula
• Fresh 1:2 in 95 percent alcohol or dried 1:5 in 50–60 percent alcohol

Syrup, Vinegar, Oxymel, Glycerite: 1 teaspoon or more as needed

Capsules/Powder: 500–2,000 mg (about ½ teaspoon) crude herb daily

Food: Peel and slice the fresh root to sauté, add to soup, broth, or ferment with veggies

Recipes: with Chai Base, page 78; Nutri-Broth, page 80; Multimineral Vinegar, page 86; Mineral-Rich "Coffee" Syrup, page 87; Bitters Spray, page 141; Gut-Healing Broth, page 153; Bitter Brew Coffee Substitute, page 158

Fresh, cultivated burdock is available in natural food stores with other weird roots and sold as "gobo" in Asian markets. Wild roots will be stronger but a bugger to dig up.

CALENDULA

Calendula officinalis

Daisy Family (Asteraceae)

Body Systems: Skin, Lymph, Detoxification, Gut, Antimicrobial, Inflammation

  annual (may self-seed)

ORNAMENTAL MEDICINAL

Calendula is among our most eye-catching commonly cultivated medicinal herbs. The blooms begin to appear in midsummer and run through late autumn, winding down after the first frost. Good soil is key for robust calendula, full sun and periodic watering with good drainage helps. I put tomato cages around my calendula because it tends to flop and take over a garden plot. Regularly harvest and deadhead the flowers to keep the plant producing. Self-seeding can be haphazard. Sow new seeds in fall or early spring, or transplant plugs. Take care to water and prevent young plants from drying up on hot days.

CAROTENOIDS, VULNERARY

Calendula's two big claims to fame are its nutrition content — the flowers boast one hundred times the carotenoids of a sweet potato by weight — and its ability to soothe and heal inflamed, irritated tissue. Calendula preparations are equally useful when applied topically on itchy, rashy skin conditions (think: eczema, allergic reactions, diaper rash, and other forms of dermatitis as well as hemorrhoids and dry skin) and when taken internally to heal the gut lining. It has mild antimicrobial properties as well. For color and nutrition, add the petals to simmering broth (hence its moniker "pot marigold") and sprinkle them into food — the flavor is quite bland and inoffensive in small quantities.

LYMPH, KINDNESS

Calendula improves lymphatic detoxification, making it a worthy component in general detox blends and for general immune support during and post infection to clear "battle debris." As a flower essence (page 68), calendula helps you be more compassionate in your communication so that you can choose kind, wise words rather than coming off as abrupt or sharp and hurting others' feelings.

FLOWER FOOD

Calendula is generally quite safe in modest to large quantities as a functional food and medicine. Occasionally people with daisy-family flower allergies react to calendula, especially if you use the whole flower head rather than the petals only.

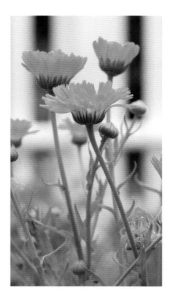

These gorgeous blooms brighten up your garden for months. Look for varieties like Alpha, Resina, and Erfurter Orangefarbige for vibrant color and potency. Farmers feed it to chickens and cows to enrich the eggs and milk with carotenoids.

Harvesting, Preparing, and Using Calendula

Pinch or snip off the entire flower head (including the green bits, called the involucre). Use fresh or dried. For food applications, pull off and use the petals. Dry in the dehydrator and ensure the middles are thoroughly dried before storing or they'll rot and mold in the jar. The flower middle and involucre taste bitter and have an unpleasant texture in food, but they offer more potent medicinal properties.

Parts Used: flower heads, petals

Tea: ¼–1 teaspoon dried herb/cup, infusion, 1–3 cups daily, or sprinkled in tea blends

Tincture: 1–3 ml, 1–3 times daily, solo or in formula
• Fresh 1:2 in 95 percent alcohol (best) or dried 1:5 in 50–60 percent alcohol

Food: Toss fresh or dried petals in soup broth, eggs, baked goods, salads, and anywhere a splash of color would be welcome

Topical: oil (preferably alcohol-intermediary plus heat), salve, cream, bath, soak, spray, liniment

Recipes: Nutri-Tea, page 79; Nutri-Broth, page 80; Infused Seltzer, Soda, and Water, page 97; Gut-Healing Tummy Tea, Take Two, page 152; Gut Healing Broth, page 153; Nettle-Peppermint-Marshmallow Tea, page 183; Calendula Oil, page 192; Calendula-Comfrey Cream, page 193; Super Skin Salve, page 198

CALIFORNIA POPPY

Eschscholzia californica

Poppy Family (Papaveraceae)

Body Systems: Nerve, Mood/Sleep, Pain, Respiratory

  annual

A LOW-FUSS BEAUTY

As you might assume, a plant that grows freely across California and the Southwest does not need to be pampered in the garden, but it does prefer warm, sunny spots without too much competition from other plants. In my Zone 4 to 5, it does best in front of the fence and near warm brick paths. Direct sow seeds in late fall (best) or early spring, or plant young plugs — it does not like being moved. Mexican poppy (*Eschscholzia californica* ssp. *mexicana*) is interchangeable.

SLEEP AND PAIN

California poppy offers nonaddictive, mild, yet effective opioid-like constituents that help relieve insomnia and pain by calming nerves. As an insomnia remedy, it promotes healthy sleep cycles and eases the swirl of thoughts that keep some people awake. Also consider when pain is a factor in insomnia. It works well for a range of types of pain and can be formulated with other herbs with different constituents for broad-spectrum pain relief. California poppy contains alkaloids that relax, sedate, and ease pain, somewhat like opioids though California poppy does not actually contain true opioids. It's nowhere near as strong as other poppy-family pain relievers like opium poppy (which is highly addictive and illegal to process for medicine), prickly poppy, and corydalis.

BANISH BRATS

For mood, it helps quell bratty behavior in children and adults. Its relaxing effects also act on the respiratory system where it can be profoundly effective for coughs, especially serious coughs that don't respond to the usual cough remedies. As a flower essence (page 68), California poppy helps ground people in their spiritual awareness and connection, reducing their attraction to flashy cultlike mentalities or escapism.

SAFE FOR CHILDREN

California poppy is one of our safest poppies and is not addictive. Nonetheless, to err on the side of caution, I would avoid it if someone already has a history of opioid, painkiller, or heroin addiction. It may or may not show a false positive on drug tests. As with any sedative or sleep herb, start with low doses and work up, especially if you're using it during the day, to determine your individual response to the herb. It may cause increased sedation if combined with sedative, mood, or painkilling medications. Once again, start low to gauge your response.

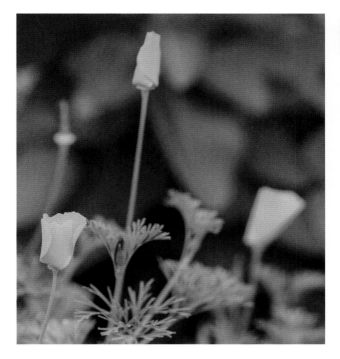

Harvesting, Preparing, and Using California Poppy

Harvest the whole plant including the translucent orange roots (the strongest part) while it is simultaneously in flower and seed. Best fresh and tinctured (especially in blends), but you can play around with other formats.

Parts Used: whole plant in flower and seeds

Tincture: 1–5 ml, before bed or 1–3 times daily, solo or in formula
• Fresh 1:2 in 95 percent alcohol

Recipes: Sleep Tinctures, page 131

California's state flower follows the sun throughout the day, opening and closing as it rises and sets, helping us to reset our own sleep cycles.

CATNIP

Nepeta cataria

Mint Family (Lamiaceae)

Body Systems: Digestive, Immune, Skin, Nervous, Mood

   perennial, Zones 3–7

LOOK WHAT THE CAT DRAGGED IN

True to its reputation, catnip may attract the unwanted attention of your cats, who could easily destroy your plant in a day. However, catnip plants grown from seed *tend* to be less tempting to felines than transplants. This herbaceous medicinal likes good soil but can be persnickety about where it's grown. It may die off yet also self-seed, then thrive and take over in its new spot. If happy, it could get weedy but is not difficult to remove. Children and adults will enjoy "petting" catnip — it's soft, though it smells a bit skunky. Note that its relatives, including cat*mint* (another *Nepeta* species), don't necessarily have the same medicinal properties.

CHAMOMILE STAND-IN

In humans, catnip is best known as a remedy for children and particularly as a mild bitter, carminative herb that improves digestive juices and function while easing colic, flatulence, bloating, and intestinal cramps and pain. For this use, it works similarly to chamomile yet it's easier to harvest in abundance and is better tolerated by a wide variety of people (those who are allergic to chamomile's daisy-family flowers). For digestion, you can use it as a tea, tincture, cordial, or glycerite. As with other herbs with skunky scents like valerian and cramp bark, catnip helps relax muscles and calm the nervous system.

FEVERS AND BUGS

Catnip also offers a shimmer of its cousin peppermint's properties. Like peppermint, catnip acts as a diaphoretic, encouraging a healthy fever response to help fight and resolve infections more quickly (another popular use for children) — use it as a hot tea with fellow pleasant-tasting diaphoretics peppermint, elderflower, and/or ginger. As a topical herb, catnip essential oil — and, to a lesser extent, crude plant preparations — repel insects.

A POPULAR CHILDREN'S HERB

Considered highly safe, catnip is a popular children's herb, though it also works for adults. To dose for a child, divide the adult dose by weight. So, assuming an adult dose for 150 pounds, a 50-pound child would get one-third the adult dose, and a 25-pound child would get one-sixth the adult dose. Do not use during pregnancy due to its emmenagogue effect. High doses may cause nausea and vomiting.

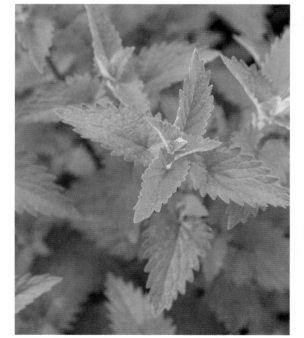

Harvesting, Preparing, and Using Catnip

Harvest any time of year — it has a long season. Use fresh or dried. Blends well with better-tasting mint-family herbs.

Parts Used: aerial parts, mainly leaves

Tea: 1 teaspoon dried herb/cup, infusion, 1–3 cups daily

Tincture: 10–60 drops (2 ml), 1–3 times daily, solo or in formula
• Fresh 1:2 in 95 percent alcohol (best) or dried 1:5 in 50–60 percent alcohol

Glycerite, syrup, oxymel: ½–1 teaspoon

Recipes: Lemon Balm–Catnip Glycerite, page 140; Chamomile-Mint Tea, page 147; Herbal Insect Repellent, page 204

Catnip may attract neighborhood cats and get them high, but it relaxes rather than stimulates people.

CAYENNE

Capsicum annuum

Nightshade Family (Solanaceae)

Body Systems: Pain, Nerve, Cardiovascular, Immune, Respiratory

  annual

FIERCE FRUITS FROM HOT CLIMATES

Cayenne, habaneros, and other hot peppers were among the first New World plants that explorers who came to the Americas introduced to Europe and other parts of the world, where they quickly became important elements of many culinary and medicinal traditions. In cold climates, start plants indoors and stick to small peppers that ripen quickly. Hot, dry conditions intensify their heat: dark or terra-cotta pots, minimal irrigation, or placement next to stone steps or a wall that radiates heat in full sun. Heat level depends on the plant's genetics as well as growing conditions. Harvest or bring peppers indoors before frost. Any hot pepper species can be used interchangeably.

HOT, HOT, HOT

Energetically, this plant is HOT. Use *small* amounts to synergize a blend. In a lab study, 1 part cayenne combined with 25 parts green tea had one hundred times the cancer-killing ability of either ingredient individually. It boosts circulation and digestion, which helps move other plants in a formula into the body. Cayenne acts as a heart tonic, thins and moves the blood (yet stops bleeding and heals wounds as a poultice), and decreases inflammation. Early American herbalists Samuel Thompson and Dr. John Christopher popularized cayenne to avert heart attacks (see cautions) and bring back spark and vitality. People who eat hot peppers and spicier food generally live longer with less heart disease. Eating large amounts of cayenne (⅓ ounce — again, see cautions) with meals may improve weight loss by boosting metabolism and thermogenesis while reducing appetite.

YOUR NERVES ON CAYENNE

Cayenne's hot constituent capsaicin topically relieves pain and nerve irritation. Capsaicin depletes substance P, a neurotransmitter that sends pain signals to the brain, which dampens the pain response. Apply regularly for arthritis, injury, and herpes zoster (shingles) infection pain relief. As a flower essence (page 68), it ignites your spark and life force — without burning your tongue.

CAUTIONS

This is a potent plant. Even a single drop of tincture diluted in a glass of water can be *incredibly* hot. Evidence suggests that cayenne could cure ulcers *or* increase ulcer pain, reflux, and gastric irritation — listen to your body. In a handful of case reports, cayenne *induced* heart attacks in otherwise healthy men taking large doses. If you use cayenne, start with a small amount and taste it as you take it. Use caution combining it with medications and toxic botanicals due to the potential for synergistic effects. When working with cayenne, use gloves and be mindful to not touch your eyes, or other sensitive spots. Topicals could burn the skin. The antidote: cold, fatty liquids like whole milk work best (not water, *especially* not hot water).

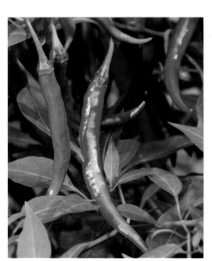

The hotter the pepper, the stronger its medicinal activity.

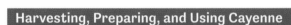

Harvesting, Preparing, and Using Cayenne

Harvest mid- or late summer when the fruits are ripe and hot. To mellow heat, remove seeds and membrane. Use fresh or dried.

Parts Used: whole pepper, seeds

Tea: 1 pinch, or to comfort level, preferably in blends

Tincture: 1 drop or less, or to comfort level, diluted
• Fresh 1:2 in 95 percent alcohol or dried 1:5 in 50–60 percent alcohol

Powder: 1 pinch, or to comfort level

Food: Enjoy liberally to taste in all manner of foods

Topical: oil (any method), salve, cream, liniment, powder poultice

Recipes: Quick Dill Pickles, page 147; Fire Cider, page 236; Fire Cider–Maple-Mustard Dressing, page 237; Thai Curry Fire Cider, page 237; Thai Curry Paste, page 237

CHAMOMILE

Matricaria chamomilla

Daisy Family (Asteraceae)

Body Systems: Digestion, Gut, Skin, Antimicrobial, Inflammation, Nervous, Mood

 annual (may self-seed)

ADORED WORLDWIDE

You'll find German chamomile tea on the shelf in almost every country in the world. Although many different types of chamomile exist and can be used somewhat interchangeably — including the perennial Roman chamomile (*Chamaemelum nobile,* formerly *Anthemis nobilis*) and petalless pineapple weed (*Matricaria discoidea*) — German remains the most popular. German chamomile has gone through several Latin name changes, including *Matricaria recutita* and *Chamomilla recutita*. Direct sow seeds or plugs in well-drained soil and harvest or deadhead regularly to keep it producing more flowers. Allow some seeds to self-sow for the next year.

CALM COLIC, BABIES

Chamomile gently calms the nerves; improves digestive juices; functions as a mild bitter and carminative; decreases gastric inflammation; eases spasms, pain, gas, and colic; and discourages pathogenic gut bacteria. These properties make it a superb, well-rounded herb for digestion and the gastrointestinal tract for both babies and adults. Its calming effects also quell anxiety, teething pain, insomnia, and fussy behavior. In fact, chamomile is specifically indicated not just for babies but also for adults who act like fussy babies. It's also fantastic where emotional tension brings digestive discomfort.

ANTI-INFLAMMATORY

Chamomile's anti-inflammatory and calming effects also help with skin irritation, making it popular in skin care as a toner, bath, or cream. For this, it also offers vulnerary healing and light antiseptic properties. As a flower essence (page 68), chamomile soothes the solar plexus belly area, quelling anxiety and digestive distress.

SAFE FOR MOST PEOPLE

Chamomile has a fantastic safety record for all ages; however, some people with daisy-family allergies may react to chamomile. (For those folks, catnip offers similar nerve-digestive benefits, page 257.)

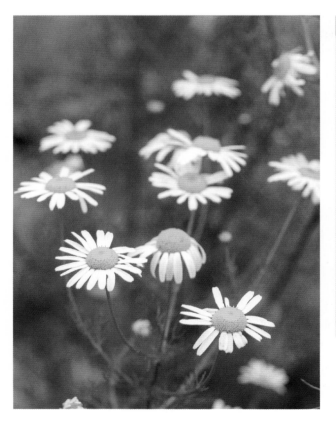

Harvesting, Preparing, and Using Chamomile

Pinch or snip off the flower heads when they're newly open and happy. Get in the mood to enjoy your garden time because it's going to take a while to harvest a decent amount. Use fresh or dried. Blueberry rakes speed the process. Almost always used as a tea.

Parts Used: flower heads

Tea: 1 teaspoon dried herb/cup, infusion, 1–3 cups daily

Tincture or Glycerite: 2–5 ml, 1–3 times daily, solo or in formula
• Fresh 1:2 in 95 percent alcohol or dried 1:5 in 50–60 percent alcohol

Topical: oil (any method), cream, soak, bath, tea spritz/toner, hydrosol

Recipes: Floral Ice Cubes, page 96; Chamomile-Mint Tea, page 147

We harvest only the small flower heads of chamomile, which means you'll need a lot of plants and time to harvest a sufficient amount. That's why good chamomile costs so much.

COMFREY

Symphytum officinale

Borage Family (Boraginaceae)

Body Systems: Skin, Gut, Bones, Inflammation, Pain, Musculoskeletal

  perennial, Zones 4–8

CHOOSE YOUR SPOT WISELY

Comfrey grows readily and rapidly almost anywhere, getting larger each year. It loves rich, semimoist soil. Those roots travel deep, break off easily, and new plants can sprout from remaining root bits — don't even think about rototilling it! So, plan carefully where you want to plant it, because once it's established, it's almost impossible to remove. As its leaves decay, it's a *fantastic* natural fertilizer and garden amendment. Plant it around fruit trees or cultivate a stand to chop and add to leaf mulch, compost piles, and make compost tea fertilizer. Use Russian comfrey (*S. × uplandicum*) similarly.

SOOTHING, SPEEDY HEALER

For wounds and bone breaks, allantoin and other compounds in comfrey rapidly get the body back on the mend and increase connective tissue integrity — sometimes *too* quickly. It can seal infection into deep or infected wounds and may encourage scar tissue as wounds heal (though it helps resolve *old* scars). Don't use it on bone breaks until they're properly set. Internal use remains controversial due to potential toxicity. Short-term, comfrey rapidly heals ulcers and other gastrointestinal lining wounds. Comfrey is soothing, slimy, and mineral-rich, historically used not only for gut healing but also for respiratory irritations, strong bones, and general nutrition, but our current knowledge of its potential toxicity makes it inappropriate for internal use, especially long term.

TOPICAL PAIN RELIEF

Topical comfrey relieves pain from a variety of sources, including sprains, back issues, osteoarthritis, and bruises. As a flower essence (page 68), comfrey provides deep healing on all levels, including the symptomatic (e.g., pain) and organic and functional (e.g., brain injury) levels. In spite its controversy, you'll fall in love with comfrey's subtle beauty and nourishing, soothing, healing vibe.

RARE BUT REAL LIVER RISK

Comfrey contains pyrrolizidine alkaloids (PAs), which have cumulative toxicity and can ultimately cause fatal veno-occlusive liver disease. Several studies confirm this. A handful of PA-related human deaths have occurred with high doses *and* very reasonable whole herb doses. You'll get more PAs in the roots, less in leaves, and the least in older leaves. But the exact amounts vary *widely* plant to plant (regardless of species), as does individual sensitivity to PAs. If you use comfrey internally, stick to low to moderate doses (e.g., ½ teaspoon of older dried leaves in tea) for no more than 1 or 2 weeks. Decoctions and oil infusions extract fewer PAs than infusions and alcohol. Liver toxicity is unlikely with local topical use or flower essence. Also see the previous cautions on using comfrey on wounds.

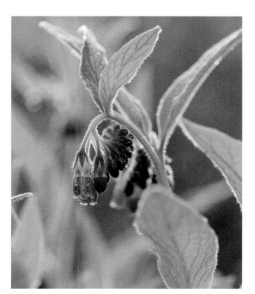

Harvesting, Preparing, and Using Comfrey

Harvest happy leaves anytime in summer, opting for older ones if you plan to use them internally. Dig up roots in spring or fall. Use fresh or dried. Allantoin extracts best in hot water.

Parts Used: leaves, roots

Tea, Tincture, Food: Not generally recommended due to toxicity. Illegal to sell for internal use

Topical: oil (any method, preferably dried leaf), double-extraction liniment (preferably root), salve, cream

Recipes: Calendula-Comfrey Cream, page 193; First Aid Simple: Comfrey Oil, page 199; Aches and Pains, Strains and Sprains Tincture/Liniment, page 220; Flower Essences for Pain, page 221

Comfrey's profound wound- and bone-healing properties come with controversy, but it's a useful garden amendment.

CRAMP BARK

Viburnum opulus

Adoxa Family (Adoxaceae)

Body Systems: Pain, Musculoskeletal, Reproductive

   perennial, Zones 2–7

AN ORNAMENTAL WILDFLOWER SHRUB

Shrubby cramp bark dots riversides across central, northern, and eastern United States and Canada. Yet it does fine without regular watering and will bloom more in the sun. It has garden-worthy attractive white flowers in a saucerlike shape that turn into trans-lucent tart-astringent red berries in the fall. Formerly categorized in the honeysuckle family (Caprifoliaceae), *Viburnum* species grow across an even wider range (except the Southwest) and tend to be used similarly by Native Americans and bioregional herbalists, particularly the closely related high bush cranberry (*V. trilobum*), black haw (*V. prunifolium*). and maple-leafed viburnum (*V. acerifolium*). It's prone to insects and disease, but you can still use it for medicine.

CRAMP BARK FOR . . . CRAMPS

True to its name, cramp bark is one of our most reliable symptomatic herbs for menstrual cramps and may also help alleviate other forms of musculoskeletal and smooth muscle tension, spasms, and pain. It contains skunky, relaxing compounds similar to valerian, but cramp bark shouldn't make you sleepy. It's most effective and fast-acting as a tincture — 2 ml every 15 minutes until the pain subsides — but you can also use it in other forms, including topical compresses or a bath. It really shines for menstrual cramps, though, and is believed to have a uterine decon-gestant property that may also help. Midwives use it to reduce cramping and early labor/miscarriage contrac-tions. It is unlikely to interfere with healthy labor.

TENSION RELEASE

Cramp bark's muscle-relaxing prop-erties may also help with asthma, coughing, gastrointestinal pain, and blood pressure. The cranberry-like berries are consiidered edible by some, mildly toxic and vomit induc-ing by others. No one (including the birds) would call them delicious. As a flower essence (page 68), cramp bark helps you feel better appreciated.

SAFE FOR TEENS AND ADULTS

While generally very safe even in acute large doses, cramp bark con-tains small amounts of aspirin-like compounds, so use caution or avoid it if you are allergic. It may also thin the blood, interact with blood thin-ning medication, and reduce blood pressure.

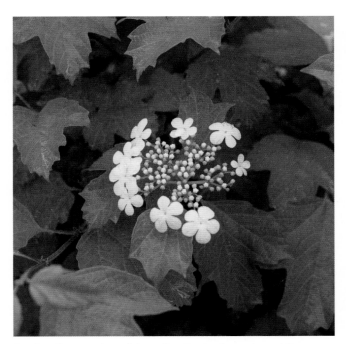

Pruning allows you to sculpt an attractive landscape tree while providing you with medicinal bark.

Harvesting, Preparing, and Using Cramp Bark

Prune branches (preferably in spring or fall), removing bark from larger branches and chopping up smaller twigs. Use fresh or dried. Dried cramp bark and cramp bark tincture lose potency within a year or two.

Parts Used: bark, twigs

Tea: 1 teaspoon dried herb/cup, decoction, 1 cup as needed

Tincture: 2 ml, every 15 minutes as needed
- Fresh 1:2 in 95 percent alcohol or dried 1:5 in 50–60 percent alcohol
- Add 10 percent glycerine to stabilize tannins and improve shelf life

Topical: compress, bath, liniment

Recipes: Cramp Bark Tincture with Glycerine, page 214; Sore Muscle Bath, page 214

DANDELION

Taraxacum officinale

Daisy Family (Asteraceae)

Body Systems: Liver, Kidney/Urinary, Detoxification, Nutritive, Immune

   perennial, Zones 3–9

LAWN WEED EXTRAORDINAIRE

Millions of Americans spray their lawn with toxic chemicals each summer to kill off the hated dandelion, yet herbalists seek it out and even cultivate it on our properties. If you're willing, let it thrive in your lawn and wild spaces of your yard. It prefers the fertile, calcium-rich soil of cow pastures and organic farm fields but will grow (less robustly) in poorer soil.

You can use young leaves and roots of dandelion's close cousin chicory similarly. Scraggly chicory (*Cichorium intybus*), with its pretty blue morning blooms, likes dry, sunny, compacted soil (median strips, abandoned lots) and won't be easy to eradicate if you come to regret planting it. Forage chicory from clean places. For regular leaf crops in the garden, consider planting Italian dandelion, a better-behaved cultivar of chicory with long, dandelion-like leaves. Milder leafy green chicory cultivars, usually grown in the dark, include endive, frisée, escarole, and radicchio.

BITTER NUTRITIOUS DETOX

The leaves and roots abound with minerals and a bitter but not entirely unpleasant flavor. The leaves pair well with strong flavors like garlic, lemon, vinegar, and olive oil. The chocolaty roots taste nice in tea and, when roasted, resemble coffee. Both the leaves and roots encourage detoxification via the liver and kidneys, with the roots favoring the liver and the leaves, the kidneys. The leaves act as a volume diuretic while the roots are subtler, sodium-leaching diuretic. As bitters (page 134), all parts stimulate digestion. Add it to hypoglycemic, skin, and hormone balancing blends for its liver/bitter benefits.

ANTIHISTAMINE DIURETIC

The fresh roots — particularly as a tincture or alcohol slurry added to hot water by the teaspoon — may function as an antihistamine for allergic reactions. Preliminary studies suggest dandelion roots act as a safe chemotherapy agent for cancer. As potassium-rich diuretics, the leaves and roots help manage hypertension. Rich in carotenoids, the flowers taste somewhat sweet and can be used topically for skin care and muscle tension. As a flower essence (page 68), dandelion releases tension to help you find joy. Chicory gives confidence and independence to needy, clingy people and animals.

SAFE FOR MOST PEOPLE

Generally quite safe, but the diuretic effect can be too much for some (the French call it *pissenlit*, or "piss the bed"). Daisy-family allergies are possible but rare. Do not harvest from contaminated soil. Use caution with medications contraindicated with diuretics or potassium.

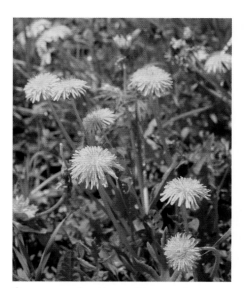

Common weed and bane of those perfect-lawn people, dandelion ranks among herbalists' most beloved plants.

Harvesting, Preparing, and Using Dandelion

Snip the young greens, preferably before it blooms (they get increasingly bitter after that). Dig roots in spring or fall. Use fresh or dried.

Parts Used: leaves, roots, flowers

Tea: 1 teaspoon dried herb/cup, infusion, 1–3 cups daily

Tincture: 1–5 ml, 1–3 times daily, solo or in formula
• Fresh 1:2 in 95 percent alcohol or dried 1:5 in 50–60 percent alcohol

Capsules/Powder: 500–2,000 mg crude herb daily

Food: Fresh and cooked leaves, pesto, flower petals for color

Topical: flower oil, salve, cream

Recipes: with Chai Base, Page 78; Multimineral Vinegar, page 86; Mineral-Rich "Coffee" Syrup, page 87; Dandelion-Violet Weed Pesto, page 88; Bitters Spray, page 141; Bitter Brew Coffee Substitute, page 158

DILL

Anethum graveolens

Parsley Family (Apiaceae)

Body Systems: Digestive

  annual, Zones 2–11

BUTTERFLY FOOD

This culinary staple has ferny foliage and gets tall quickly, producing yellow flowers that go to seed then die. Dill is one of the *easiest* herbs to direct sow from seed, preferring a sunny garden bed with moderate moisture. Remove mulch, rough up the soil, sprinkle the seeds, then gently rake them in and tamp the soil down. Wait until the seedlings are well established as young plants to mulch around them. If you see a brightly colored "monarch" caterpillar munching on your dill (or parsley, fennel, carrot) leaves, it's actually the swallowtail. They can do some serious munching! Let them be or cut the branch it's chewing and bring the caterpillar over to some Queen Anne's lace, golden alexander, or other abundant parsley-family food alternative.

DIGESTIVE CARMINATIVE

As with most parsley-family culinary herbs (particularly seeds), dill is a fantastic, safe carminative herb that improves digestive function while also easing gas, bloating, and intestinal spasms. Dill and its close relative fennel favor sensitive stomachs in particular, which is why we pair dill (and pickles) with rich, fatty and protein-dense foods like egg salad, tuna salad, potato chips, burgers, and meaty sandwiches. It provides flavor contrast and helps you better digest your meal. Use other parsley-family culinary seeds the same way, choosing your favorite flavor — dill, fennel (page 267), anise, cumin, caraway, lovage, angelica, coriander . . .

ANTINAUSEA

Among the culinary seeds, dill or fennel tend to best settle the stomach and ease nausea — a reason for those pregnancy cravings! Small amounts of dill weed (mild) or seed (stronger) in food lend an herbaceous, tangy, salty flavor. I make my own ranch dip mix to stir into yogurt for veggies. Grind together 12 parts dry buttermilk powder, 3 parts parsley, 2 parts garlic powder, 2 parts onion powder, 1 part dried dill weed, 1 part dried minced onion, ¾ part salt, ¼ part black pepper. Then stir 1 tablespoon into 1 cup of Greek yogurt or sour cream. As a flower essence (page 68), dill calms the solar plexus (the part of the stomach just below the ribs) and eases agitation from sensory overload.

SAFE FOR MOST PEOPLE

Dill is quite safe, even for babies, in the modest doses in which it's typically used. In larger doses, dill can be diuretic, another feature common to the parsley family.

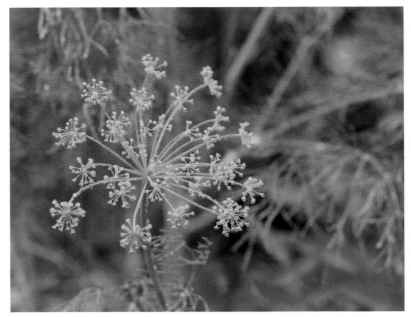

Plant dill and fennel in different areas of the garden. They can interbreed and self-seed new plants that taste like a blend of fennel and dill.

Harvesting, Preparing, and Using Dill

Snip off fresh greens as you need them. Harvest seed heads as the plant is dying back but before it turns completely brown. Use fresh or dried.

Parts Used: aerial parts, seeds (strongest)

Tincture: 10–30 drops, 1–3 times daily as needed
- Fresh 1:2 in 95 percent alcohol or dried 1:5 in 50–60 percent alcohol

Food: nibble, add to all manner of foods, pickles, pickle juice

Recipes: Quick Dill Pickles, page 147, Ranch Dip Mix, above

ECHINACEA

Echinacea spp.

Daisy Family (Asteraceae)

Body Systems: Immune, Lymph, Detoxification, Skin, Respiratory, Antimicrobial

  perennial, Zones 3–9

SHOWY MEDICINAL WILDFLOWER

Echinacea radiates with beauty when its pink-purple flowers are in bloom, catching the eye of people and pollinators. Although the wild, overharvested *E. angustifolia* root may be more potent, the more robust-looking *E. purpurea* can be used similarly and takes much better to cultivation. Popular for landscaping, it likes nice soil and full sun but does not need regular watering. Considered a very easy plant to grow for almost anyone, this one challenges me personally: my subterranean rodent population likes to eat the roots. If you decide to try *E. angustifolia*, place it in poorer, somewhat dry soil.

IMMUNE AND LYMPH STIMULANT

Echinacea has a range of uses related to fighting infections and improving lymph detoxification. Take high doses regularly at the first sign of infection to thwart a cold or flu (better combined with ginger) and to help manage bacterial infections and prevent sepsis. Many different compounds and actions aid infection response. Echinacea boosts white blood cells and macrophage activity, clears "battle debris" via the lymph, and inhibits the enzyme hyaluronidase that some pathogens (and venom) use to break into and infect cells.

ANTIMICROBIAL ALTERATIVE

Echinacea acts as an alterative lymph mover, historically used as a "blood cleanser" for skin conditions, sepsis, and general detoxification. Its numbing, antimicrobial activity makes it useful on wounds, bites, and sore throats. As a flower essence (page 68), echinacea helps with fundamental healing and the restoration of vital force, particularly after illness, abuse, or trauma.

USUALLY SAFE

Echinacea (unnervingly, but harmlessly) numbs the tongue and increases salivation. While generally safe for children and adults, people with daisy-family flower allergies may react to it, particularly if using the flowers. As an immune stimulant, it *occasionally* triggers autoimmune disease flare-ups.

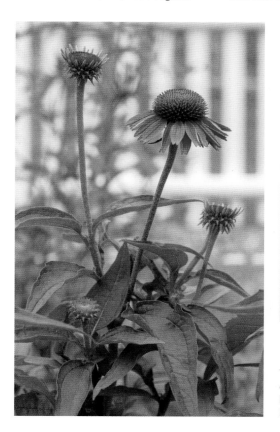

Harvesting, Preparing, and Using Echinacea

Harvest roots in fall of the third or fourth year. Leave some broken taproots or a section of the root crown in place for future growth. Harvest aerial parts when the plant is in flower. Fresh works best. Feel free to combine root and aerial preparations.

Parts Used: root (strongest), aerial parts in flower

Tea: 1 teaspoon dried herb/cup, infusion, 1–3 cups daily or more.

Tincture: 3–5 ml, frequently (6–12 times/day) at the onset of illness
• Fresh 1:2 in 95 percent alcohol (or substitute glycerite or vinegar)

Capsules/Powder: 500–1,000 mg crude herb 6–12 times/day at onset

Topical: liniment

Recipes: Echinacea Tincture, page 169

The original "snake oil salesman," Dr. Meyer, demonstrated echinacea's potency by getting bit by venomous snakes onstage, then curing himself with the herb.

ELDER

Sambucus nigra

Adoxa Family (Adoxaceae)

Body Systems: Immune, Respiratory, Antiviral, Musculoskeletal

   perennial, Zones 3–9

ROBUST FLOWERING SHRUB

In the wild, this robust shrub thrives in damp, rich soil along drainage ditches and waterways, preferring the edge between open and wooded areas, yet it's content in a garden landscape with less moisture. It may take a few years to begin producing flowers and fruit, which will be more prolific in full sun. The huge flat-topped clusters of white flowers in early summer will help you find the shrub in the wild. Berries ripen in late summer or early fall. Act quickly — the birds swoop in to gobble them up, and ripe berries also fall easily off the stem. Wild American black (*S. canadensis*) and blue (*S. cerulea*) elder are now considered subspecies of European black elder (*S. nigra*) and used interchangeably, but avoid the toxic red elder (*S. racemosa*).

TOP ANTIVIRAL MEDICINE

Elderberries stop oncoming viral infections in their tracks by blocking viruses out of cells, limiting their ability to replicate, spread, and damage the body. Elder also activates the immune system for swift action against germs. Take the berries when you know you're likely to be exposed to more germs (traveling, parties, when you're run down or around others who are sick) or at the first sign of infection (tickle of a sore throat, achy flu feeling, exhaustion). Hot elderflower tea encourages a healthy fever response to more quickly resolve infections and break the fever, and flower extracts also ease allergies with mild anti-inflammatory, antihistamine action.

TOPICAL ARNICA SUBSTITUTE

Topically, elder leaves — which are toxic internally — can be applied and used like arnica for bumps and bruises. As a flower essence (page 68), elder brings renewal, joy, and revitalization.

SAFE WHEN PROPERLY PREPARED

Elderflowers and elderberries are extremely safe — even for children — when cooked or dried, preferably in formulas where the berry's seeds are strained (tea, syrups). Fresh elder and its seeds can be *horribly* nauseating and may also contain small amounts of potentially toxic cyanide-like compounds. Avoid internal use of the leaves and stems as well as all parts of red elder, which are even more nauseating and toxic.

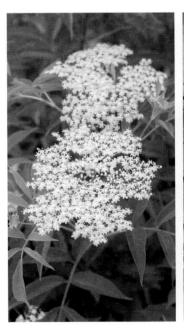 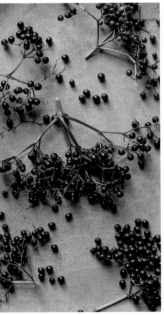

Not just a mythical wand in *Harry Potter and the Deathly Hallows*, this shrub has been shrouded in lore for centuries, associated with fairies, protection, birth, death, and the spirit realm.

Harvesting, Preparing, and Using Elder

Clip off clusters of freshly opened flowers or ripe berries, which you can remove later with a fork. It's okay if a *few* tiny stems remain. Use dried (my preference) or cooked only — not fresh.

Parts Used: berries, flowers

Tea: 1 teaspoon dried herb/cup, infusion, 1–3 cups daily

Tincture: 1–3 ml daily or every few hours in an acute infection
• Dried 1:5 in 50–60 percent alcohol

Syrup, Glycerite, Oxymel: ½–1 teaspoon daily or every few hours in an acute infection

Food: jam, cordial

Topical: leaf oil, ointment, salve, compress

Recipes: Darcey Blue's Elderberry Syrup, page 168; Elder–Rose Hip Oxymel (and tea variation), page 169

ELECAMPANE

Inula helenium

Daisy Family (Asteraceae)

Body Systems: Respiratory, Immune, Digestive, Antimicrobial

   perennial, Zones 4–9

WOODLAND SUNFLOWER

Elecampane is among the many wild sunflower relatives, but it has the distinction of producing unique aromatic medicinal roots. In the first year, the scrappy rosette with its large, flat leaves could easily be mistaken for a docklike weed. It looks *completely* different in its blooming years, reaching 4 to 7 feet tall with robust leaves and branching stalks of yellow blossoms. It prefers damp, rich loamy soil yet tolerates garden beds without irrigation.

WARMING, LUNG OPENER

Elecampane has a potent, complex flavor with bitter, aromatic/perfumey, balsam, and pungent notes. In the respiratory system, it moves mucus, warms and opens the lungs, and fights infections, particularly in cold, stagnant, congested states. Perfect for cough syrup.

BITTER, ANTIMICROBIAL

Although best known as a lung herb, elecampane also makes a superb digestive bitter, stimulating digestion while fighting chronic dysbiosis and intestinal infections. It has a unique reputation as a warming bitter (most bitters, like artichoke leaf, are considered energetically cold). It also contains inulin, a starch that feeds beneficial bacteria. Elecampane can be added to animal feed as an antimicrobial and deworming agent. As a flower essence (page 68), elecampane helps facilitate the transition into spiritual growth spurts.

SAFE YET POTENT

This is not a plant for high doses, which may cause nausea, yet it is quite safe in low to moderate amounts. People with gastric irritation or who are already hot and dry may not be a good fit for elecampane unless it is formulated with cool, moist herbs like mullein or marshmallow.

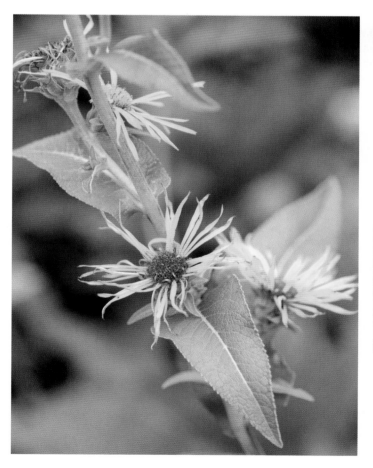

Harvesting, Preparing, and Using Elecampane

Harvest roots in its second or third year in spring or fall with a garden fork. Use fresh or dried.

Parts Used: roots

Tea: 1 teaspoon dried herb/cup, infusion, 1–3 cups daily

Tincture: 1–3 ml, 1–3 times daily, solo or in formula
- Fresh 1:2 in 95 percent alcohol or dried 1:5 in 50–60 percent alcohol

Syrup, Glycerine, Oxymel, Vinegar: ½–1 teaspoon as needed

Recipes: Bitters Spray, page 141; Darcey Blue's Elderberry Syrup, page 168. Also try it in cough syrup

This tall sunflower relative produces potent large bitter, pungent, balsam-y roots relatively quickly. In its first year, the basal rosette looks like a weed.

FENNEL

Foeniculum vulgare

Parsley Family (Apiaceae)

Body Systems: Digestion, Gut, Respiratory

  perennial, Zones 4–9

GO FOR THE BRONZE

All types of fennel can be uses similarly. Bronze fennel (*F. vulgare* var. *purpureum*) offers a sweeter Good & Plenty candy flavor and fun color, but no bulb. Plant this someplace in your garden bed where it won't have too much competition and where it will thrive and provide color and texture. It can reach several feet tall when it blooms. When I lived in Bisbee, Arizona, during herb school, huge stands of wild fennel grew throughout the town, wafting a sweet aroma through the air at night.

CARMINATIVE DIGESTIF

All parts stimulate healthy digestive function and ease spasms, cramps, bloating, and gas, but the seeds have the strongest antispasmodic activity. Fennel shares similar properties with parsley-family culinary herbs, including anise, dill, chervil, coriander, cumin, lovage, and angelica. All these carminatives balance digestive bitters in a formula, improve the flavor, and provide complementary actions for digestive function and upsets. In acute episodes of flatulence and intestinal cramps, fennel seeds are my go-to, useful for colicky babies and adults.

SOOTHING AND DELICIOUS

Fennel has an affinity for the lungs and is perfect for soothing and easing spasms and flavoring and enhancing a formula for coughs and respiratory irritation. And, of course, fennel is delicious in food and drink — whether you stuff the fronds into fish or snip them into salads; mix fennel into a salad dressing for beets or into goat cheese; use it to flavor teas; infuse the seeds into seltzer, soda, or a Sambuca-like cordial; or add them to Italian stews, meat sauces, sausage, and meatballs. Bronze fennel fronds make beautiful colors — light purple seltzer, violet glycerite, and magenta-red vinegar. As a flower essence (page 68), fennel helps you become more decisive and focused, including in group work.

SAFE FOR MOST PEOPLE

Very safe for all ages in low to moderate doses — whether you add fennel to food, chew on a few seeds, or brew a cup of fennel tea. Large therapeutic doses of the seeds may not be appropriate for infants or during pregnancy or nursing; it contains mild phytoestrogens.

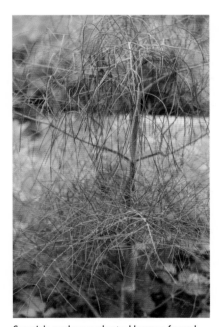

Spanish explorers planted bronze fennel along the King's Highway, also known as El Camino Real, in California, where it now grows as a weed.

Harvesting, Preparing, and Using Fennel

Trim fronds and dig bulbs to use fresh when they're lush. Gather green, plump seed heads to use fresh or dry.

Parts Used: seeds (strongest), fronds, bulb

Tea: ½–1 teaspoon dried herb/cup, infusion, 1–3 cups daily

Tincture: 5–30 drops (1 ml), 1–3 times daily, solo or in formula
• Fresh 1:2 in 95 percent alcohol or dried 1:5 in 50–60 percent alcohol

Glycerite, Vinegar, Oxymel, Honey, Syrup: 1 teaspoon as needed

Cordial: 1 ounce sipped as a medicinal treat

Seeds: Nibble a few fresh or dried, as needed

Food: Crush or grind seeds to add to recipes. Use fronds and bulb in seltzer, soda, infused water (see culinary tips above)

Recipes: Floral Ice Cubes, page 96; Infused Seltzer, Soda, and Water, page 97; Bitters Spray, page 141; Fennel and Korean Mint Seltzer, page 146; Sweet Fennel Liquor, page 146; Bronze Fennel Vinegar, page 146; Fennel Seed Chews, page 146; Gut-Healing Tummy Tea, Take One, page 152; Soothing Lung Tea, page 176; Allergy Tincture Blend, page 182; Lady Tea, page 243

GARLIC

Allium sativum

Amaryllis Family (Amaryllidaceae)

Body Systems: Immune, Respiratory, Cardiovascular, Skin, Digestive, Antimicrobial, Metabolic

  perennial, Zones 4–9

FEED YOUR MEDICINE

Garlic's a heavy feeder that prefers well-prepared beds with plenty of organic matter, good drainage, mulch, and minimal pressure from weeds or other plants. Get seed garlic from local organic growers, opting for big, healthy bulbs and cloves. Hard-neck varieties generally store better and are more potent medicinally. Plant the individual cloves point-side-up in late fall (crack the skin a bit, but not the clove itself) and mulch well. Pull back mulch and top-dress with compost in spring. Harvest when the stalks turn yellow in summer. Other *Allium* species including onions, shallots, chives, and walking onions have similar, milder medicinal properties.

A PUNGENT MOVER

Garlic's strong aroma and flavor generally indicate its potency. It helps thin the blood and boost circulation; decreases cardiovascular inflammation; improves digestion, libido, and sexual function; stimulates the immune system; acts as an expectorant, moving and clearing mucus from the respiratory tract; fights a wide range of pathogens not only locally in pretty much every system (e.g., gut, skin, lungs) but also systemically; lowers blood sugar; and feeds good bacteria in the gut. As an antimicrobial, consider it as part of a Lyme or pneumonia treatment protocol. Other *Allium* species — onions, shallots, chives, leeks — have similar but milder action.

FOOD AND MORE

Of course, garlic is also a delicious food crop! Garlic bulbs sometimes turn vinegar teal blue while magenta chive blossoms lend a pink hue. You can also make sprays for your garden to fend off pests and vermin. Eating garlic regularly may ward off biting insects, ticks, parasites — our modern-day vampires. As a flower essence (page 68), garlic cleanses and strengthens the vital force, banishing fear and parasites.

STINKY AND STRONG

Garlic breath is no myth — therapeutic doses make not only your breath but also your whole body stink. A FODMAP, it may cause gas and bloating in people with SIBO, IBS, and dysbiosis. The juices can irritate sensitive tissue, including sensitive stomachs and when applied topically (ear oil, vaginal suppository). The use of garlic in animals is controversial; it may cause hemolytic anemia, particularly in large doses.

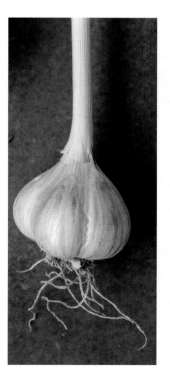

Harvesting, Preparing, and Using Garlic

Pull up bulbs in summer when the tops turn yellow. Use immediately or cure it for storage: spread out or hang to dry out of direct sunlight with good airflow until the tops turn brown. Chop and let sit 10 to 15 minutes before proceeding with your recipe.

Parts Used: bulbs/cloves

Tincture: 1–3 ml, 1–3 times daily, solo or in formula
• Fresh 1:2 in 95 percent alcohol

Honey, Syrup, Vinegar, Oxymel: 1–3 teaspoons as needed

Capsules/Powder: 500–2,000 mg crude herb daily

Food: use liberally fresh (stronger) or dried, minced/puréed in pesto and hummus. Also enjoy the milder aerial scapes

Topical: oil, compress, poultice, soak (may irritate)

Recipes: Dandelion-Violet Weed Pesto, page 88; Fire Cider, page 236; Heart Tonic Tincture Blend, page 237; Fire Cider-Maple-Mustard Dressing, page 237; Thai Curry Fire Cider, page 237. Also try it in broth

Get the most out of garlic by chopping it 10 to 15 minutes before you eat it or add it to a recipe.

GOLDENROD

Solidago spp.

Daisy Family (Asteraceae)

Body Systems: Respiratory, Immune, Kidney/Urinary, Detoxification

   perennial, Zones 3–9

GOLDEN FIELDS AND MEADOWS

You'll recognize goldenrod in late summer — its yellow clusters of flowers erupt across fields and meadows and along woodland edges just when allergy season hits. Inconspicuous ragweed hides among the goldenrod, blooming at the same time, causing the bulk of those allergies. Goldenrod spreads quickly by underground root runners and seed, and its tall stature crowds out more sensitive plants. It's easily foraged and can be cultivated in less-maintained edges of the property alongside fellow weedy brutes like bee balm and wild raspberry. Goldenrod grows everywhere in North America, with multiple species present. It's tricky to key out, but most species appear interchangeable. The most common medicinal species are Canada goldenrod (*S. canadensis*) and anise-scented (*S. odora*, "at risk" in some areas). Europeans use *S. virgaurea*.

WATER-MOVER ANTIHISTAMINE

Considering how prolific and useful this plant is, it's amazing how overlooked goldenrod tends to be in herbal medicine. Think of goldenrod as a "water mover" — improving the flow of water in and out of the body — both as a diuretic and for mucus congestion. It contains mild toning, astringent, antihistamine properties for mucosal lining that ease allergies and acute respiratory complaints, including hay fever, sinus congestion, and sinusitis, and is helpful as an adjunct in asthma. During a monthlong "cold from hell" that ended with a painful sinus infection, I threw *everything* at it to no avail and was surprised when goldenrod and bee balm tinctures *finally* moved it out. It's now a regular ingredient in my allergy, sinus, and lung formulas. Goldenrod also acts as a diuretic and kidney tonic, particularly as a tea.

AND MUCH MORE

Look into goldenrod's rich history across the world, particularly among Native Americans and Europeans, and you'll learn its many uses: a carminative for digestion, gas, and bloating; a mild antimicrobial for respiratory and urinary infections; an anti-inflammatory; a diuretic for hypertension formulas; a rich source of bioflavonoids for blood vessel health; and more. As a flower essence (page 68), goldenrod helps people find their "spine," or resolve against fear and others' influence.

SAFE FOR MOST PEOPLE

Goldenrod's pretty safe, but as a diuretic, it might be inappropriate before bedtime and should be used with caution alongside pharmaceuticals contraindicated with diuretics such as blood pressure medications.

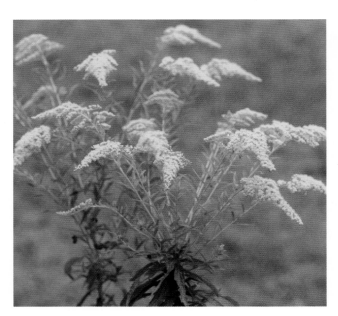

An eye-catching weed, goldenrod is often wrongly accused of causing allergies, yet may actually help relieve them.

Harvesting, Preparing, and Using Goldenrod

Trim the top one-third to two-thirds of the plant's leaves and flowers, just as the blooms are about to open. For tea, use while in bud or just before it blooms to avoid the flowers turning into puffballs (if they do, you can still use it). Use fresh or dried.

Parts Used: aerial/leaves and flowers

Tea: 1 teaspoon dried herb/cup, infusion, 1–3 cups daily

Tincture: 1–5 ml, 1–3 times daily, solo or in formula
• Fresh 1:2 in 95 percent alcohol (best) or dried 1:5 in 50–60 percent alcohol

Vinegar, Oxymel: 1 teaspoon as needed

Recipes: Floral Ice Cubes, page 96; Allergy Tincture Blend, page 182

GOLDENSEAL

Hydrastis canadensis

Buttercup Family (Ranunculaceae)

Body Systems: Immune, Digestive, Skin, Blood Sugar, Antimicrobial

   perennial, Zones 3–8

AT-RISK WOODLAND WILDFLOWER

This shy northeastern woodland wildflower has become the mascot for the United Plant Savers, a non-profit dedicated to medicinal plant conservation and sustainability. Even though goldenseal is the most commonly available berberine-rich herb in commerce, it's increasingly scarce in the wild and often unsustainably wild harvested for the industry. Though slow-growing, it propagates easily from young roots. It thrives in dry shade gardens or in the forest among its friends wild ginger, ginseng, trillium, bloodroot, black cohosh, violet, and Solomon's seal. Other herbs (see page 271) can be used similarly.

BITTER ANTIMICROBIAL BERBERINE

Goldenseal contains berberine, a bitter-tasting, somewhat acrid, bright yellow alkaloid. Berberine is most prevalent in the roots, which are the most common part used for medicine. However, the leaves contain some berberine as well as additional constituents that improve the efficacy of the roots. As a bitter (page 134), goldenseal and other berberines stimulate digestive juices and improve gastric function, but they have the additional benefit as antimicrobials that are particularly well suited to fight intestinal infections, chronic diarrhea, dysbiosis, and small intestinal bacterial overgrowth (SIBO). As a flower essence (page 68), goldenseal helps clear out the old to make room for the new.

NOT *EXACTLY* ANTIBIOTIC

Goldenseal fights infections only on contact — in the digestive tract when consumed, nasal passages in a nasal spray or wash, on the throat as a spray, and topically on the skin. It works particularly well in this way for a variety of bacterial and fungal

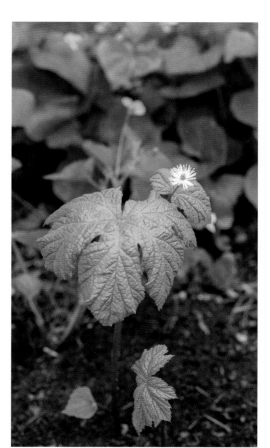

Harvesting, Preparing, and Using Goldenseal

Harvest roots in fall from mature plants (at least 5 years old). Use fresh or dried. Goldenseal is stronger and more precious than other berberines; you can blend it with others.

Parts Used: roots (strongest), aerial parts

Tea: ⅛–½ teaspoon dried herb/half cup, decocted, ¼–½ cup 1–3 times daily

Tincture: 0.5–2 ml, 1–3 times daily, solo or in formula (up to 10 ml for acute care)
• Fresh 1:2 in 95 percent alcohol (best) or dried 1:5 in 50–60 percent alcohol

Capsules/Powder: 500–1,000 mg crude herb, 1–3 times daily

Topical: oil (preferably alcohol-intermediary, using leaf), salve, liniment

Recipes: Bitters Spray, page 141; Allergy Tincture Blend, page 182. Also blend with echinacea as a throat or topical spray

Welcome the sensitive wildflower goldenseal into shady woodland gardens or seek out its more abundant analogs barberry and Oregon grape root.

infections. Contrary to its use in viral infections with echinacea, goldenseal really isn't useful as an antiviral or systemic antibiotic. Systemically, the goldenseal *does* tighten and tone mucous membranes and has an antihistamine-like action, drying up "catarrh" or excessive mucus discharge and buildup, helpful in acute allergies.

STRONG MEDICINE

Goldenseal is generally safe in high doses short term or low doses as part of a long-term formula if needed. High doses as a single herb may be too drying and generally inappropriate long term (more than 2 weeks). Do not use it in pregnancy. Never wildcraft goldenseal. Berberine improves the efficacy of antibiotics but may also interact with some pharmaceuticals by altering liver clearance.

Other Berberine-Rich Plants

Many plants contain berberine and can be used relatively interchangeably with goldenseal. Collectively, I refer to all berberine-rich herbs as "berberines." These substitute herbs are useful considering goldenseal's threatened status in the wild and its slow-growing nature. Barberry (*Berberis* spp.) and Oregon grape root (*Mahonia* spp., sometimes categorized as a *Berberis* species) are more prolific and common.

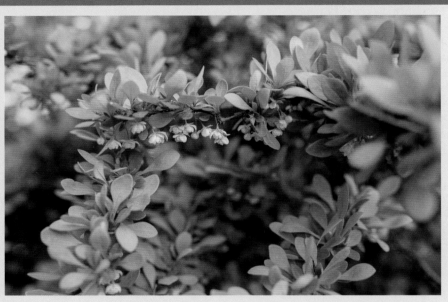

Barberry. This invasive shrub is widely cultivated in landscapes across most of North America. Covered in tiny barbs (not so fun during harvesttime), it produces attractive berries that persist through winter. The roots — especially the root bark — as well as the inner bark of aerial parts are richest in berberine, though the leaves can also be used. It's been well studied by Middle Eastern scientists.

Oregon grape root. As its name suggests, this plant grows prolifically throughout Oregon and the rest of the West Coast; it's also cultivated as landscape shrub. It has hollylike leaves with thorny tips and fruits that resemble grapes when ripe. Although often prolific, be mindful when wildcrafting, because some species may be threatened. You can use the roots and leaves for medicine.

Additional berberine-rich plants. These include *tiny* goldthread (*Coptis* spp.), herbal medic Sam Coffman's favorite algerita (*Mahonia trifoliolata*) in Texas, and yellow root (*Xanthorhiza simplicissima*) in the south/central/eastern United States, with several others growing throughout the world.

How to use berberines. See the goldenseal profile for more on how to use these berberine-rich herbs. They are a bit milder (that's not necessarily a bad thing) but otherwise similar, more sustainable, and easier to harvest in large quantities. Going back to the bitter properties, berberine-rich herbs also lower blood sugar and encourage liver detoxification, bile excretion, fat digestion, and healthy skin (particularly for acne) as "blood cleansing" alteratives. Because of their gentler nature, barberry and Oregon grape root are even more appropriate for this than goldenseal.

GOTU KOLA

Centella asiatica

Parsley Family (Apiaceae)

Body Systems: Nervous/Adrenal, Heart, Skin, Cognition/Brain

   tender perennial, Zones 8–11

SOGGY, RICH SOIL

This leafy Indian herb prefers to grow as a creeping ground cover in *extremely* rich, soggy soil in warm dappled sunlight. Heat brings out more adaptogenic constituents, but gotu kola tolerates cooler temps, containers, full sun, and the indoors. Grow it in nearly 100 percent compost and water daily, being attentive to hanging pots. It sends out runners that root in water or soil at the nodes. The inconspicuous flowers put out seed with low germination rates.

BRAIN AND HEALING TONIC

Gotu kola has many benefits across various body systems. Key uses include as a nervine, calm energy adaptogen, brain tonic, vulnerary, and circulation enhancer. Consider it for gut healing, memory enhancement, ADHD, anxiety, protection and healing from nerve injury, and circulatory issues like varicose veins and vascular insufficiency. Use water, oil, or alcohol extracts topically for wounds, hemorrhoids, scars, and gum health. High doses and long-term use work best; it can take a few months for effects to build. As a flower essence (page 68), it helps you remember and understand who you are and what you are meant to do in the world.

EDIBLE GREENS

This is also an edible green raw, cooked, and juiced with a bland seaweedy or watercress-like flavor. Though not exciting tasting on its own, gotu kola blends well with mint, holy basil, spinach, garlic, or onions. Add powdered gotu kola to smoothies, nut butter–honey balls, and other foods.

SAFE FOR MOST PEOPLE

Gotu kola is very safe and foodlike for children and adults. It may inhibit conception and should not be used during pregnancy. Market quality is poor; plants are often contaminated with fecal bacteria. Reports of cancer are unfounded. Reports of liver damage are based on its presence in adulterated weight-loss products in Argentina. Research suggests *anti-cancer* activity.

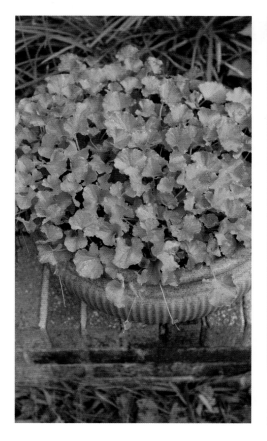

Harvesting, Preparing, and Using Gotu Kola

Trim back tendrils and older leaves to the ground node, leaving at least one-third of the leaves intact. Use fresh or dried.

Parts Used: leaves/aerial parts

Tea: 1 teaspoon dried herb/cup, infusion, 1–3 cups daily. Add to super infusions as well as simmering broths.

Tincture: 2–5 ml, 1–3 times daily, solo or in formula
• Fresh 1:2 in 95 percent alcohol (best) or dried 1:5 in 50–60 percent alcohol

Capsules/Powder: 500–5,000 mg (up to 1 teaspoon) crude herb daily

Food: nibble a few leaves, up to 1 cup packed as a leafy green, smoothie, juiced

Topical: liniment, oil (preferably alcohol-intermediary), salve, cream, bath

Recipes: Brain-Boosting Tincture, page 112, Minty Memory Tea, page 113, Super Skin Salve variation, page 198, Heart Tonic Tincture Blend, page 237

I grow gotu kola in pots and hanging planters to keep it out of reach of hungry woodchucks and to allow me to bring this Indian herb indoors for winter.

HAWTHORN

Crataegus spp.

Rose Family (Rosaceae)

Body Systems: Heart, Cardiovascular, Nervous, Mood

   tree, Zones 3–9

LONG-TERM REWARDS

It takes *several* years for a young hawthorn to become fruitful, but plant this lovely tree if you know you'll be there for a while and have an interest in heart health. Depending on pruning and the species, you can grow it as a graceful specimen tree or a shrubby hedge of thorns, food, and medicine. *Crataegus* means "strong." Established trees withstand harsh conditions and hardscrabble locations, living to be hundreds of years old. It prefers well-drained, slightly acidic soil. The more sun, the more fruitful it will be. It is prone to diseases of fellow rose-family fruit trees — see Michael Phillips's *The Holistic Orchard* for tips.

SUPREME HEART TONIC

No other herb has more of an affinity for the human heart and cardiovascular system than hawthorn, which works via a variety of mechanisms as a daily tonic with foodlike safety. It can take several weeks, even months, for the effects to build. Hawthorn strengthens the heart's pumping ability, helps protect against and repair damage, and is often used in heart attack prevention and long-term postattack care. It improves the quality of blood vessel lining, reducing inflammation, fighting oxidative stress with antioxidant constituents, and dilating blood vessels to reduce blood pressure with ACE-inhibitor-like action. It gradually eases palpitations, tachycardia, arrhythmias, and angina, and it's been researched most for its role in managing congestive heart failure. Its effect on cholesterol is subtle but beneficial. Commercial hawthorn solid extract works well, but homemade forms are also useful.

HEART'S REACH

Hawthorn also works on the emotional heart, gladdening and lifting the spirits, easing grief, heartache, and trauma. Because it improves circulation, it has tangential benefits as a supportive herb in cognitive health and for managing diabetes, inflammation, stroke, and other conditions. As a flower essence (page 68), this plant opens the heart and helps it heal emotionally, physically, and spiritually.

FOODLIKE SAFETY

Hawthorn is among our safest herbs, but remember that it is not strong, fast, and druglike, so it's less useful in acute conditions. It may increase the effects of a few medications, particularly certain blood pressure medications.

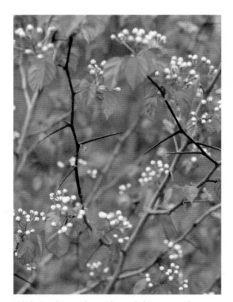

With its thorny branches, delicate apple blossom–like flowers, and deep red berries, this small tree evokes emotion, lore, and deep medicine when incorporated into the landscape.

Harvesting, Preparing, and Using Hawthorn

Pinch off buds, newly opened flowers, and young leaves in early spring, and the berries in fall (remove individually or prune branches off to process at a table). Watch for the long, sharp thorns; consider wearing thick gloves. Use fresh or dried. Dry berries in the dehydrator and ensure they're *completely* hard and dried before storing.

Parts Used: berries, leaves, flowers (often combined)

Tea: 1 heaping teaspoon dried herb/cup, infusion, 1–3 cups daily

Tincture: 3–5 ml, 2–3 times daily, solo or in formula
• Fresh 1:2 in 95 percent alcohol or dried 1:5 in 50–60 percent alcohol

Oxymel, Glycerite, Syrup, Electuary: 1 teaspoon, 2–3 times daily

Capsules/Powder: 1,000–5,000 mg (up to 1 teaspoon) crude herb daily

Food: berry jam, jelly, cordial, powder in smoothies, honey–nut butter balls

Recipes: Hawthorn Tincture, page 230; Peaceful Heart Tea, page 231; Heart Tonic Tincture Blend, page 237. Also consider adding to the Elder–Rose Hip Oxymel, page 169

HOLY BASIL

Ocimum sanctum

Mint Family (Lamiaceae)

Body Systems: Nervous/
Adrenal, Mood, Blood Sugar,
Cognition/Brain, Inflammation,
Pain, Immune, Digestive,
Cardiovascular, Antimicrobial

  annual

HEAT-LOVING AROMATIC

Holy basil (also called tulsi) jumps
for joy when everything else in your
garden bows in submission to hot-as-
Hades midsummer temps and begins
rapidly producing useful medicine,
provided you're watering it enough in
good, well-drained garden soil. This
plant comes from India, and several
varieties (even a few species) are
used somewhat interchangeably.
"Kapoor" or "temperate" tulsi thrives
and produces best in temperate
gardens. If your seed catalog offers
one type and does not specify the

variety, it's probably kapoor, which
may also self-seed. Some types are
perennial in warm zones or if brought
indoors. Also called sacred basil and
O. tenuifolium. Kapoor tulsi produces
nonstop flowers, which you can trim
regularly (to use for tea, water, medicine) to encourage growth.

CALM-ENERGY ZEN

Inhaling and consuming this aromatic herb reminds me of doing
yoga, meditating, or surrounding
myself with incense. The intense,
sweet flavor hints of clove, mint, and
basil. As an adaptogen and nervine,
holy basil both calms and energizes
the spirit, quells anxiety and grief,
and brings clarity and focus to the
mind. As a cortisol modulator, it not
only eases stress but also reduces
blood sugar, bad cholesterol, tri-
glycerides, and sugar cravings. As an
anti-inflammatory COX-2 inhibitor,
it helps fight many chronic diseases
and eases pain, especially when combined with other anti-inflammatory
herbs like turmeric, ginger, rosemary,
and ashwagandha.

GREAT PROTECTOR

Holy basil is associated with the
Hindu god Vishnu and is used for
medicinal protection in Ayurveda.
It fortifies the immune system to
fight infection, increases digestive
function and juices, and protects
against ulcers and radiation. It may
stimulate anticancer activity and
fights both oxidative stress and
inflammation with its antioxidant and
anti-inflammatory properties. Holy
basil could take a spot in almost every
garden in this book — it's that kind of
plant. As a flower essence (page 68),
holy basil brings sacred sensuality.

SAFE FOR MOST PEOPLE

Holy basil is safe for adults and
children and rarely interacts with
medications. Some may find its
digestive effects too stimulating. If
you're prone to hypoglycemia, take it
with meals or lightly sweetened with
honey. A few people paradoxically
feel anxious with holy basil or simply
don't like it.

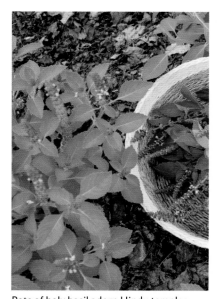

Pots of holy basil adorn Hindu temples,
creating sacred space and bringing prayers
to heaven with its Zen-like aroma.

Harvesting, Preparing, and Using Holy Basil

Regularly trim the top one-half to two-thirds of the flowers and leaves, which
will keep the plant happy, producing more vital growth. Use fresh or dried.

Parts Used: aerial in flower

Tea: 1 teaspoon dried herb/cup, infusion, 1–3 cups daily

Tincture: 1–3 ml, 1–3 times daily, solo or in formula
• Fresh 1:2 in 95 percent alcohol (best) or dried 1:5 in 50–60 percent
  alcohol

Honey, Oxymel, Glycerite, Syrup: 1 teaspoon as need (heavenly!)

Capsules/Powder: 500–2,000 mg crude herb daily

Also: cordial, infused water, seltzer/soda, hydrosol

Recipes: Yummy Teas, page 94; Infused Seltzer, Soda, and Water, page
97; Holy Rose Water, page 107; Stress Support Tincture Blend, page 107;
Brain-Boosting Tincture Blend, page 112; Holy Basil Beverages, page 124;
Mellow Me Glycerite, page 125

HOREHOUND

Marrubium vulgare

Mint Family (Lamiaceae)

Body Systems: Respiratory, Immune, Digestive

  perennial, Zones 3–8

A PLANT FOR DRY PLACES

We use horehound for damp, stagnant health conditions, yet it prefers dry, sunny spots in the garden. I would brush by horehound that was growing along the roadside on my morning walks in herb school in Arizona. Here in my Northeast garden, I've finally found dry, semisandy spots where it doesn't get too waterlogged in winter and spring. Its fuzzy, wrinkled, silvery herbaceous foliage adds nice texture to the garden layout. Rosemary, thyme, and lavender prefer similar conditions.

MOVES MUCUS, CONGESTION

Horehound tops the charts of herbs sold in the mainstream market because it's a common ingredient in many brands of cough syrup and drops, including Ricola. Most famous for clearing wet coughs, horehound is stellar whenever mucus secretions are too thick, stagnant, or drippy. I love this plant for postnasal drip and mucus-y allergies and often combine it with the antihistamine herb goldenrod. It thins mucus so you can move and expectorate it. Michael Moore used horehound capsules alongside echinacea tincture and passionflower tea as a synergistic trio for asthma in children, which he found helped reduce trips to the hospital during cold and flu season. Store-bought horehound tends to be rubbish.

OTHER USES

It's quite bitter and can be used to stimulate digestion. As a flower essence (page 68), horehound helps you more clearly express yourself and has an affinity for the throat.

GENERALLY SAFE BUT SO BITTER

Children and adults can use horehound safely as needed, but it is contraindicated in pregnancy and with some cardiac conditions and drugs. It's *terribly* bitter tasting! This makes it nauseating in moderate to large doses, and it may lower blood sugar — take it sweetened or with food.

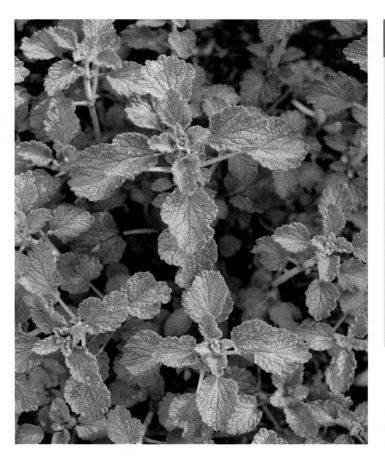

Harvesting, Preparing, and Using Horehound

Harvest leafy growth when it's happy, preferably in spring or fall. Use fresh or dried. Have I mentioned it's *bitter*? Most people prefer tincture or capsules for this reason.

Parts Used: aerial/leaves

Tincture: 1–2 ml, 1–3 times daily, solo or in formula
• Fresh 1:2 in 95 percent alcohol (best) or dried 1:5 in 50–60 percent alcohol

Syrup, Honey, Glycerite, Cough Drop: ½–1 teaspoon or 1 cough drop as needed

Capsules/Powder: 250–1,000 mg crude herb daily

Recipes: Horehound Cough Syrup, page 177; Allergy Tincture Blend, page 182

This silvery wildflower of sunny, dry places moves mucus like no other.

HORSETAIL

Equisetum arvense

Horsetail Family (Equisetaceae)

Body Systems: Skin, Bones, Nutritive, Musculoskeletal, Inflammation, Connective Tissue, Pain, Gut, Kidney/Urinary

 perennial, Zones 2–9

LOVE OR HATE IT

Once this Jurassic-era weed settles in the garden, it's difficult to eradicate; however, it serves many purposes and does little harm in semiunkempt beds on the edges of your property. A plant of watersheds, ensure water and soil quality before harvesting. Other plants gladly grow alongside horsetail, including nettle and elder. Other species of *Equisetum* likely have similar properties. The more ornamental, formidable scouring rush (*E. hyemale*) — popular in Asian gardens — may be less soluble in tea, though it can still be used.

SILICA STRENGTH

Rich in minerals in general, horsetail earns bonus points for its silica content. Horsetail blows oatstraw out of the water with three times the silica content. Silica helps maintain the strength and flexibility of connective tissues, including bones, hair, skin, and nails, as well as their constituents keratin and elastin. For a supportive treatment for bone breaks and osteoporosis, blend it with other mineral-rich herbs like oatstraw and nettle. Horsetail is underrated for its benefits in wound healing, gut repair, joint health, and arthritis relief. In a study of patients taking medications for rheumatoid arthritis, adding horsetail brought treatment to 80 percent efficacy versus just 17 percent without the herb. In another study, horsetail ointment applied for 10 days post-delivery reduced pain (to one-sixth of what the placebo group felt) and improved healing of episiotomy wounds (4.4 times better than in the placebo group).

KIDNEYS TO COMPOST

Horsetail tonifies the kidneys and acts as a diuretic. According to organic orchardist Michael Phillips, fermented horsetail "compost tea" sprayed on plants fights fungal pathogens, strengthens plants, and promotes beneficial microbes. (Nettle and comfrey leaf are nice additions in your compost tea, too. It smells like rotten eggs when it's ready.)

A FEW CAUTIONS

Horsetail's avoidable dangers stem from a few concerns. First, it accumulates toxins, particularly nitrogenous ones, in contaminated soil and watersheds. Avoid areas downstream from big farms, factories, and chemical plants. Also, the fresh plant contains an enzyme called thiaminase that reduces vitamin B_1, which is why it's toxic to grazing animals. Drying or tincturing should denature the enzymes, and, given the small quantities of horsetail we consume, the risk of toxicity is negligible. If you grind dried horsetail, use a mask in a well-ventilated area to avoid dangerous silicosis.

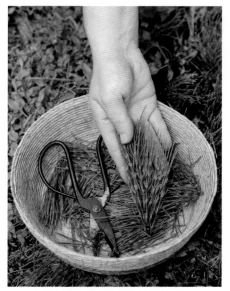

Horsetail prefers damp, rich soil along riverbeds and in gardens where it can get weedy.

Harvesting, Preparing, and Using Horsetail

Harvest the green "tails" in springtime when bright green and upright. The plant breaks easily at the joints, making it simple to process. Silica is best extracted as tea, but the (silica-free) tincture also works. Use dried, cooked, or tinctured.

Parts Used: aerial sterile green growth

Tea: 1 heaping teaspoon dried herb/cup, decoction or long infusion, 1–3 cups daily

Tincture: 5–60 drops, 1–3 times daily, solo or in formula
• Fresh 1:2 in 95 percent alcohol or dried 1:5 in 50–60 percent alcohol

Capsules/Powder: 500–1,000 mg crude herb daily

Food: broth (strain before eating)

Topical: oil, ointment, salve, cream, glycerite, vinegar, liniment

Recipes: Nutri-Tea, page 79; Nutri-Broth, page 80; Gut Healing Broth, page 153; Aches and Pains, Strains and Sprains Tincture/Liniment, page 220

KOREAN MINT AND ANISE HYSSOP

Agastache rugosa and
A. foeniculum

Mint Family (Lamiaceae)

Body Systems: Immune,
Respiratory, Digestive,
Inflammation, Nervous, Mood,
Antimicrobial

   perennial,
Zones 4–10

LOVELY SELF-SEEDING BLOOMS

Korean mint and anise hyssop are
nearly indistinguishable and completely interchangeable. I prefer
Korean mint, which I inherited from
the previous owner of my home, for
its softer fennel-honey flavor even
though anise hyssop is more widely
available. These short-lived perennials tolerate a range of conditions,
but they do best in decent, moderately moist (not necessarily regularly
watered) soil. They self-seed rampantly (look for purple-green babies
with scalloped leaves) but are easy
to pull out or move. They reach 4 to
5 feet in their second and third years.
Both produce gorgeous, long-lasting
purple spikes in mid/late summer.
Korean mint is hard to find — I'm
on a mission to get more people
growing it!

INCREDIBLY DELICIOUS

Most famous as tea, *Agastache* gives
a sweet, bright fennel-mint flavor
fresh or dried and holds its flavor
well in storage. The dried leaves
stand in nicely for fennel seeds in
Mediterranean and Asian cuisine.
Freshly snipped, the leaves blend well
in salads, surprising guests with their
pleasant flavor (think: Italian sausage and meatballs, fresh Thai spring
rolls, seafood, and other dishes that
benefit from fennel-like flavor). The
herb-infused honey tastes divine in
tea, marinade, and salad dressing or
drizzled into seltzer and enjoyed by
the spoonful. For a delicious Asian
fusion dipping sauce/dressing, mix
1 tablespoon each Korean mint honey
and chive blossom vinegar with 1 teaspoon toasted sesame oil. The flowers
add color appeal to dried tea blends
and can be used fresh in seltzer and
infused water — combining Korean
mint with vanilla extract evokes a
posh, sugar-free root beer flavor. Use
it to flavor medicinal blends.

UNDERRATED MEDICINAL

It's easy to overlook *Agastache*'s rich
medicinal value. Michael Moore
recommends the antioxidant, anti-
inflammatory mint-family herbs,
rich in rosmarinic acid, for general
well-being and cooling on a hot
day. In traditional Korean medicine,
Korean mint relieves summer damp-
ness without being overly drying, acts
as a carminative and mild digestive
(a cross between mint and fennel's
medicine), eases nausea and vomiting, settles the stomach, and can
be added to formulas for respiratory infections and the stomach flu.
Larken Bunce uses anise hyssop as
a mild nervine and for people who
feel like they have a lump ("plum
pit") stuck in their throat. As a flower
essence (page 68), these plants bring
sweetness back to life.

QUITE SAFE

No known contraindications. Some
people don't like the licorice-like
flavor.

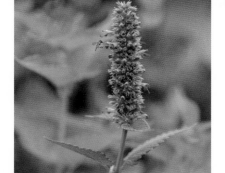

These are two of the most beautiful and
delicious herb species you can grow. Sure,
they're medicinal, but I savor them for the
joy they bring to life, drink, and food.

Harvesting, Preparing, and Using Korean Mint

Harvest aerial parts before or once the plant has flowered. It has a long
season. Use fresh or dried.

Parts Used: aerial/leaves and flowers

Tea: 1 teaspoon dried herb/cup, infusion, 1–3 cups daily

Glycerine, Oxymel, Honey, Syrup: 1 teaspoon as desired

Food: Fresh or dried as a culinary herb, chopped in cheese, seafood, salad,
dressings, marinades, dipping sauce, flower sprigs in water, seltzer, soda,
and cordials

Recipes: Floral Ice Cubes, page 96; Infused Seltzer, Soda, and Water,
page 97; Bitters Spray, page 141; Fennel and Korean Mint Seltzer, page
146; Sweet Fennel Liquor, page 146; Gut-Healing Tummy Tea, Take One,
page 152; Asian Fusion Dipping Sauce, above

LADY'S MANTLE

Alchemilla vulgaris, A. mollis

Rose Family (Rosaceae)

Body Systems: Reproductive, Gut, Skin

  perennial, Zones 3–8

DEWDROP FOLIAGE

Lady's mantle's chartreuse early-summer flowers have subtle beauty, but the silvery green leaves really catch your eye when grown en masse — crinkled umbrellas with scalloped leaves that catch the morning dew and so soft to the touch. Lady's mantle does best in a spot that feels like Ireland. Not too hot, dry, or sunny. It forms a lovely mound or edge to the garden but doesn't compete well when crammed in with other plants.

ROSE-FAMILY ASTRINGENT

Lady's mantle is what Michael Moore would call a YARFA (yet another rose-family astringent) gentle enough for regular use. As with its fellow cousins rose petal and red raspberry leaf, lady's mantle is helpful for uterine issues — tightening and toning boggy or prolapsed tissues and drying excessive secretions, bleeding, or discharge. Also consider adding it to blends for healing ongoing intestinal problems (e.g., leaky gut, chronic diarrhea), and as a background herb in beverages. Most often used as tea, it has a light, tannic flavor similar to green or white tea (without the caffeine). It blends nicely with light, subtle flavorful herbs like rose petals, Korean mint, lemongrass, lemon verbena, and linden, or with a wedge of lemon.

OF MYTH AND BEAUTY

Much lore surrounds the dewdrops that cling to its leaves — alchemists believed that the collected dew would help them find the Philosopher's Stone. Drinking or applying the dew to the skin was said to attract love and bestow everlasting beauty. As a flower essence (page 68), lady's mantle helps ground and connect your heart to the green world and heal female reproductive trauma or disease.

SAFE FOR MOST PEOPLE

Lady's mantle is quite safe but not generally recommended during pregnancy (use raspberry leaves instead). It is quite astringent and drying, so large amounts could irritate sensitive stomachs and people who are already too dry or constipated.

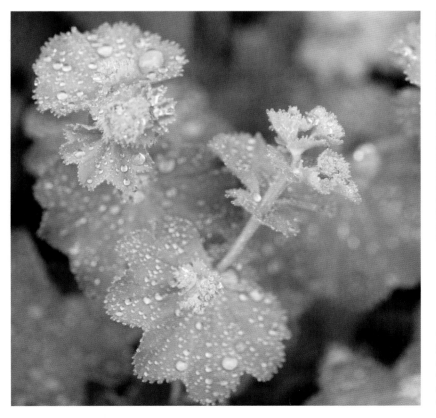

Harvesting, Preparing, and Using Lady's Mantle

Harvest individual leaves with or without flowers before it blooms or just as blooms open — the flowers go by very quickly. Use dried.

Parts Used: leaves, flowers

Tea: 1 teaspoon dried herb/cup, infusion, 1–3 cups daily

Recipes: Lady Tea, page 243; more tea tips above

The Irish hold lady's mantle in high esteem, and it does best in a landscape similar to Ireland's with dreary, cool, moist, shady spots where the dewdrops cling magically to its graceful leaves.

LAVENDER

Lavandula angustifolia

Mint Family (Lamiaceae)

Body Systems: Nervous, Mood, Pain, Skin, Digestive, Antimicrobial

  perennial, Zones 5–8

MEDITERRANEAN HILLSIDE

A fragrant hedge of silvery lavender dotted with those tiny buds immediately evokes calm and connection to the plant world. Lavender has become the poster plant for medicinal herbs, aromatherapy, self-care, relaxation, and the French hillsides. When planting lavender, seek seedlings and root divisions from varieties known to thrive in your region, then find a sunny, warm spot with somewhat dry, sandy, well-drained soil. Lavender tends to rot out in your standard pampered, watered, mulched garden bed.

POTENT NERVE TONIC

Lavender essential oil has the most research and traditional use — inhaled to relieve stress and aid sleep or topically applied to repel insects and heal irritated skin, wounds, and burns. But you'd need 16 pillow-sized pounds of lavender buds and fancy distillation equipment to make the essential oil at home. Less concentrated homemade lavender preparations also work well, and even in this less potent (yet more complex) state, lavender is still plenty strong in small doses. Lavender has moving, carminative, dispersive, pain-relieving, sedative-antidepressant properties. Try it for anxiety, tension headaches, and nervous indigestion, solo or in blends.

A MULTITUDE OF USES

Oh, the many ways you can use lavender! This is a *supreme* skin herb for almost anything you can think of — bug repellent, bug bite care, irritated skin, sensitive skin, rashes, acne, dry skin, oily skin, aging skin, infections, burns, poison ivy. Lavender's antioxidant and antimicrobial properties also help preserve formulas. As a flower essence (page 68), lavender calms the spirit and the mind — one of my favorites for client formulas!

SAFE FOR MOST PEOPLE

Lavender is a strong plant that doesn't agree with everyone. Don't ingest it while pregnant. The flavor can be too soapy for some. Studies found lavender essential oil (which is far more concentrated than homemade preparations) has phytoestrogenic and antiandrogenic effects, implicated in breast development in boys.

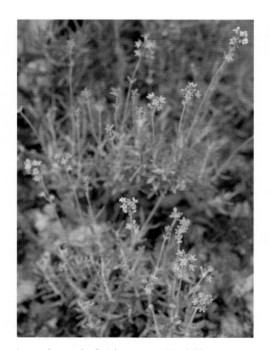

Lavender can be finicky to grow. Much like horehound, thyme, and rosemary, it prefers dry, sunny, sandy spots without a lot of competition.

Harvesting, Preparing, and Using Lavender

Cut stems to dry and process to remove the buds, ideally before the buds open. For aromatic remedies, you can include leaves and stems. Use fresh or dried. You just need a bit — use it as a synergist in blends. Homemade liniment, infused oil, and/or hydrosol can be substituted for the essential oil.

Parts Used: buds, flowers

Tea: ½ teaspoon dried herb/cup, infusion, 1–3 cups daily

Tincture: 0.5–1 ml, 1–3 times daily, solo or in formula
• Fresh 1:2 in 95 percent alcohol or dried 1:5 in 50–60 percent alcohol

Glycerite, Syrup, Honey, Oxymel: ¼–½ teaspoon as needed

Food: Add a few buds to sugar, shortbread, chocolate, and in herbs de Provence blends

Topical: oil (preferably alcohol-intermediary), salve, cream, hydrosol, liniment, soak/bath, compress, glycerite, essential oil

Recipes: Calendula-Comfrey Cream, page 193; Super Skin Salve, page 198; First Aid Simple: Lavender Essential Oil or Hydrosol/Liniment, page 199; Herbal Insect Repellent, page 204

LEMON BALM

Melissa officinalis

Mint Family (Lamiaceae)

Body Systems: Nervous, Mood, Digestive, Immune, Cardiovascular, Skin, Antiviral, Metabolic, Cognitive

   perennial, Zones 4–9

PAMPERED MEDITERRANEAN

Our oldest written herbals extol the virtues of lemon balm, including Dioscorides's *De Materia Medica* and Avicenna's *Canon of Medicine*. Lemon balm hails from the Mediterranean but thrives in moist, well-drained rich soil and dappled sunlight. It spreads by underground root runners and occasionally self-seeds. It may get rambunctious in its favorite spots, but it's not as bad as spearmint and apple mint. It propagates well from root division.

UPLIFTING CALMING NERVINE

Lemon balm could be featured in almost every garden in this book, it's so useful! It supports the nervous system — calming anxiety and aiding sleep without oversedating. The lemony aromatics lift the spirit, ease mild to moderate depression (especially in combination with St. John's wort or holy basil), gladden the heart, and quell heart palpitations. Consider an evening cup of lemon balm and holy basil tea for insomnia, nightmares, anxiety, and hypervigilance. Lemon balm is a popular, safe children's herb, too.

DIGESTION, MEMORY

Lemon balm's aromatic, carminative, and mild bitter properties ease digestive distress and improve digestive function and also improve blood sugar and heart health. The essential oil and tannins have direct antiviral — particularly antiherpes — action when applied topically. Try a squirt of tincture internally and dabbed on the area at the first tingle of a cold sore, or blend the tincture with St. John's wort oil to apply topically. It improves calm focus and cognitive abilities, increasing levels of the important neurotransmitter acetylcholine. As a flower essence (page 68), lemon balm relaxes and restores, especially during headaches or after being stretched too thin.

SAFE FOR MOST PEOPLE

Lemon balm is one of the safest herbs. Sensitive folks might find it a tad too drying or stimulating for digestion (stomach upset, nausea), or hypoglycemic — especially if taken as a strong tea on an empty stomach. A little honey, a shorter steep, the addition of other herbs, or taking it with food helps. Lemon balm loses its potency quickly once dried.

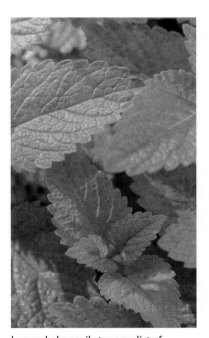

Lemon balm easily tops my list of favorite garden herbs. You can't help but rub and inhale the spirit-lifting lemon aroma of its leaves as you walk by.

Harvesting, Preparing, and Using Lemon Balm

Harvest aerial parts, preferably before it flowers, several times throughout the season. Use fresh (best) or freshly dried. Great in blends.

Parts Used: aerial/leaves

Tea: 1–2 teaspoons dried herb/cup, infusion, 1–3 cups daily

Tincture: 1–5 ml, 1–3 times daily, solo or in formula
• Fresh 1:2 in 95 percent alcohol

Glycerite, Honey, Syrup, Vinegar: 1 teaspoon as needed

Capsules/Powder: 500–3,000 mg crude herb daily

Food: Add fresh to pesto, infused water, cordials, smoothies, or cake

Topical: liniment, oil (freshly dried), cream, bath/soak, poultice/compress

Recipes: Nutri-Tea, page 79; Dandelion-Violet Weed Pesto, page 88; Yummy Teas, page 94; Stress Support Tincture Blend, page 107; Brain-Boosting Tincture Blend, page 112; Minty Memory Tea, page 113; Happy Tea, page 118; Lemon-St. John's Wort Pick-Me-Up, page 118; Good Mood Tincture, page 119; Holy Basil Beverages, page 124; Mellow Me Glycerite, page 125; Sleep Tea, page 130; Lemon Balm–Catnip Glycerite, page 140; Bitters Spray, page 141; Peaceful Heart Tea, page 231

LEMON VERBENA AND LEMONGRASS

Aloysia citrodora and *Cymbopogon citratus*

Verbena Family (Verbenaceae) and Grass Family (Poaceae)

Body Systems: Mood, Nervous, Digestion, Gut, Antimicrobial

 perennial, Zones 8–11

TROPICAL LEMONY GOODNESS

These tender perennials will perish in cold winters, but they provide tropical lemony goodness throughout the summer. Just one or two seedlings will easily stock your pantry and freezer by fall. Grow them in warm, sunny plush garden beds or large well-tended containers with rich, moist soil and not too much competition from other plants. Harvest throughout the season, cutting everything down before the first frost unless you plan to bring it indoors. They go dormant in winter. Lemon verbena will look dead. You'll have more success overwintering lemongrass.

BRIGHT, UPLIFTING FLAVOR

Compared to perennial lemony herbs like lemon balm and lemon thyme, lemon verbena and lemongrass offer far superior aroma, flavor, and shelf life. They're still best fresh, but fresh lemongrass stalks freeze very well, and the dried chopped tops will hold their lemon flavor for at least a year. Lemongrass hints of Thai cuisine, zinger tea, and Froot Loops. Lemon verbena evokes lemon cake, especially if you combine it with vanilla, and lasts 6 to 12 months when dried. Both lemongrass and lemon verbena are most prominently used for their delicious flavor and aroma; however, any lemon-scented herb uplifts and calms the spirits. These two have modest stimulating and antimicrobial properties for the digestive and respiratory systems when taken internally as well as for the skin when applied topically. Their essential oils are far more potent. In one study, diffusing lemongrass and geranium essential oils in the air of a hospital burn unit reduced airborne bacteria, including methicillin-resistant *Staphylococcus aureus* (MRSA), by 89 percent!

FOR THE LOVE OF FOOD

These herbs bring joy when you rub their leaves (especially lemon verbena's) or smell and taste them. Fresh or fresh-frozen lemongrass stalks are delicious simmered in soups, infused into seltzer, and in cordials. Chop and purée them into homemade fire cider or Thai Curry Paste (pages 236, 237). Fresh and freshly dried lemon verbena sprigs are a delightful addition to tea — especially green, white, or lady's mantle or with vanilla. Pack the fresh leaves in sugar, infuse them in honey, or place them on the bottom of a pan before you pour in vanilla or yellow cake batter.

QUITE SAFE

These are perfectly safe plants in the quantities in which they're typically consumed. Sensitive stomachs might find them too stimulating to digestion (aggravating nausea, reflux) in large quantities or if overbrewed. Fresh lemongrass's sharp edges grip clothes and slice fingers like papercuts.

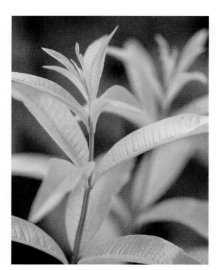

I treat these delicious tropical tender perennials as annuals, but you can also pot them to overwinter (in dormancy) indoors.

Harvesting, Preparing, and Using Lemon Verbena and Lemongrass

Trim lemon verbena down, leaving a few sets of leaves — new stems will grow at each leaf in the whorl where you cut. For lemongrass, trim the tops back as desired or cut the largest stalks at the base as you need them (no more than half the plant), then cut it all at the end of the season. Use fresh (best) or dried. Leave lemon verbena leaves whole and cut dried lemongrass tops into small pieces with sharp scissors.

Parts Used: leaves, stalks

Tea: 1 teaspoon dried herb/cup, infusion, 1–3 cups daily

Honey, Glycerite, Syrup: ½–1 teaspoon as desired

Food: seltzer, soda, cordial, curry, poached fish, desserts, soup

Recipes: Yummy Teas, page 94; Infused Seltzer, Soda, and Water, page 97; Happy Tea, page 118; Thai Curry Fire Cider, page 237; Thai Curry Paste, page 237

LINDEN

Tilia spp.

Mallow Family (Malvaceae)

Body Systems: Nerve, Heart, Mood

 tree, Zones 3–7

FLOWERING ORNAMENTAL TREE

If you have the time to plant and wait for a tree to grow, consider linden. Various species are used interchangeably, but littleleaf *T. cordata* has a nice compact structure, silver *T. tomentosa* is popular for its foliage but will get bigger, and you can forage the wild basswood *T. americana* — it will eventually get too tall to reach unless you prune it carefully. Linden trees are popular along city streets, parks, and yards because they're lovely and aromatic and require little maintenance. They prefer rich, moist soil but will tolerate much less favorable soil conditions.

CALM AND GLADDEN THE HEART

Europeans enjoy sipping linden tea after a meal to calm and uplift the spirit, gladden the heart, and aid digestion. It's a great nightcap or cocktail alternative (that said, it *does* make a great cordial, sweetened with honey, sipped straight or with seltzer). The light flavor is reminiscent of honey and amaretto. A sensual evening cup brings relaxed joy to dinner guests. Linden has the reputation as a heart tonic and mild hypotensive for blood pressure and though little research has been done, the relaxing aromatics and diuretic effect likely play a role. The irregularly heart-shaped leaves serve as a doctrine of signatures to remind you of their cardiovascular benefits.

TILLEUL IN AROMATHERAPY

The French adore the aroma of linden, also called *tilleul*, for soaps and perfumery — it's divine, though most of the commercial products you'll find are synthetic knockoffs. Energetically, linden is intensely aromatic, mildly carminative, gently cooling, and lightly astringent and mucilaginous. Yet, drunk hot, it acts as a diaphoretic to help break a fever. Foragers eat young leaves as a salad green. As a flower essence (page 68), linden calms emotional turmoil and anxiety, releases tension, and helps rewire us so that we can let go of old patterns to embrace the new.

SAFE FOR MOST PEOPLE

Very safe. Some might find it too floral.

Graceful linden trees line American and European city streets and grow near woodland creeks. The blooms fill the air with a honey-vanilla-cherry aroma that intoxicates bees and humans alike.

Harvesting, Preparing, and Using Linden

When the blooms open, pinch off the flower and bract (the unusual "leaf" attached to the flower). The heart-shaped leaves can also be used but aren't quite as potent. Use fresh or freshly dried, mainly in tea.

Parts Used: flowers with bracts

Tea: 1 teaspoon dried herb/cup, infusion, 1–3 cups daily. Great iced, too.

Tincture: 1–3 ml, 1–3 times daily, solo or in formula
- Fresh 1:2 in 95 percent alcohol (best) or dried 1:5 in 50–60 percent alcohol
- Add 10 percent glycerine to stabilize tannins and improve shelf life

Honey, Syrup, Glycerite: 1 teaspoon as desired

Cordial: 1 ounce as a treat, use honey as a sweetener

Food: foraged young leaves and ripe fruit seeds

Recipes: Peaceful Heart Tea, page 231; Linden-Honey Cordial, page 231

MARSHMALLOW

Althaea officinalis

Mallow Family (Malvaceae)

Body Systems: Digestive, Gut, Skin, Respiratory, Kidney/Urinary

   perennial, Zones 5–8

SOFT LEAVES, PRETTY FLOWERS

Marshmallow can reach 5 feet or higher in bloom, with stalks of delicate pale pink flowers. Use the root and/or leaves for medicine. Mallow (*Malva* spp.) leaves and flowers can be used interchangeably and can grow in Zones 3 to 10, including the ornamental high mallow (*M. sylvestris*) and musk mallow (*M. moschata*).

SOOTHING SLIME

Mucilaginous herbs turn into mucus-like slime in water, our purpose for using mallows. In teas, this lends a velvety mouthfeel, eases dry mouth, and relieves dehydration better than water. Add a splash of juice and pinch of salt for a home-made electrolyte drink. In stronger infusions — particularly overnight root and powder infusions in cold water — the consistency can begin to resemble snot. Not very palatable, but immensely soothing and healing for dry, inflamed, irritated gastrointestinal lining or skin. Mallows fabulously soothe and heal reflux, ulcers, gastritis, gastroparesis, and leaky gut. These soothing properties also translate to the lungs (supportive in tea and cough syrup blends), sore throats, and irritated kidney-urinary conditions. Marshmallow doesn't fight infections, so combine it with antimicrobial herbs and spices if one is present. Mucilage, the slimy starch, provides food for good gut flora.

SPECIAL STARCHES

Marshmallow root contains a gentle immune stimulant compound called xylan. And, yes, you *can* make marshmallows from the root (not quite the modern confection). Forager John Kallas uses mallow's immature seed head "peas" as a thickener for gumbo and to make "egg whites." As a flower essence (page 68), marshmallow softens our feelings toward one another, fostering friendliness.

SAFE BUT STARCHY

Mallows are supersafe and foodlike, but the mucilage — particularly from marshmallow root powder — may bother people with candidiasis, dysbiosis, and small intestinal bacterial overgrowth (SIBO), potentially "feeding" pathogenic bacteria or yeasts. Leaf and flower infusions are usually fine. If you feel worse (e.g., experience gassiness, reflux, flare-ups) when you take root preparations, back off, switch to the leaf, or stop taking them.

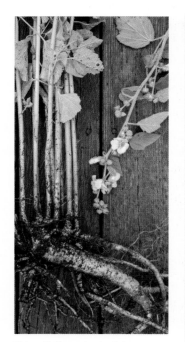

This tall, flowering herb is soothing, slimy, and soft.

Harvesting, Preparing, and Using Marshmallow

Harvest happy leaves and freshly opened flowers to dry for tea in summer. Dig up the marshmallow roots in spring or fall — large plants may be ready within the first season. Best dried. Mucilage loves water and repels alcohol. Cold infusions extract purer mucilage.

Parts Used: roots, leaves, flowers

Tea: 1 heaping teaspoon dried herb/cup, infusion, 1–3 cups daily. Long infusions and long cold infusions work best

Syrup, Glycerite, Decoction Tincture: 1 teaspoon as needed, best simmered or cold infused for several hours or overnight. No more than 30 percent alcohol as a preservative

Powder: Up to 1 teaspoon crude root powder in water, oatmeal, or smoothies

Food: Mild edible leafy green, fresh flowers decorate food and infused water; "peas," leaves, and roots thicken

Topical: bath/soak (best), glycerite, decoction liniment

Recipes: with Chai Base, page 78; Nutri-Tea, page 79; Gut-Healing Tummy Tea, Take One, page 152; Gut-Healing Broth, page 153; Soothing Lung Tea, page 176; Nettle-Peppermint-Marshmallow Tea, page 183

MEADOWSWEET

Filipendula ulmaria

Rose Family (Rosaceae)

Body Systems: Pain, Inflammation, Gut, Musculoskeletal

 perennial, Zones 3–9

QUEEN OF THE MEADOW

Meadowsweet grows wild in meadows, drainage ditches, and swampy spaces, and in the garden. It prefers rich, consistently moist soil and full sun. Don't confuse *this* meadowsweet with the abundant wild *Spiraea* species. Though closely related to *Filipendula ulmaria*, *Spiraea* species lack their cousin's wintergreeny flavor and don't have the same benefits. Harvest before the Japanese beetles descend.

GENTLE PAIN RELIEF

Meadowsweet, along with white willow, inspired the creation of aspirin. It contains small amounts of aspirin-like constituents called salicylates, including salicin and methyl salicylate. Compared to fellow "herbal aspirins" like willow, meadowsweet is much gentler on the stomach and less apt to promote ulcers and bleeding. In fact, meadowsweet flowers contain mucilaginous and soothing properties that help heal the gut, and it is often incorporated into *healing* tea blends for ulcers, leaky gut, reflux, and gastritis to soothe pain and inflammation. It also lacks the "chewing on aspirin" bitter flavor and has only a hint of the sweet wintergreen flavor found in much larger amounts in wintergreen and black birch. Meadowsweet eases pain and tension in sore muscles — make a jug of strong meadowsweet tea to add to the bath. Consider it for other types of pain including headaches and arthritis, but remember that it's generally slower acting and milder (though far safer) than willow and NSAID drugs like aspirin and ibuprofen. As a flower essence (page 68), meadowsweet helps you feel whole, safe, and connected with the earth.

SAFE FOR MOST

Meadowsweet's our safest "herbal aspirin," but use caution if you're allergic to aspirin, and avoid using it for children's fevers, in cases of kidney or liver disease or bleeding disorders, or with medications contraindicated with NSAIDs, including blood thinners. Using leaves without flowers produces a more tannin-rich, astringent, bitter tea that's a tad harder on the stomach.

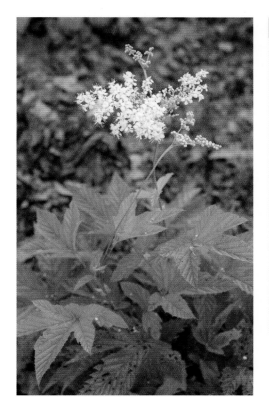

Harvesting, Preparing, and Using Meadowsweet

Harvest meadowsweet tops (leaves and flowers) just as the flowers come out, and be quick — they go by within *days*. Typically used dried.

Parts Used: aerial leaves and flowers

Tea: 1 teaspoon dried herb/cup, infusion, 1–3 cups daily

Tincture: 1–5 ml, 1–3 times daily, solo or in formula
- Fresh 1:2 in 95 percent alcohol (best) or dried 1:5 in 50–60 percent alcohol
- Add 10 percent glycerine to stabilize tannins and improve shelf life

Food: Add finely chopped leaves to fruit salad or a sprig to infused water for flavor

Topical: bath/soak

Recipes: Gut-Healing Tummy Tea, Take Two, page 152; Sore Muscle Bath, page 214

True to its name, meadowsweet tastes sweet, reminiscent of wintergreen, watermelon, and cherry, making a delightful tea.

MIMOSA

Albizia julibrissin

Legume Family (Fabaceae)

Body Systems: Mood, Nerve

   tree, Zones 6–9

INVASIVE BUT USEFUL

The mimosa tree — also called albizia and silk tree — doesn't get enough credit in Western herbal medicine even though it grows easily (sometimes *too* easily) across most of the United States. It's a *fantastic* mood-elevating plant. Check its status in your region and avoid planting it if it's invasive. It sprouts vigorously from seed. Wildcraft where it's overabundant. The leaves close at night and a little when you touch them. As girly as the pink blossoms appear, the fiber-opticlike filaments are not actually petals but a slew of stamens, the male reproductive part of the plant.

CALM AND HAPPY

True to its "collective happiness" name, mimosa may be the most broadly effective, fast-acting herb to lift the spirits, ease depression, and calm anxiety. Research on it is slim — highly preliminary lab and animal studies confirm antianxiety effects — but it has a long history of use in traditional Chinese medicine. Landscapers introduced it to America long ago, and herbalists David Winston and Michael Tierra are gradually raising awareness of its usefulness. The bark is more potent — fresh or freshly dried — though the delightful aromatic flowers can be used similarly. As a flower essence (page 68), mimosa improves your intuition, understanding, and sensitivity.

SAFE AS FAR AS WE KNOW

Mimosa has a long history of use in China and appears to be safe. Little modern data exists to determine whether it's safe alongside medications, including antidepressants and sedatives, so use caution.

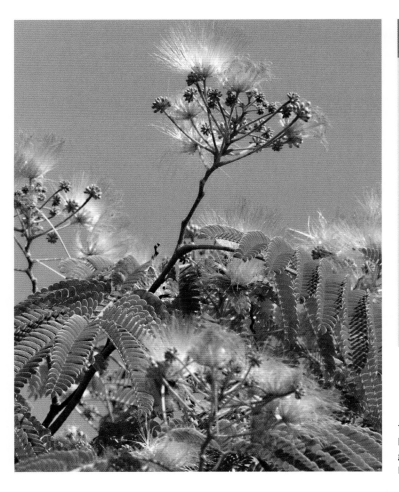

Harvesting, Preparing, and Using Mimosa

Prune and process the bark (page 25), preferably in spring or fall. Harvest flowers just as they open, taking care to dry them quickly and store carefully to keep them from turning brown. Use fresh or freshly dried.

Parts Used: bark (strongest), flowers

Tea: 1 teaspoon dried herb/cup, infusion, 1–3 cups daily

Tincture, Glycerite: 1–5 ml, 1–3 times daily, solo or in formula
- Fresh 1:2 in 95 percent alcohol (best) or (freshly) dried 1:5 in 50–60 percent alcohol

Recipes: Happy Tea, page 118; Good Mood Tincture, page 119

This stunning "tree of collective happiness" from Asia grows quickly into a graceful medium-sized tree with fragrant powder-puff pink blossoms.

MINT

Mentha spp.

Mint Family (Lamiaceae)

Body Systems: Digestive, Gut, Respiratory, Pain, Musculoskeletal, Mood, Nervous/Adrenal, Cognition/Brain

   perennial, Zones 5–9

LOVE-HATE HERB

Mint's so delicious, and abundant — sometimes *too* abundant. The root runners run rampant, getting messy and pushing out sensitive plants. Try growing it in a large pot with good soil and moisture. Or plant it out of the way where it can run amok or get mowed back. Peppermint (*M. x piperita*) and its variety chocolate mint are rich in menthol and most medicinal, but spearmint (*M. spicata*) and apple mint (*M. suaveolens*) offer milder medicine and earthy flavor. Most cultures have a favored mint, including my grandfather's mint from Italy or herb grower Lior Sadeh's beloved "nana" spearmint from Israel.

MENTHOL

Mint essential oils take center stage, particularly the abundant menthol in peppermint and chocolate mint. Menthol releases spasms, gas, pain, bloating, and muscle tension. Peppermint essential oil capsules reduced pain by 70 percent in children with irritable bowel syndrome. It also eases coughs and expectorates mucus. As a steam or air spray, it clears the sinuses and relieves sinus headaches. Apply topically to nix itches and ease headaches, back, foot, and neck pain. All mints increase digestion.

FLAVOR PUNCH

Aside from all their medicinal uses, we love mint for its flavor. Delicious on its own or improving the flavor of less-tasty herbs in blends. Mints also lift the spirits and improve cognitive function whether they're inhaled or consumed. Preliminary studies on spearmint tea found that it helped block excessive androgen production to lessen facial hair as well as polycystic ovary syndrome (PCOS) in women. As a flower essence (page 68), peppermint invigorates the mind and spirit while spearmint aids gentle detoxification.

USUALLY SAFE, WATCH REFLUX

Peppermint can aggravate reflux and heartburn because it kicks up digestive juices while relaxing the lower esophageal sphincter. Yet it *relieves* reflux for some — you'll know quickly which camp you're in. Go easy when using it for gastritis.

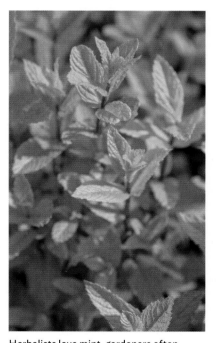

Herbalists love mint, gardeners often hate it. You've *got* to grow some, but put thought into how and where you want to plant it.

Harvesting, Preparing, and Using Mint

Harvest leafy growth anytime. Use fresh or dried. Peppermint tincture is strong — just use a little bit.

Parts Used: aerial/leaves

Tea: 1 teaspoon dried herb/cup, infusion, 1–3 cups daily

Tincture: 1–5 drops, 1–3 times daily, solo or in formula
• Fresh 1:2 in 95 percent alcohol

Glycerite, Syrup, Honey, Oxymel: 1 teaspoon as needed

Capsules/Powder: 500–2,000 mg crude herb daily

Food: with chocolate, lamb, jelly, fruit salad. Fresh in cocktails, cordials, seltzer, infused water. In various types of ethnic cuisine

Topical: liniment, bath/soak, compress, diluted essential oil, hydrosol

Recipes: Nutri-Tea, page 79; Yummy Teas, page 94; Floral Ice Cubes, page 96; Infused Seltzer, Soda, and Water, page 97; Brain-Boosting Tincture Blend, page 112; Minty Memory Tea, page 113; Sleep Tea, page 130; Chamomile-Mint Tea, page 147; Bee Balm-Mint Tea, page 171; Soothing Lung Tea, page 176; Nettle-Peppermint-Marshmallow Tea, page 183; Plantain-Yarrow Bite Rub, page 205

MOTHERWORT

Leonurus cardiaca

Mint Family (Lamiaceae)

Body Systems: Nervous, Mood, Reproductive, Cardiovascular

   perennial, Zones 3–8

MISCHIEVOUS SELF-SEEDER

Motherwort self-seeds rampantly and has a tendency to pop up unexpectedly in the garden where you did not plant it. Meanwhile it might not thrive where you *did* want it to grow. That said, it's easy to grow (and pull out), preferring good soil and moderate moisture. Mine does best in partial shade, but with the right soil, it's happy in full sun.

LION-HEARTED MOOD CARE

Motherwort's bitter, grounding energy provides excellent anxiety and panic attack relief. (I also love kava, but unless you live in Hawaii, it's not a backyard herb.) The Latin name translates to "lion hearted," which sums up motherwort's uses nicely. In anxiety and panic, it fosters courage, grounding the nerves and quelling overreactions within 10 to 15 minutes. Taken daily, it takes the edge off worry, frustration, and emotional rampages that occur when you're faced with never-ending demands, a lack of appreciation, and other people's messes. This is particularly common for mothers — Rosemary Gladstar says motherwort is for "mothers and people who need a little mothering" — though certainly its usefulness ranges across a broader audience. As a flower essence (page 68) and a tincture, motherwort helps you develop healthy boundaries so you can tend to your *own* care while still being warm and loving with others. I use it in formula for people with depression and those who have lost their spark for life — it blends well with other herbs in the Energy and Relaxation chapter (page 99). It does not appear to interact with antidepressant and antianxiety medications.

BRANCHING OUT

Motherwort also provides "lion-hearted" care by bridging cardiac-mood conditions. Consider it for panic attacks that feel like heart attacks, anxiety that you feel in the heart (tightening, palpitations, racing heartbeat), as well as mild cardiac conditions with a nervous component. For example, when hypertension, angina, or palpitations are mild and stress related, combining well with more overt heart tonics like hawthorn. It also works well alongside lemon balm and bugleweed to quell hyperthyroid disease including Graves' disease (this dangerous condition also requires a doctor's supervision). For the reproductive system, motherwort is a mild phytoestrogen that helps cool hot flashes and mood swings in perimenopause and PMS.

SAFE BUT BITTER

While generally safe, even for children, motherwort's strong bitter flavor makes it undesirable in tea and potentially nauseating in large doses. Don't use while pregnant due to its emmenagogue effect. In spite of its use in hyperthyroid disease, it's generally fine in hypothyroid conditions.

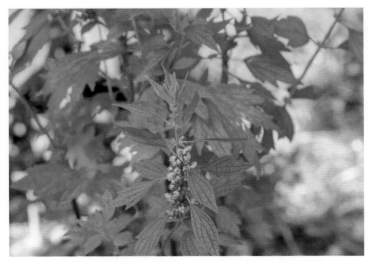

Motherwort looks scraggly, but when you get close up to its beautiful flowers, you'll feel its fierce, loving energy that takes the edge off anxiety and frustration.

Harvesting, Preparing, and Using Motherwort

Harvest aerial parts as it begins to bloom (it goes by quickly!), though you can also harvest it prebloom to add to another in-bloom batch. Vastly superior fresh. Best tinctured.

Parts Used: aerial/leaves and flowers

Tincture: 1–3 ml, 1–3 times daily, solo or in formula
• Fresh 1:2 in 95 percent alcohol

Glycerite, Syrup, Vinegar, Oxymel: 2–5 ml as needed

Recipes: Good Mood Tincture, page 119

MULLEIN

Verbascum thapsus

Figwort Family (Scrophulariaceae)

Body Systems: Respiratory, Immune, Musculoskeletal, Connective Tissue, Kidney/Urinary/Bladder, Prostate

  biennial, Zones 3–9

A COMMANDING PRESENCE

When in bloom, mullein is one of the easiest herbs to identify and attracts attention with its tall yellow flowering spike. It grows wild in fields and along roadsides and will plant itself in your garden and walkways, moving year to year. Buy seeds to sprinkle and introduce or save a few dead seed heads to shake around the yard during fall cleanup. Similar-looking species can be used interchangeably. Greek mullein (*V. olympicum*) and dense-flowered (*V. densiflorum*) both sport candelabra-style inflorescences, which make the tedious flower harvest somewhat easier.

SUPREME LUNG TONIC

Mullein moistens and opens irritated lungs, soothing inflammation in the respiratory tract. There's hardly a respiratory condition that wouldn't benefit from mullein leaf: use it to address everything from coughs, asthma, and irritation from things you shouldn't have inhaled to bronchitis, pneumonia, allergies, and chest colds. Mullein flower oil ear drops (often combined with St. John's wort, calendula, and possibly garlic) ease the pain of earaches, and the flowers can also be used as a respiratory tonic. I don't condone smoking herbs as a habit, but inhaling a smudge of mullein leaf quickly stops cough spasms. Place a leaf in your shoes to relieve sore feet, a trick I learned from Julie Bruton-Seal. The leaves also make serviceable toilet paper on camping trips, provided you don't get a skin rash from its hairs. As a flower essence (page 68), mullein connects people to their honesty and integrity, helping them make wise choices during moral dilemmas.

ROOT MEDICINE

Mullein root improves the integrity and "proper stretch" of connective tissue including tendons, ligaments, joints, the bladder, and the pelvic floor. Consider it internally and externally for tendonitis, arthritis, back pain, and dislocations — especially with Solomon's seal and horsetail. It's specific for pelvic floor weakness and incontinence (so is physical therapy), as well as benign prostatic hyperplasia (BPH), potentially combined with horsetail, saw palmetto, and/or corn silk.

SAFE, CORRECTLY IDENTIFIED

Mullein is extremely safe. Some people find the hairs irritating; strain well through a coffee filter, fine-woven cloth, or tea bag. Do not confuse mullein with the deadly foxglove plant. They look similar before they flower.

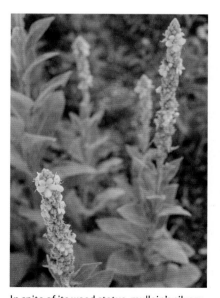

In spite of its weed status, mullein's silvery rosette of leaves and tall flowering stalk look lovely in the garden landscape.

Harvesting, Preparing, and Using Mullein

Harvest different parts — leaf, flowers, root — of this biennial herb in different stages of its life cycle. Snip happy leaves any time. Dig up roots before it sets a flower stalk, preferably in spring or fall. Bigger plants have bigger roots. Pinch off new flowers. Use fresh or dried.

Parts Used: leaves, flowers, root

Tea: 1 teaspoon dried leaves herb/cup, infusion, 1–3 cups daily. Strain hairs well.

Tincture: 2–5 ml leaf/flower or 0.5–2 ml root, 1–3 times daily, solo or in formula
• Fresh 1:2 in 95 percent alcohol (best) or dried 1:5 in 50–60 percent alcohol

Glycerite, Syrup: ½–1 teaspoon as needed, solo or in formula

Topical: flower oil ear drops, root liniment, leaf poultice

Recipes: Soothing Lung Tea, page 176; Allergy Tincture Blend, page 182; Aches and Pains, Strains and Springs Tincture/Liniment, page 220

NETTLE

Urtica dioica

Nettle Family (Urticaceae)

Body Systems: Nutritive, Bones, Reproductive, Kidney/Urinary, Detoxification, Respiratory

  perennial, Zones 5–9

NUISANCE OR BELOVED?

Stinging nettle may be the bane of gardeners and hikers when it hits them with fire ant–like venom from its stinging hairs. Yet it's a beloved tonic and a nutritious foodlike medicinal herb. Nettles spread via root runners and seed in damp, rich soil and dappled sunlight on stream-banks, pastures, and compost piles. Wildcraft or cultivate it in moist, rich soil in an out-of-the-way spot. Caterpillars love to munch on nettles in summer — more reason to harvest leaves early. The leaves (but not the roots) of other *Urtica* species can be used relatively interchangeably.

VITAL GREEN MINERALS

Once dried, cooked, or frozen, nettle loses its sting and transforms into a superfood green. It's one of the most mineral-dense plants on the planet, conveniently devoid of antinutrients like oxalic acid. Per ounce, nettle supplies approximately 100 percent of your recommended daily intake of calcium and 60 percent of the magnesium you need, as well as some potassium, iron, and silica and a good dose of green-power chlorophyll with amazingly better bioavailability than dairy and most wild greens. Nettle makes a good base for simmered herbal chai spices, broths, and flavorful infusions with peppermint, lemongrass, or holy basil.

ADDITIONAL PERKS

A notable antihistamine, nettle is often used as a fresh leaf tincture for acute and chronic allergies or sipped in a dried leaf tea for long-term support. Its gentle astringency and mineral content address heavy menstrual bleeding. As a diuretic kidney tonic, it flushes wastes, including uric acid, out of the kidneys, helping with gout. The roots tone the prostate, bladder, and pelvic floor. Use them in formula with saw palmetto and pumpkin seeds for benign prostatic hyperplasia (BPH) in men. Blend the root with horsetail, saw palmetto, mullein root, and/or yellow pond lily root tinctures to strengthen the bladder and pelvic floor in cases of incontinence. Try seeds as food for nervous-adrenal and kidney support. Whacking sore joints with the fresh plant (stings!) relieves arthritis pain temporarily (once the hives go away) by boosting the body's anti-inflammatory response. As a flower essence (page 68), it creates healthy boundaries and protects us in toxic situations and relationships.

SAFER THAN SPINACH

Treat nettle as food, even in large doses. That said, it doesn't agree with everyone. Some find the diuretic effect too drying or the spinachy flavor too vegetal (try oatstraw, marshmallow leaf, or violet leaf instead). Idiosyncratic negative responses happen periodically. Stick to spring nettle greens; leaves harvested after nettle flowers may *irritate* the kidneys.

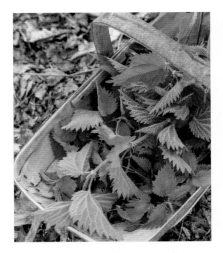

Nettle's name comes from the medical term for hives ("urticaria"), which is what it will inflict on your skin if you let its fresh syringelike hairs zap you.

Harvesting, Preparing, and Using Nettle

Harvest carefully or wear thick gloves and long sleeves and pants to avoid getting stung. Gather tops in spring before they flower. Dig roots in fall.

Parts Used: Leaves, roots, seeds (different uses)

Tea: 1 teaspoon to ¼ ounce of leaves per cup, steeped or simmered 15 minutes to several hours, 1–4 cups per day.

Tincture: 0.5–2 ml, 1–3 times daily, solo or in formula
- Fresh leaves or roots 1:2 in 95 percent alcohol
- Dried roots 1:5 in 50–60 percent alcohol

Powder/Capsules: up to 30 g (1 ounce) powdered leaves in food, including smoothies and honey–nut butter balls

Recipes: Chai Base, page 78; Nettle-Oat Super Infusion, page 78; Nutri-Tea, page 79; Nutri-Broth, page 80; Multimineral Vinegar, page 86; Mineral-Rich "Coffee" Syrup, page 87; Nutri-Detox Tea, page 159; Allergy Tincture Blend, page 182; Nettle-Peppermint-Marshmallow Tea, page 183

OAT

Avena sativa

Grass Family (Poaceae)

Body Systems: Nervous/Adrenal, Nutritive, Bones, Skin, Connective Tissue

 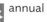 annual

A COVER CROP WITH PURPOSE

Oats offer three forms of herbal medicine — grain, milky oat seed, and oatstraw — each with different applications, yet sharing the same ability to nourish and soothe. People rarely grow it in the garden (and processing oatmeal is too tedious for most gardeners), but it's a great cover crop that doubles as medicine. Consider growing oat in a new or old garden bed, or behind shorter plants in the landscape. After the threat of frost, rough up the soil surface, and thickly scatter the seeds. (I use a 5-pound bag for the previous year's 25-by-25-foot chicken run.) Tamp them in lightly. Water periodically if you don't have regular rainfall. Oats will die off in winter and enrich the soil.

NOURISHING AND RESTORATIVE

Milky oat seed nourishes the adrenal-nervous system to soothe, calm, rebuild, and nourish. Think of it as food for the nerves, and take it in regular moderately high doses for months to get the best effects. It's specifically indicated for when you feel burnt out, wired, and tired, and it combines well with calm-energy adaptogens and gentle nervines in blends. As a flower essence (page 68), oat helps restless souls convert tentative ideas into direction and find a meaningful path in life.

Oatstraw is about four times more nutrient-dense than oatmeal, providing calcium, silica, magnesium, and potassium. Use it for healthy hair, skin, and nails and to heal broken bones, and as a pleasant lightly sweet haylike background flavor for delicate yet flavorful herbs like lemongrass and Korean mint.

SAFE, BUT CELIACS BEWARE

Milky oat seed and oatstraw are safe and foodlike, often used in high doses. Oats do not contain gluten, and when you grow your own, you don't need to worry about gluten contamination. That said, oats contain glutenlike proteins called avenins that some people may react to. If you know you react to oatmeal, skip all forms of oat.

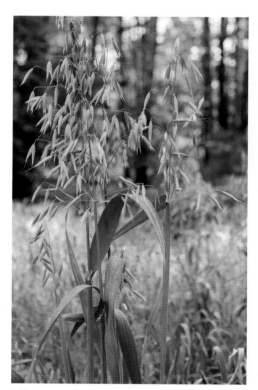

Milky oat seeds are ready only for a few days of the year. White latex should spurt out when you squish and pop them.

Harvesting, Preparing, and Using Oats

Milky Oat Seed: Squeeze a few in the plot to ensure they're ready — they should pop and exude a milky latex. Then run your hands up each stalk so the seeds slide off between your fingers. To extract the seeds, whir them in a blender with alcohol, vinegar, glycerine, or water. Fresh only. Once dried, they're more like oatstraw.

Oatstraw: When the plant is vital, green, and happy (perhaps directly after you harvest the milky seeds), cut one-third to two-thirds of the grassy tops. Dry. Then use sharp, sturdy scissors to chop it into pieces. Extract vastly more minerals by simmering or making a super infusion.

Tea (Oatstraw): 1 teaspoon to ¼ ounce dried herb/cup; infusion, super infusion, or decoction, 1–4 cups daily. Nice in super infusions as well as simmering broths

Tincture (Milky Seed): 2–5 ml, 1–3 times daily, solo or in formula
• Fresh 1:2 in 95 percent alcohol or vinegar (best) or glycerine

Recipes: Nettle-Oat Super Infusion, page 78; with Chai Base, page 78; Nutri-Tea, page 79; Nutri-Broth, page 80; Milky Seed–Milky Oats Tincture, page 106; Stress Support Tincture Blend, page 107; Mellow Me Glycerite, page 125

OREGANO

Origanum vulgare

Mint Family (Lamiaceae)

Body Systems: Immune, Respiratory, Digestive, Gut, Skin, Antimicrobial

   perennial, Zones 4–8

MEDITERRANEAN HEAT LOVER

The use of oregano as an integral medicinal and culinary herb originated in the Mediterranean region and eventually spread around the world. Many cultivars exist, and growing conditions also influence the flavor and potency. Nibble a leaf — you want a hot, spicy, pungent bite. You can grow oregano in a pampered garden bed, but a sunny, semidry spot bumps up the potency. Here in New Hampshire, where the heat of summer doesn't last long, I find it challenging to grow really strong oregano.

PUNGENT ANTIMICROBIAL

Winter savory, summer savory, and bee balm (especially *M. fistulosa*) can stand in for oregano and tend to be more reliably potent. (Marjoram, while closely related, lacks the antimicrobial punch.) Bee balm (page 249) remains my favorite due to its beauty and prolific growth, and medicinally it's more of a mix between oregano and thyme. Likewise, you can use oregano as a general aromatic antimicrobial. All these herbs open, warm, and disinfect the lungs, relieve sinus infections, address stomach bugs and yeast infections, and can also be applied topically to treat infections, wounds, and fungus.

CULINARY QUEEN

Being half Sicilian, I go through more oregano in my kitchen than any other culinary herb. It's not only essential for southern Italian cuisine and pizza but also Latin American and Middle Eastern fare. It pairs well with ground meat, sausage, lamb, chicken, and grilled fish like sea bass, as well as white beans, chili, tomatoes, hot peppers, eggplant, curdito, feta, garlic, cumin, and paprika. Simultaneously antimicrobial and antioxidant-rich, oregano preserves food and extends its shelf life and improves the digestibility of old meat and fatty dishes. Oregano and friends boost digestion in general and help with gas and bloating — perhaps that's why it's so popular in bean chili.

SAFE BUT HOT AND DRY

Oregano and friends are safe for most people, children, and animals. It's often used as an essential oil — far more potent — but crude herbal formulas work extremely well with even greater safety. That said, it's a hot, dry herb more suited for sluggish, cold, damp, stagnant conditions and people and less for hot and dry circumstances where it might irritate instead (for example: respiratory conditions, gut health).

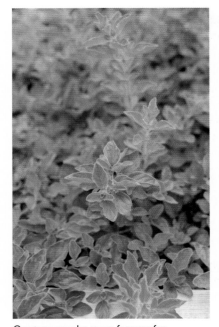

Oregano may be more famous for medicine, but bee balm makes an equally effective and more prolific substitute.

Harvesting, Preparing, and Using Oregano

Trim happy aerial parts, preferably before it flowers. Taste your plant periodically to see when it's most pungent — likely after a hot, dry spell. Use fresh or dried.

Parts Used: aerial/leaves

Tea: ½–1 teaspoon dried herb/cup, infusion, 1–3 cups daily

Tincture: 1–3 ml, 1–3 times daily. solo or in formula
- Fresh 1:2 in 95 percent alcohol (best) or dried 1:5 in 50–60 percent alcohol

Syrup, Honey, Vinegar, Oxymel, Glycerite: 1 teaspoon as needed

Capsules/Powder: 500–2,000 mg crude herb daily

Food: liberally in food (see above), broth, pesto, hummus

Topical: oil (preferably alcohol-intermediary), bath/soak, compress, liniment, vinegar

Recipes: Dandelion-Violet Weed Pesto, page 88; Bee Balm-Mint Tea, page 171; Ick Stick Thuja Salve, page 199

PASSIONFLOWER

Passiflora incarnata

Passionflower Family
(Passifloraceae)

Body Systems: Nervous, Mood,
Cardiovascular, Respiratory

   perennial,
Zones 6–9

OTHERWORLDLY TROPICAL

Passionflower rambles somewhat invasively across the southeastern states, putting forth stunning blooms and edible maypop passionfruit. Many species exist, but trust only *P. incarnata* for medicinal use — other species may lack the safety and benefits. It has white petals, a purple crown, and three-lobed leaves. Seek the plant from a trustworthy source. I've seen it labeled incorrectly even by herb growers, but you can trust Strictly Medicinal Seeds for spring-shipped seedlings. Protect it in winter in Zone 6 (the very edge of its range). Plant in a protected spot or bring it indoors where it does nicely in a pot, blooming through winter.

NATURAL SEDATIVE

As one of our most reliable, safe sedatives, passionflower brings deep sleep. In studies, it was more effective and broad-acting for insomnia compared to other popular sleep herbs, particularly in blends. It's specific for people who can't shut off their brains due to mind chatter. People prone to anger, frustration, and frenetic energy usually find it a lovely calming, cooling remedy. It can be useful for anxiety solo or in formula, but it may make some people too sleepy, sluggish, or even depressed.

CALMING ALL OVER

Passionflower gently calms many body systems and can be employed for digestive, cardiac, and respiratory issues related to tension, anxiety, stress, or agitation — for example, stress-induced asthma and hypertension. Perfect for formulas. As a flower essence (page 68), passionflower helps connect you to the divine within yourself and follow your creative passions. Simply staring at the mandala-like flower will help you relax and find peace.

SAFE SEDATIVE

While safe for children, adults, and elders, you'll want to start with low doses to gauge your personal response and ensure it's not *too* sedating (making you groggy, sluggish, depressed, or sleepy during the day).

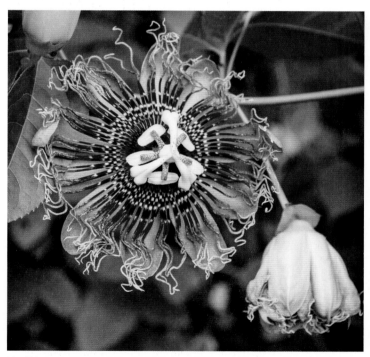

You'll be mesmerized by passionflower's otherworldly blooms and heavenly aroma. Its name originated with Spanish missionaries in the New World who used the parts of the flower to illustrate their teachings about the Passion of Christ.

Harvesting, Preparing, and Using Passionflower

Cut back aerial parts, preferably while in flower. Use fresh or freshly dried.

Parts Used: aerial/vine, leaves, flowers

Tea: 1 teaspoon dried herb/cup, infusion, 1–3 cups daily or at night

Tincture: 1–5 ml, 1–3 times daily, solo or in formula
• Fresh 1:2 in 95 percent alcohol (best) or dried 1:5 in 50–60 percent alcohol

Syrup, Glycerite, Oxymel: 1 teaspoon as needed

Capsules/Powder: 250–1,000 mg crude herb as needed

Recipes: Mellow Me Glycerite, page 125; Sleep Tea, page 130; Sleep Tinctures, page 131; Soothing Lung Tea, page 176; Peaceful Heart Tea, page 231

PLANTAIN

Plantago major

Plantain Family (Plantaginaceae)

Body Systems: Respiratory, Gut, Skin, Immune

  perennial, Zones 3–10

WHITE MAN'S FOOTPRINT

European explorers intentionally and unintentionally brought this medicinal potherb weed with them to the Americas; however, native species were already here. Plantain likes to grow where people walk — along pathways, in lawns, through sidewalks. The better the soil, the bigger the leaves will grow. With its stringy-veined wide basal leaves and upright seed stalk, this first aid plant helps children quickly learn to identify it. Interchangeable plantain species include Northeast native (*P. rugelii,* often confused with *P. major*) and the almost ornamental English plantain (*P. lanceolata*).

FIRST AID CARE

Best known for first aid, the fresh leaf poultice quickly and effectively draws out venom, splinters, and irritation when applied quickly to bug bites, bee stings, and poison ivy. It may even avert an allergic reaction (but still use your EpiPen). The infused oil, vinegar, or low-alcohol tincture spray has a subtler anti-itch effect for poison ivy and rashes. Alder leaf (*Alnus* spp.) can be substituted.

DEMULCENT ASTRINGENT

Underrated for its other uses, plantain leaf has gentle demulcent and astringent properties without being overly slimy. It's perfect in gut healing teas, and lung soothing recipes, including broth. The leaves make serviceable food — ground into pesto, cooked, baked like kale chips — if you can get past the stringy veins (similar to celery's). The seed heads can be dried and ground for soluble fiber and a grainlike substance much like its relative psyllium, but it's tedious to harvest.

VERY SAFE

This plant agrees with almost everyone and is safe as food. Be sure of what you're harvesting. Before it blooms, English plantain is less distinctive looking than other species and could be mistaken for several other plants, including a deadly narrow-leafed foxglove.

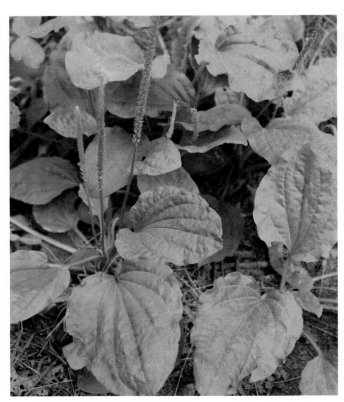

This underrated weed pops up in lawns and pavement cracks. It does far more than quell bug bites and bee stings.

Harvesting, Preparing, and Using Plantain

Harvest happy leaves anytime. Use fresh or dried.

Parts Used: leaves

Tea: 1 teaspoon dried herb/cup, infusion, 1–3 cups daily

Tincture: 2–5 ml, 1–3 times daily, solo or in formula
- Fresh 1:2 in 95 percent alcohol or dried 1:5 in 50–60 percent alcohol

Glycerite, Syrup: 1 teaspoon as needed

Food: in broth, as a cooked or raw green (not amazing)

Topical: poultice (especially fresh), oil, salve, liniment, vinegar, bath, compress

Recipes: Soothing Lung Tea, page 176; Nettle-Peppermint-Mallow Tea, page 183; Super Skin Salve, page 198; Plantain Salve, page 198; First Aid Simple: Plantain Oil, page 199; Plantain Poultice, page 205; Plantain-Yarrow Bite Rub, page 205

RASPBERRY

Rubus idaeus

Rose Family (Rosaceae)

Body Systems: Reproductive, Gut, Skin, Mouth, Nutritive

   perennial, Zones 4–8

BRAMBLE BERRY

Raspberries amble easily via underground root runners that are a bane in the garden but not so bad in the wilder edges of your property. It has fine bristly "thorns," pinnately compound leaves, and red berries with a hollow center. For medicine, use wild raspberry, which does not produce a lot of fruit — it has better leaves. Perennial roots put forth biennial canes. Harvest leaves from the first-year canes in late spring/early summer: bright, happy leaves, green stems. The stems get woodier as they enter the second year, which is when they produce flowers and fruit. Good raspberry leaves have a fruity tang when you nibble them.

ROSE-FAMILY TONER

A gentle tonic plant — yet another rose-family astringent — raspberry leaves contain mild tannins that tighten, tone, and astringe the tissues. Like the leaves of many in the rose family (strawberry, blackberry, lady's mantle, cinquefoil), raspberry leaf makes a tea that tastes a bit like true tea but comes without the caffeine and was common in "Liberty Tea" blends during the American Revolution. Raspberry improves the muscle tone of the uterus and lining. Considered a tonic at any stage of a woman's life, it facilitates childbirth and recuperation after pregnancy. It tones the skin, gut, mouth, gums, and possibly the prostate, and helps stanch diarrhea, vaginal discharge, heavy menstrual flow, and mild (non-life-threatening) gastrointestinal or uterine bleeding. Many plants in the *Rubus* genus can be used as astringents with varying strength. Blackberry (*R. fruticosus* and *R. allegheniensis*) roots help stanch diarrhea in dysentery and cranky bowel flare-ups. It's quite nice infused in blackberry brandy or wine!

NUTRITIVE TEA

Raspberry leaves contain appreciable levels of vitamin C, bioflavonoids, iron, and calcium and make a nice nutritive tea base, particularly for women. Of course the edible, often delicious, *Rubus* berries are loaded with antioxidants. As a flower essence (page 68), raspberry brings forgiveness while blackberry manifests thoughts and desires into reality.

SAFE BUT ASTRINGENT

Generally very safe, even in modest doses (not super infusions) during pregnancy and for children. However, the astringency may upset sensitive stomachs, especially without food or sweetener, and could be mildly constipating if drunk in excess. Theoretically, the tannins might reduce mineral absorption. Although blackberry root is excellent for both acute and chronic diarrhea, note that diarrhea may serve a purpose (flushing out pathogens) or need to be examined by a medical doctor so that the root cause can also be addressed.

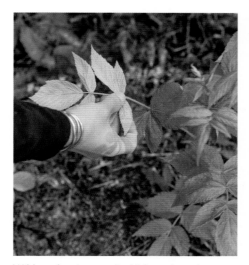

Wild raspberries grow in thickets along the edges of forests and yards. The leaves can easily be harvested in abundance. Note the white underside of the leaf.

Harvesting, Preparing, and Using Raspberry

Trim leaves from first-year canes (described above). Wearing gloves is advised to avoid splinters from the prickles, especially when processing the dried herb. Use as tea. For blackberry roots, trim back the plant so you can access the soil, then dig up the long, thin root runners. Often extracted as a tincture or similar extract.

Parts Used: raspberry leaves, blackberry root, berries

Tea (leaves): 1 teaspoon or more dried herb/cup, infusion, 1–3 cups daily

Tincture, Glycerite, Syrup, Cordial (roots): 1–5 ml, 1–3 times daily, solo or in formula
- Fresh 1:2 in 95 percent alcohol or dried 1:5 in 50–60 percent alcohol
- Add 10 percent glycerine to stabilize tannins and improve shelf life

Food: Enjoy the berries!

Recipes: Nutri-Tea, page 79; Lady Tea, page 243

RED CLOVER

Trifolium pratense

Legume Family (Fabaceae)

Body Systems: Reproductive, Lymph, Detoxification, Immune

   perennial, Zones 5–9

COVER CROP WEED

Red clover grows wild in lawns, fields, and meadows and along sunny woodland paths, and farmers plant it as a cover crop to fix nitrogen and bring nutrients into the soil. Red clover has purple-magenta blossoms, hairy stems, and green leaves often grouped in threes, with a greenish white triangle or V on each leaf. It's easy to wildcraft, but you can also plant it in your lawn on the edge of the property (it won't produce flowers if you mow it) or incorporate it into areas sown with milky oats. Unlike oats, clover won't die in winter and will need to be plowed into the soil if you need to clear it for a future garden bed.

MINERALS, PHYTOESTROGEN

Red clover blossoms contain phytoestrogenic isoflavones including biochanin A as well as daidzein and its metabolite equol, which are not as potent as soy phytoestrogens but serviceable. Phytoestrogens — common in legumes — bind preferentially to estrogen receptor sites, blocking the production of natural estrogen but are much weaker (possessing less than 1 percent of the strength of your body's natural estrogen), making them useful for managing an overabundance of estrogen and as a minor source of estrogen during postmenopause, when levels would be low. With long-term use, it relieves hot flashes, night sweats, and tender breasts (mastalgia). As a phytoestrogen *and* a source of calcium and other nutrients, it's added to nourishing infusions for strong bones. Studies show that red clover isoflavones prevent bone from breaking down as quickly during postmenopause and improve the efficacy of calcium, magnesium, and calcitrol. Gut bacteria improve the potency, and some research suggests that taking probiotics helps, too.

LYMPH MOVER, CANCER FIGHTER?

As a tea or tincture, red clover and other clovers improve lymph flow, draining edema, lymph swellings, and clearing skin conditions via "blood purification." It's added to alterative detoxification blends for this reason. Perhaps related to this (many immune cells reside in the lymph), red clover has a long-standing reputation for fighting cancer. It appears in several controversial formulas including Hoxey's and some variations of Essiac. Highly preliminary lab studies support its use as an antiproliferative that also induces cancer cell death. Some studies suggest red clover inhibits breast cancer cells while others find that it fuels them. As a flower essence (page 68), red clover helps people think for themselves in the face of group influence or mob mentality.

PREPARATION PROBLEMS

Dried red clover is generally safe for most people. Its effects in estrogen-dependent cancer are unclear. Proper harvesting and drying is important. Red clover forms toxic coumarins if it dries too slowly or ferments, and clover infected with black patch fungus may contain the mycotoxin slaframine. Both can be deadly to grazing animals but human exposure to toxic doses rarely occurs. See drying tips below to limit these risks.

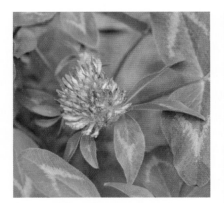

Pretty red clover blossoms taste pleasant in tea and look lovely in dried blends. Home-harvested clover surpasses anything you can buy.

Harvesting, Preparing, and Using Red Clover

Pinch off the colorful young flowers with the top leaves, preferably in the morning. Only use happy-looking red clover. Process fresh immediately for tinctures. Dry thoroughly and quickly in the dehydrator.

Parts Used: flower heads with top three leaves

Tea: 1 tablespoon dried herb/cup, infusion, 1–3 cups daily

Tincture: 1–5 ml, 1–3 times daily, solo or in formula
• Fresh 1:2 in 95 percent alcohol (best) or dried 1:5 in 50–60 percent alcohol

Food: fresh flowers taste nice as a garnish

Recipes: Nutri-Tea, page 79; Lady Tea, page 243

ROSE

Rosa spp.

Rose Family (Rosaceae)

Body Systems: Nutritive, Mood, Nerve, Cardiovascular, Gut, Skin, Reproductive

 perennial, Zones 2–7 (depending on species)

FINDING A GOOD ROSE

There are *hundreds* of rose species. Opt for wild and heirloom species with fragrant flowers and/or plump, red hips. Favorites include seaside (*R. rugosa*), dog rose (*R. canina*), Damask (*R. damascena*), apothecary (*R. gallica* var. *officinalis*), and cabbage (*R. centifolia*). Forage invasive multiflora rose (*R. multiflora*), but don't plant it. Roses do best in full sun with periodic pruning or thinning. Hedge roses can get invasive, so keep them on the edge of your yard or sprawling along a wall.

ASTRINGENT AROMATIC

The leaves and flowers of this family (raspberry, lady's mantle, strawberry) contain gentle astringent tannins, safe enough for regular use to tighten and tone tissues, mucous membranes, skin (toner), and the gut (leaky gut, diarrhea). They're employed in midwifery in various stages of pregnancy and labor to prepare the uterus for birth, stanch bleeding, and help lady bits heal. Rose additionally offers aromatic essential oils that nourish and relax irritated or damaged tissues (uterus, skin) while calming the mind, gladdening the heart, and uplifting the spirits. Rose's aromatics foster self-love and heal the heart after trauma. Sprinkle petals in tea, cold water, honey, or glycerine in cool, long-term infusions to maximize aromatics. Alcohol and hot water extract more of the bitter, astringent tannins.

ANTIOXIDANT FRUITS

Much like its relatives (raspberry, strawberry, apple, hawthorn), roses also produce nutritious antioxidant- and bioflavonoid-rich fruits. Rose hips may taste fruity, tart, slightly sweet, or tomatoey. Fresh, they provide ample vitamin C, but vitamin C dissipates with drying, cooking, and storage. You'll retain 45 times more vitamin C in a jam than tea. Bioflavonoids persist well and help you get more out of the vitamin C. Together, they support immune function, connective tissue repair, and wound healing. They also promote heart health and decrease inflammation. In flower essences (page 68), the blossoms help workaholics stop and smell the roses, aid healing from traumatic experiences, and heal the emotional heart.

SAFE FOR MOST PEOPLE

Roses are quite safe, but strongly brewed flowers may be too astringent and drying for some, leading to constipation or nausea. Some people simply don't like the aroma.

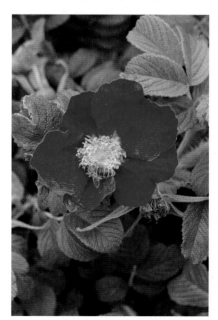

Fancy roses are prone to disease and hardier ones ramble out of control, but they nonetheless remain the most eye-catching, beloved herbs in the landscape.

Harvesting, Preparing, and Using Rose

Use flowers and hips fresh or dry (in a dehydrator). Pinch off blooms or pull petals, preferably in the morning. Gather rose hips in fall when they're ripe and tasty. Check for bugs. Dry whole small or cut large hips. Once they're cut, you'll need to scoop out seeds or strain through a fine cloth.

Parts Used: flowers, petals, hips (different uses)

Tea: ½–1 teaspoon dried herb/cup, infusion, 1–3 cups daily

Glycerite, Syrup, Honey, Oxymel, Vinegar, Hydrosol: 1 teaspoon

Food: Hips as jam, jelly, juiced. Flowers as a garnish and infused in water

Topical (Flowers): glycerite, hydrosol, tea spritz, bath/soak

Recipes (Flowers): Yummy Teas, page 94; Infused Soda, Seltzer, and Water, page 97; Holy Rose Water, page 107; Stress Support Tincture Blend, page 107; Happy Tea, page 118; Good Mood Tincture, page 119; Rose Glycerite, page 119; Mellow Me Glycerite, page 125; Gut-Healing Tummy Tea, Take One, page 152; Rose Hydrosol, page 192; Calendula-Comfrey Cream, page 193; Lady Tea, page 243

Recipes (Rose Hips): Darcey Blue's Elderberry Syrup, page 168; Elder–Rose Hip Oxymel, page 169

ROSEMARY

Rosmarinus officinalis

Mint Family (Lamiaceae)

Body Systems: Cognition/
Brain, Inflammation/Pain,
Nerve, Immune, Respiratory,
Cardiovascular, Digestive, Skin

  tender perennial,
Zones 8–11

FINICKY BUT WORTH IT

Rosemary's one of the more finicky
herbs to grow, yet we love it so much
that almost *everyone* still plants it
each spring. It grows wild along the
Mediterranean coast and likes hot,
dry conditions (overwatering rots
it as does high humidity). Plant it
in a sunny, well-drained, minimally
watered bed — perhaps alongside
cayenne, lavender, horehound, or
California poppy — or in a container.
Terra-cotta pots look great and help
achieve its favored growing conditions. Harvest it all or bring it indoors
before frost. Do not overwater, but
consider misting it periodically.

INVIGORATING AROMATIC

Rosemary works for the immune
and respiratory systems, like thyme,
bee balm, and oregano, with a hint
of eucalyptus. Yet it leans in other
directions for which it's better known:
anti-inflammatory COX-2 inhibi-
tion for pain relief and heart health,
circulation support, and cognition
enhancement. Studies show that
inhaling the herb or consuming small
foodlike doses perks up memory,
focus, and mental clarity, confirming
a long history of use of "rosemary for
remembrance."

STIMULATING BY NATURE

Rosemary's stimulating in nature
(not like caffeine but because it
turns on the body's systems) and
profoundly antioxidant, making it an
excellent culinary and tea ingredient
to improve digestion, particularly with
heavy, fatty, or protein-rich meals.
Topically it also invigorates, improves
circulation, repels insects, and helps
relieve pain. As a flower essence
(page 68), rosemary perks up the
brain and brings zest and joy to life.

SAFE IN LOW DOSES

This is safe but potent and best as
a synergist in blends (1 to 5% of the
formula), or enjoy one or two fresh
sprigs per day in food or tea.

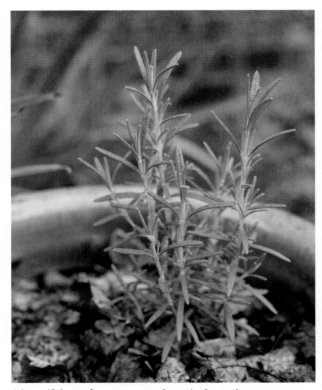

A beautiful pot of rosemary stands out in the garden, prevents
the plant from getting too wet, and makes it easy to bring it
indoors for winter.

Harvesting, Preparing, and Using Rosemary

Harvest any time via "heading" or "thinning" cuts
(page 25) depending on how you want to affect
its growth pattern. If the stems are woody, remove
them during processing. Best fresh, vaguely
serviceable dried.

Parts Used: aerial/leaves

Tea: 1 teaspoon dried herb/cup, infusion,
1–3 cups daily

Tincture: 1–5 drops, 1–3 times daily, solo or in formula
• Fresh 1:2 in 95 percent alcohol

Capsules/Powder: 200–750 mg crude herb daily

Food: fresh sprig or two daily in food, drink

Topical: oil (preferably alcohol-intermediary), liniment, soak/bath, compress, vinegar

Recipes: Dandelion-Violet Weed Pesto, page 88;
Stress Support Tincture Blend, page 107; Brain-
Boosting Tincture Blend, page 112; Minty Memory
Tea, page 113; Rosemary-Lemon Tea, page 113; Herbal
Insect Repellent, page 204; Heart Tonic Tincture
Blend, page 237

SAGE

Salvia officinalis

Mint Family (Lamiaceae)

Body Systems: Cognition/Brain, Digestive, Immune, Antimicrobial, Reproductive, Skin, Respiratory

  perennial, Zones 4–8

A GARDEN GUARDIAN

Herbalists plant sage in their gardens not only for culinary and medicinal purposes but also for its long-held reputation for bringing wisdom and protection to the property. Native to the Mediterranean, sage likes it warm and dry and will do well near "like-minded" herbs including lavender, horehound, thyme, and rosemary. It may die off after a few years, especially if it gets too cold or damp. Older happy plants produce beautiful purple flowers throughout most of the growing season. Several other species of sage have similar properties but are rarely winter-hardy.

DRY, ANTIMICROBIAL, AROMATIC

Sage shares medicinal benefits with close relatives lavender, rosemary, oregano, and thyme, yet it has its own special affinities. It's profoundly drying and helps with conditions of excess secretions: heavy perspiration from stress, daytime hot flashes, or overactive sweat glands; night sweats; and postlactation leaking. It affects hormones by providing plant estrogen and inhibiting prolactin. As an antimicrobial, it's useful in a variety of forms: a gargle for sore throats, a foot powder for sweaty feet and fungus, an antiseptic vinegar spray for countertops. As an aromatic, whether you take it internally or inhale its aroma, sage provides wisdom by perking up cognitive function and helping to fight the effects of aging on the brain. Anti-inflammatory aromatic properties also make it useful for cold, achy joint pain and arthritis, especially with lemon and ginger. Sage, a bitter carminative, improves digestion, fights intestinal pathogens, and makes it easier to digest fat.

AUTUMN CUISINE

Most people recognize sage as a culinary herb, yet it often sits unused in most herb gardens and spice racks. To be fair, it's pretty potent. Just a little bit brings an earthy-herbaceous-aromatic flavor to chicken, turkey stuffing, and other poultry dishes. I recommend frying the fresh leaves in a little butter or olive oil. This mellows and transforms the flavor. It tastes *amazing* with autumn cuisine: winter squash, bread, mushrooms, white beans, eggs, butternut ravioli, creamy soups, and chowder. As a flower essence (page 68), sage brings wisdom and understanding of the lessons of the planet.

LOW-DOSE HERB

This potent herb is best used in low to modest quantities or occasional use. Its hormonal influences may not always be appropriate, and there is concern over its thujone content, a controversial constituent that may be toxic to the kidneys and liver in large quantities and will be more concentrated in the essential oil. (Some say Spanish sage [*S. lavandulaefolia*] — also studied for cognitive benefits — contains minimal thujone. Not exactly, but it has about half that of garden sage.)

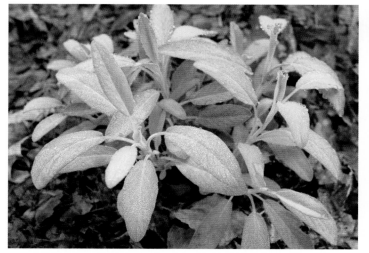

Almost everyone grows sage in their herb gardens, but people often feel challenged in how to use it.

Harvesting, Preparing, and Using Sage

Trim fresh sprigs of leaves. Use fresh or dried.

Parts Used: leaves

Tea: ¼ teaspoon dried herb or 1 small sprig/cup, infusion, 1–2 cups daily

Tincture: 5–20 drops, 1–3 times daily, solo or in formula
• Fresh 1:2 in 95 percent alcohol (best) or dried 1:5 in 50–60 percent alcohol

Food: Fresh, fried, or dried (see above)

Topical: oil, salve, bath/soak, powdered, vinegar, liniment

ST. JOHN'S WORT

Hypericum perforatum

St. John's Wort Family
(Hypericaceae)

Body Systems: Mood, Nervous,
Pain, Immune, Antiviral

  perennial,
Zones 3–8

PLANT OF THE SUN

Everything about St. John's wort revolves around the sun. Its yellow flowers grow in dry, hot, sunny spots in compact soil, bloom near summer solstice (and the feast of St. John), and will be most potent harvested after a hot-as-Hades week. Rub a fresh bud to see the maroon smear and get an idea of the plant's potency. Put your oil or tincture in the sun, where it will macerate, activating the hyperforins, red pigments from the plant that will gradually turn your extract from yellow to blood red and intensify its therapeutic properties. The redder the better. Hold the leaves up to the sun and look *very* closely to see the "perforation" of light and black dots. Although it'll grow in part shade, St. John's wort prefers and will be more potent in full sun. It tolerates drought and is considered invasive in some states. In the garden, it moves around, self-seeding and dying off, alternating boom and bust years. Find baby plants in early spring in untended spots (e.g., neglected lawns, abandoned lots) to move into your garden.

SUNNY MOOD, NERVE TONIC

St. John's wort brings the sun in. Best known as an antidepressant, it acts much like an selective serotonin reuptake inhibitor (SSRI) drug to slowly boost levels of serotonin and other neurotransmitters that uplift mood. It works best in seasonal affective disorder and mild to moderate depression and can be combined with other treatment protocols for major depression. Expect results to kick in after 2 to 6 weeks of taking substantial doses of a high-quality product two or three times a day. St. John's wort also acts as a nervine; heals nerve damage and irritation topically and internally; and is broadly useful for treating poststroke and postaccident nervous system damage, including brain injuries and sciatica.

ANTIVIRAL AND TOPICAL HERB

As an antiviral in herpes outbreaks including shingles, St. John's wort limits the severity, relieves symptoms (pain, itching, numbness), and gradually repairs nerve damage. Use the oil as a light sunscreen; it may not be strong enough for fair-skinned folks. Topically, it promotes wound healing and helps relieve and prevent bedsores, rashes, and scars. As a flower essence (page 68), St. John's wort brings light-filled protection, useful for nightmares and times when you feel overly vulnerable to the influence and energies of others.

CAUTION WITH MEDICATIONS

St. John's wort is quite safe, but it increases the production of the CYP450 enzymes in the liver, including CYP3A4, which speeds clearance of many medications. Used in conjunction with serotonin-boosting medications, the herb may increase the risk of serotonin syndrome, a condition that causes uncomfortable and potentially dangerous symptoms including confusion, fever, and rapid heartbeat. In *rare* cases, fair-skinned individuals ingesting St. John's wort develop a phototoxic sun rash — a greater risk in grazing animals. Topical use does not pose drug interaction, sun rash, or other safety concerns. It may inhibit thyroid function.

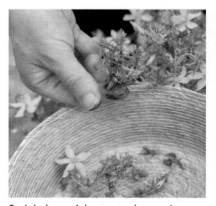

St. John's wort's lore not only associates it with the Christian saint but also with warding off hexes, witchcraft, evil spirits, and nightmares with light-filled protection.

Harvesting, Preparing, and Using St. John's Wort

Snip off the flower tops, focusing on flowers and buds (it's fine if a few leaves sneak in). Best fresh, almost useless dried. A deep red hue indicates its strength; it will turn brown and lose potency over time. Refresh your tincture every few years.

Parts Used: flowers, buds

Tincture: 2–5 ml, 3 times daily, solo or in formula
• Fresh 1:2 in 95 percent alcohol

Topical: oil (fresh maceration), salve, cream, liniment

Recipes: Lemon–St. John's Wort Pick-Me-Up, page 118; Calendula-Comfrey Cream, page 193; St. John's Wort Oil, page 215

SKULLCAP

Scutellaria lateriflora

Mint Family (Lamiaceae)

Body Systems: Mood, Nervous, Musculoskeletal, Digestion, Pain

   perennial, Zones 4–8

ALONG THE RIVER'S EDGE

Skullcap's persnickety in the garden — booming one year, gone the next. In the wild, you'll find various skullcap species, used interchangeably, growing along a riverbank or at the edges of lakes, often alongside wild mint and bugleweed. In the garden it prefers rich, consistently moist but well-drained soil, particularly in spring, and minimal competition. Make plenty of medicine in boom years so you have it during the bust.

SEDATIVE NERVINE

Skullcap "caps the skull" when you're anxious, wired, and tired. It brings sleep, calms nerves, relaxes muscles, and eases pain. Use it in a formula for headaches, sciatica, and back pain. What makes it special is its ability to turn down an overly reactive nervous system for people who get irritated and overwhelmed by incoming stimuli such as lights, sound, or touch. This makes it useful not only for insomnia and anxiety but also agitation, hyperactivity, and attention deficit disorder in children and adults alike. It works quickly, nourishing and supporting the nervous system.

MILD BITTER DIGESTIVE

Skullcap has a mild bitter flavor with minty undertones and can be employed as a bitter to promote relaxation and aid digestion. As a flower essence (page 68), skullcap relaxes and opens the flow of positive energy, particularly between the healer and recipient.

GET THE REAL DEAL

Skullcap is easily identified by its hooded lipped flowers, the "scute" (dishlike) projection on the top of the calyx, and its unidirectional flowers — yet it's *often* mismarked and adulterated in commerce. Get your seeds or seedlings from a reputable source, then double-check the identity when it blooms. True skullcap is quite safe except that it may cause oversedation or aggravate depression and melancholy in rare, sensitive people. Be cautions using it alongside sedative and pain medications — it may synergistically oversedate.

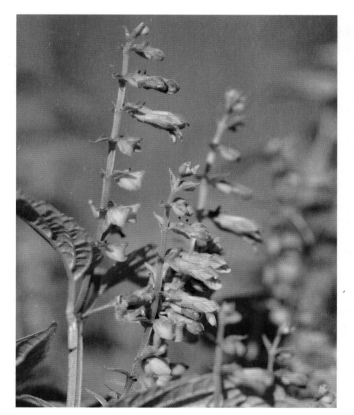

Harvesting, Preparing, and Using Skullcap

Harvest happy blooming plants to confirm identity before it goes by. In good years you may get multiple harvests. Fresh works best. Dry carefully in a single layer for tea. It loses potency quickly. Refresh your tincture every 1 to 3 years.

Parts Used: aerial/leaves, flowers

Tea: 1 teaspoon dried herb/cup, infusion, 1–3 cups daily

Tincture: 1–5 ml, 1–3 times daily, solo or in formula
• Fresh 1:2 in 95 percent alcohol

Glycerite: ½–1 teaspoon as needed

Recipes: Mellow Me Glycerite, page 125; Sleep Tea, page 130; Sleep Tinctures, page 131

Skullcap sold in stores tends to be low potency and adulterated with liver-toxic germander. Grow your own to ensure quality and identity.

SOLOMON'S SEAL

Polygonatum biflorum

Asparagus Family (Asparagaceae)

Body Systems: Musculoskeletal, Pain, Inflammation, Connective Tissue

   perennial, Zones 3–8

EASTERN WOODLAND NATIVE

Solomon's seal grows wild in rich, damp woodland habitats — the kind of special spot where you might find fiddleheads and linden, fancying the thought of woodland fairies all around. Easily cultivated, Solomon's seal is distinguished by a graceful, robust appearance that evokes a quiet old garden. Plant it in full- to partial-shade spots with soil that is naturally rich or has aged manure worked in. It proliferates quickly, providing plenty of medicine without a long wait. Other species likely offer similar properties. The herb becomes slimy and mucilaginous as you process it.

TOP-NOTCH FOR INJURIES

Much of what I've learned about Solomon's seal comes from herbalists Jim McDonald and Matthew Wood. The white knobby roots of Solomon's seal resemble the joints of a spinal column, a good doctrine of signatures of its use. It shines for its ability to heal joints and connective tissue injuries, including tendons and ligaments. Use it for sprains, strains, back pain, slipped disks, tendonitis, and other musculoskeletal injuries. The effects are often remarkable when taken internally or applied topically. It blends well with horsetail and mullein root (targeting joints, bones, and connective tissue), St. John's wort (add nerve support), boswellia (anti-inflammatory), topical comfrey or arnica (aches and bruises), and other pain herbs. Being prone to nasty spills, I keep a sprain formula on hand and use it topically and internally along with homeopathic arnica. After a bad sprain, I got lax once things felt *almost* normal and stopped using the herbs. A month later, I realized I hadn't improved since then, resumed the herbs, and was back in tip-top shape in a week.

TECHNICALLY EDIBLE

Foragers dig and cook Solomon's seal root like potatoes. I value it too much as medicine to waste it on food — maybe I'd reconsider if I had an overabundance and was hungry enough. It's worth combining with horsetail in gelatin-rich bone broth for joint and arthritis support. As a flower essence (page 68), Solomon's seal brings mercy, forgiveness, and humility for yourself and others.

LIKELY SAFE

Little safety data exists but considering its use as food and the fact that high doses aren't necessary for it to work, Solomon's seal appears safe.

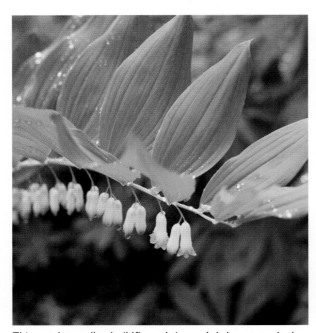

This stately woodland wildflower brings subtle beauty to shade gardens. The rhizomes spread quickly and help heal sprains, strains, and joint injuries.

Harvesting, Preparing, and Using Solomon's Seal

Dig up the roots in spring or fall. Leave or replant some of the roots in the stand. In the wild or where it's limited, harvest the back section of the root and leave the plant itself with a root section in the ground for future growth. Fresh preferred, but dried works.

Parts Used: rhizomes, roots

Tea or Broth: ½–1 teaspoon dried herb/cup, decoction, 1–3 cups daily

Tincture: 5–60 drops, 1–3 times daily, solo or in formula
• Fresh 1:2 in 95 percent alcohol (best) or dried 1:5 in 50–60 percent alcohol

Food: boiled and eaten like potatoes

Topical: oil, salve, cream, liniment, bath/soak, compress

Recipes: Aches and Pains, Strains and Sprains Tincture/Liniment, page 220

THUJA

Thuja occidentalis

Cedar Family (Cupressaceae)

Body Systems: Immune, Skin, Antimicrobial

   perennial, Zones 2–7

EVERGREEN NATIVE

Thuja grows wild across most of the northeastern United States and is often cultivated along yard borders for privacy. It grows wild in northern, swampy forests and prefers some moisture — I see a lot of brown arborvitae planted in poor soil in dry, sunny spots. On the West Coast, western red cedar (*T. plicata*) and other *Thuja* species can be used similarly. Local extension offices that sell trees often offer packs of young bare-root arborvitae trees for $1 per tree. These take many years to grow, but that's fine if you've just moved in, plan to stay for decades, or are in no big rush.

POTENT ANTIMICROBIAL

Thuja is one of our *most* reliable herbs to apply topically to icky skin conditions, particularly fungal, viral (warts), and some sexually transmitted infections. I've seen it clear ringworm in a few days, though with any fungal condition, you should continue applying herbs for at least a week or two after it clears, since fungus has a way of creeping back. Foot fungus, fungal rashes under sweaty breasts, jock itch, you name it. Use it externally as needed and internally in low doses or homeopathically for warts. But my *favorite* wart remedy is greater celandine (*Chelidonium majus*), a common semitoxic weed with bright orange juice. Apply the fresh leaf poultice at night — the warts usually disappear within 1 to 3 days!

IMMUNE STIMULANT

European herbalists have long used thuja in *low doses* internally as a deep immune tonic for everyday infections, chronic low immune function, and as an adjunct in cancer. A classic remedy for colds combines thuja with baptisia and echinacea. I add thuja to tincture formulas as a low-dose synergist for chronic fungal and yeast conditions. It reportedly addresses parasites. Dried thuja makes a nice, sweet-smelling incense, too.

LOW-DOSE INTERNALLY

Topically, thuja is pretty safe. Internally as a tincture; use it only short term or in low doses due to its thujone content and potential liver/kidney toxicity. That story about Cartier's team drinking arborvitae tea for vitamin C? While thuja *does* contain some vitamin C, historians now believe there was a mix-up and Native Americans more likely gave the them (much safer) white pine needle tea. Do not use thuja internally during pregnancy due to abortifacient properties. Many different plants are called "cedar," so check the Latin name.

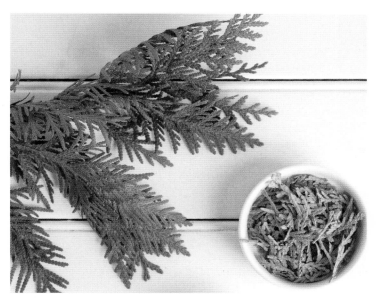

Also known as arborvitae, thuja was called the "tree of life" because it was credited as saving explorer Jacques Cartier's crew from scurvy during the Canadian winter.

Harvesting, Preparing, and Using Thuja

Harvest the needles any time of the year. Use fresh or dried.

Parts Used: needles

Tea: ½–1 teaspoon dried herb/cup, infusion, 1 cup daily short term

Tincture: 1–15 drops, 1–3 times daily, solo or in formula (keep dose on the low side when using long term)
• Fresh 1:2 in 95 percent alcohol (best) or dried 1:5 in 50–60 percent alcohol

Topical: oil (alcohol-intermediary), salve, cream, liniment, vinegar, soak/bath, compress, poultice

Recipe: Ick Stick Thuja Salve, page 199

THYME

Thymus vulgare

Mint Family (Lamiaceae)

Body Systems: Immune, Respiratory, Digestive, Gut, Skin, Antimicrobial

  perennial, Zones 5–9

MEDITERRANEAN MEDICINE

Yet another Mediterranean culinary herb packed with medicinal punch, thyme is a dense, low, herbaceous ground cover with small leaves and little spikes of pinkish white flowers. Popular in English, French, and Italian garden design, it prefers dry spots. If planted in a rich garden bed, thyme might thrive at first but eventually rot. Grow it alongside sage, lavender, horehound, and oregano. Use various thyme species interchangeably, including lemon thyme (*T. citriodorus*, variegated varieties add visual interest to the garden) and creeping (*T. serpyllum*). Let creeping thyme take over dry, sunny lawns — aromatherapy while you mow!

RESPIRATORY REMEDY

Medicinally, thyme offers properties similar to those of oregano and bee balm — yet another aromatic, antimicrobial mint-family herb. Thyme has the strongest affinity for the respiratory system, particularly the lungs. Its dry, moving, warming properties work well for damp, stagnant congestion. Thyme moves out phlegm, disinfects the lungs, and opens the airways. Combine it with ginger, lemon, and honey in tea, or other lung herbs for coughs, colds, bronchitis, asthma, and pneumonia (alongside conventional care, as needed).

DISINFECTANT AND ANTISEPTIC

You might recognize the flavor of thyme as one of the prominent ingredients in Listerine (thymol). Thyme's powerful antifungal and antibacterial disinfecting properties are useful in a wide variety of different formats, ranging from a mouthwash, steam, foot spray, or wound compress to a counter cleaner. As a flower essence (page 68), thyme helps you live in the now, especially when there doesn't seem to be enough time.

SAFE FOR MOST PEOPLE

Generally very safe. Therapeutic doses are not recommended in pregnancy. Since thyme is warm and dry, use caution with hot, dry conditions, though it might be fine balanced with moist, cooling herbs like marshmallow and mullein leaf.

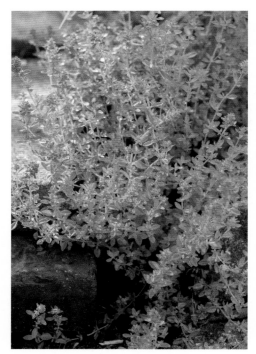

This aromatic creeping ground cover does nicely in dry spaces, cascading from stone walls or tucked along walkways.

Harvesting, Preparing, and Using Thyme

Thyme is like a minihedge — shear it to harvest and promote happy new growth. Fresh tends to be stronger, but dried works well, too.

Parts Used: aerial/leaves

Tea: ½–1 teaspoon dried herb/cup, infusion, 1–3 cups daily

Tincture: 10 drops to 5 ml, 1–3 times daily, solo or in formula
• Fresh 1:2 in 95 percent alcohol (best) or dried 1:5 in 50–60 percent alcohol (optional 10 percent glycerine)

Glycerite, Syrup, Honey, Oxymel, Vinegar: 1 teaspoon as needed

Capsules/Powder: 500–2,000 mg crude herb daily

Food: Mediterranean culinary herb fresh and dried in savory dishes, especially with lemon

Topical: oil (alcohol-intermediary), salve, liniment, vinegar, bath/soak, compress

Recipes: Bee Balm-Mint Tea, page 171; Soothing Lung Tea, page 176; Allergy Tincture Blend, page 182

VALERIAN

Valeriana officinalis

Honeysuckle Family
(Caprifoliaceae)

Body Systems: Nervous,
Mood, Musculoskeletal, Pain,
Cardiovascular

   perennial,
Zones 4–7

SWEET FLOWER, STINKY ROOT

Also called garden heliotrope, valerian's a lovely tall flower in the garden, easily reaching 4 to 6 feet tall. The pinkish white flowers catch your eye, wafting a honeysuckle-like aroma throughout the garden. The robust divided leaves and thick stems resemble lovage. Valerian's mass of small white roots reek of skunk, perfume-y dirt, and stinky feet, which gets worse as they dry, sit out, or are exposed to heat. This plant self-seeds rampantly and tolerates many soil types but really takes over in moist, manure-rich soil. More than once, organic farmers have called me over to dig up ill-behaved plants. When I filled my trunk, they said, "That's *all* your taking?" In my dry, sandy gardens, it's far better behaved. Be sure your region permits planting valerian.

HERBAL VALIUM

In spite of the urban myth, the sedative drug Valium is *not* made from valerian; however, the herb's effects are somewhat similar to the drug's. It is nonaddictive and much safer. Best known for insomnia, valerian sedates, brings sleep, eases anxiety, relaxes muscles, and relieves pain related to muscle tension. Studies support its ability to improve sleep latency, which is how quickly you fall asleep. It can improve quality of sleep as well. However, it does not agree with everyone — some people find that it agitates like coffee (never a happy discovery when you're already sleep-deprived) while others feel groggy the next day. Sleep herbs like passionflower, skullcap, and California poppy tend to work more reliably for a broader audience. Studies have shown that when taken solo and in blends, passionflower is more effective for insomnia relief than other sleep herbs such as valerian. The "valerian type" tends to be cold, anxious, and thin-framed, with muscular tension. This describes me well, and valerian was one of the first herbs I ever used (successfully, I might add).

PAIN RELIEF AND PEACE

Valerian promotes muscle relaxation, which makes it useful for muscle pain including tension headaches and back pain (it will probably make you sleepy). Valerian mildly reduces hypertension by relaxing and dilating the blood vessel lining. As a flower essence (page 68), valerian brings deep peace regardless of whether or not someone is a "valerian type" or on medications.

A FEW WORDS OF CAUTION

Remember, this is a sedative herb. Don't drive or operate heavy machinery after taking it. Many medications (antianxiety, sleep, antidepressant, pain) may synergistically increase sedation alongside herbal sedatives including valerian. Slowly introduce the herb, gradually increasing the dose to make sure it agrees with you and doesn't oversedate. Not everyone feels good with valerian.

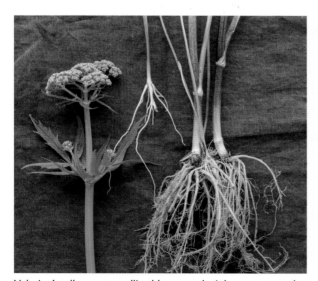

Valerian's tall, sweet-smelling blooms and stinky roots may take over meadows, pastures, and gardens with rich, damp soil.

Harvesting, Preparing, and Using Valerian

Pull up the roots in spring or fall. Usually you can simply grab the whole plant at the base and pull. Spray off dirt, then scrub well with a bristle brush (watch for earthworms). Bigger, older plants have bigger roots. Two-year-old and older plants are preferred, but you can use babies as you weed them out. Best fresh. You can make tea, but it tastes funky and is even more apt to disagree with sensitive people than the tincture.

Parts Used: roots

Tincture: 1–5 ml, before bedtime or in formula
• Fresh 1:2 in 95 percent alcohol

Glycerite: ¼–1 teaspoon as needed

Recipes: Sleep Tinctures, page 131

VIOLET

Viola spp.

Violet Family (Violaceae)

Body Systems: Lymph, Detoxification, Gut, Nutritive, Respiratory, Colon

    perennial, Zones 3–8

TINY MEDICINE

These small shy, sweet flowers dot the spring landscape. Popular medicinal species include sweet violet (*V. odorata*), common blue violet (*V. sororia,* including an escaped white cultivar with blue streaks), and multicolored heartease pansy (*V. tricolor*), but many others are likely useful, particularly those with white or blue flowers and tender heart-shaped leaves. They're perfect for planting in shady corners or edging garden beds and sunny lawns. With more than 500 species worldwide, a few different types of violets are likely to turn up near you. Some wild species may be at risk of becoming endangered.

MOISTENING NUTRITION

Most of our nutritives greens tend to be diuretic and drying in nature. Violet leaves and flowers not only pack in the nutrition (calcium, magnesium, potassium, carotenoids, vitamin C), but also have mucilaginous, demulcent, moistening properties. This gives tea a velvety mouthfeel and favors people who are already dry by nature. Add the leaves and flowers to respiratory and gut formulas for its soothing, healing, moistening properties. Plus, violets taste nice. Happy green, lightly sweet, with a hint of wintergreen — and those adorable flowers really perk up a recipe! Foragers note that violet leaves are among the few wild greens that taste good throughout the growing season, making them perfect not only for tea but also as a cooked or salad green and in smoothies and pesto.

LYMPH AND COLON SUPPORT

Violets gently and effectively support lymph flow, draining edema, improving immune function, and clearing toxins and infection "battle debris." Long reputed as useful for cancer treatment support, violet also helps break up benign fatty cysts when taken internally and applied topically. Due to its mucilaginous property, it helps keep waste moving through the colon and may be mildly laxative if taken in large doses. As a flower essence (page 68), violet fosters confidence in groups for shy people who appear aloof.

FOODLIKE

Violet leaves and flowers are extremely safe in therapeutic doses for people as well as animals of all ages. Large doses can be mildly laxative. Leaves contain a *little* salicylates, which *might* pose a problem for people with aspirin allergies. Herbalist David Winston avoids yellow violets, because of their acridity.

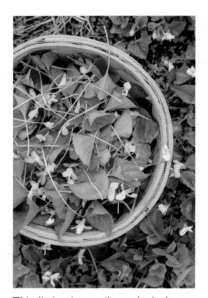

This diminutive, easily overlooked wildflower makes wonderful teas and remedies — nutritious, mucilaginous, gently detoxifying, and tasty.

Harvesting, Preparing, and Using Violet

Harvest leaves and flowers at any time, primarily spring. Use fresh or dried.

Parts Used: leaves, flowers

Tea: 1 teaspoon or more dried herb/cup, infusion, 1–3 cups daily

Tincture: 2–5 ml, 1–3 times daily, solo or in formula
• Fresh 1:2 in 95 percent alcohol (best) or dried 1:5 in 50–60 percent alcohol

Glycerite, Syrup, Vinegar, Oxymel: 1 teaspoon as desired

Powder: ½–1 teaspoon daily

Food: Leaves in salad, juiced, pesto, cooked, smoothies. Flowers as garnish, candied, to decorate tea, infused water, seltzer. Blue flowers (tedious to harvest) make a *gorgeous* purple syrup, popular for cocktails and tea parties

Topical: oil (for lymph massage, fatty cysts)

Recipes: Nutri-Tea, page 79; Multimineral Vinegar, page 86; Dandelion-Violet Weed Pesto, page 88; Infused Seltzer, Soda, and Water, page 97; Nettle-Peppermint-Marshmallow Tea, page 183

WILD CHERRY

Prunus serotina

Rose Family (Rosaceae)

Body Systems: Respiratory, Immune, Nervous, Mood

   perennial, Zones 3–9

TREE MEDICINE

Wild black cherry grows wild across most of the United States. Chokecherry *(P. virginiana)*, a serviceable substitute, grows everywhere. Both wild black and chokecherry thrive in recently disturbed or logged areas, often on the edge of open and forested spaces. White lenticels speckle the young shiny brown bark. Both species smell like amaretto when scratched and are prone to pests and diseases, including black knot fungus and tent caterpillars. Drooping white flower raceme clusters give way to red-black fruit. Wild black cherry eventually becomes a tall tree whereas chokecherry remains short and shrubby. You can easily wildcraft this plant, but if you want to introduce it to the landscape, go for black cherry, pruning it regularly to keep the bark within reach.

COUGH REMEDY

Artificially cherry flavored cough drops and syrup are likely a remnant of wild cherry bark's history as a cough suppressant, lung-soothing remedy. It calms, eases spasms and irritation, and opens up the airways. Turn to cherry bark for dry, irritated, spastic unproductive coughs. (For mucus gunk in need of expulsion, use horehound instead.) Combine cherry bark with honey to increase its the cough-soothing properties. Consider cherry bark for dry asthma and lungs tight from dry winter air, wood smoke, or wildfires — it combines well with mullein leaf, which soothes and moistens. Bonus: cherry bark tastes delicious, like amaretto and maraschino cherries.

CALM, FOOD, CREATIVITY

The bark has a mild calming effect on the nervous system, especially alongside passionflower, helpful when anxiety, trauma, and stress trigger or are triggered by respiratory distress. The fruits are edible. Wild cherry tastes better, but chokecherry is vastly easier to reach and appears more prominently in Native American food history, including pemmican meat-fat-fruit "energy bars." Woodworkers prize lumber from wild cherry. As a flower essence (page 68), wild cherry aids creative expression, new ideas, and thinking outside the box. Chokecherry helps to illuminate your understanding of yourself and others, improving clarity.

CYANIDE?

As with many rose-family fruit trees, the bark, leaves, and pits contain varying amounts of prunacin, or prussic acid, which breaks down into weak cyanide as it wilts. This substance can be lethal to browsing animals but poses less risk to humans using low doses of cherry bark for medicine. Once dried (and possibly if perfectly fresh), the cyanide content in the bark and twigs really isn't a concern. Other cherries, including pin cherry, do not share the medicinal properties.

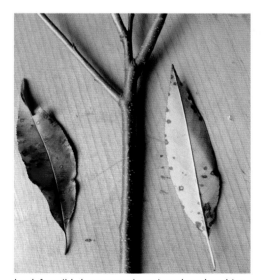

Look for wild cherry trees in spring when the white clusters of flowers bloom, or scan treetops for tent caterpillars. Harvest in late summer or fall.

Harvesting, Preparing, and Using Wild Cherry

If given the choice, go for black cherry. Prune branches up to 1 inch in diameter, then shave the bark and chop up twigs per page 25. With larger branches, remove the outer bark, using only the green inner bark. Always dry first. Glycerine or honey helps stabilize the tannins to prevent tinctures from getting gloppy over time. Excessive heat will make cherry bark less effective.

Parts Used: bark, twigs

Tea: 1 teaspoon dried bark/cup, infusion, 1–3 cups daily (use not-quite-boiling water)

Tincture: 1–3 ml, 1–3 times daily, solo or in formula
• Dried 1:5 in 50–60 percent alcohol with 10 percent glycerine

Raw Honey, Syrup, Glycerite, Cordial: 1 teaspoon as needed (dried bark, cold process)

Recipes: Soothing Lung Tea, page 176; Raw Wild Cherry Honey, page 177

YARROW

Achillea millefolium

Daisy Family (Asteraceae)

Body Systems: Skin, Immune, Digestion, Gut, Antimicrobial, Cardiovascular

   perennial, Zones 3–9

STEALTHY WILDFLOWER

For budding herbalists studying wild plants, yarrow ranks in the top 10 easy-to-identify, incredibly useful plants to know. The flattopped clusters of white flowers catch your eye — look closely and you'll see each cluster has five petal-like structures each with two notches, and a cluster of *tiny* yellowish white true flowers in the center. Notice the ferny, soft, finely divided "million leafed" leaves. Glance around, and you'll realize those leaves are *everywhere* interspersed with grass and other plants. Yarrow's widespread in fields, meadows, roadsides, edges between forest and field, and sunny garden beds that don't get watered.

Favor the white yarrow medicinally even though other colors exist in cultivation.

WOUNDWORT AND MORE

Yarrow offers complex, multifaceted medicine. It improves structural integrity of mucosal lining, blood vessel lining, and connective tissues while increasing function and "juice flow." Taken hot, it's moving; cold, more toning. Pack wounds with the fresh mashed leaves to stop bleeding, reduce the risk of infection (antimicrobial), and quickly heal the injury (vulnerary) with minimal scarring. Use the liniment on cuts and scrapes for infection and healing, diluted tincture or glycerite as a mouthwash, in low-alcohol formats for hemorrhoids, and as a sitz bath to tone (astringent), disinfect, and heal lady bits. Even though it improves clotting and stanches bleeding, it also thins the blood, promotes healthy circulation, and stimulates other juices in the body including stomach acid and digestive enzymes (an aromatic, carminative, warming bitter). Drunk hot, it acts as a diaphoretic to break a sweat and a fever and is often combined with tastier diaphoretics elderflower, peppermint, and ginger. Also consider it for gut healing and dysbiosis.

BUG AND NEGATIVITY PROTECTION

A low-alcohol yarrow tincture rivals and may surpass essential oils as a tick and mosquito repellent, bonus points for being relatively odorless and safe. The long, straight stems from yarrow flowers are cut into sticks and used for I Ching divination. As a flower essence (page 68), yarrow protects so that a person can heal. White yarrow offers all-purpose protection against pollution, allergens, other people's energy. Think pink for the heart, specifically not absorbing others' emotions. Yellow, to protect from others' anger and frustration.

DAISY-FAMILY FLOWER

Yarrow is very safe, but as a member of the daisy family it can cause allergic reactions with respiratory or topical symptoms in some people. Wear a mask if processing lots of dried flowers.

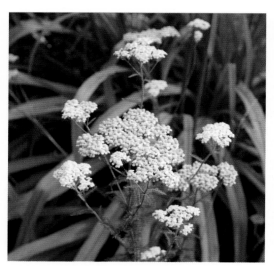

Legend tells us that the Greek soldier Achilles used yarrow as a battlefield woundwort. The finely divided, feathery "million leafed" leaves are easy to identify.

Harvesting, Preparing, and Using Yarrow

Pinch off individual leaves from the ground anytime. Harvest aerial parts in flower. Use fresh or dried. Feel free to try nonalcohol formats, too.

Parts Used: aerial leaves, flower

Tea: 1 teaspoon dried herb/cup, infusion, 1-3 cups daily

Tincture: 2-5 ml, 1-3 times daily, solo or in formula
• Fresh 1:2 in 95 percent alcohol (best) or dried 1:5 in 40–50 percent alcohol

Topical: poultice (preferably fresh), oil, salve, cream, liniment or vinegar, spray, bath/soak, compress, sitz bath

Recipes: First Aid Simple: Yarrow Poultice, page 199; First Aid Simple: Yarrow Liniment, page 199; Herbal Insect Repellent, page 204; Plantain-Yarrow Bite Rub, page 205

YELLOW DOCK

Rumex crispus

Buckwheat Family (Polygonaceae)

Body Systems: Colon, Detoxification, Liver, Skin, Nutritive, Digestion, Gut, Antimicrobial

   perennial, Zones 4–8

ROADSIDE WEED

Yellow dock's rust-colored seed heads dot abandoned waste areas, fields, and roadsides. The long, wavy-curly leaves resemble horseradish — hence its name "curly dock." This weed won't win any horticultural awards, but let it grow on the unkempt edges of the yard or wildcraft it. The wider-leafed, burdock-y broad dock (*R. obtusifolius*) is often misidentified as yellow dock but can be used similarly.

LIVER-COLON BITTER

Like fellow weeds dandelion and burdock, yellow dock also has bitter, liver-moving, detoxification-enhancing properties that improve digestion and help clear chronic skin issues like acne. But it's got a few more tricks up its sleeve. All bitters indirectly stimulate elimination through the colon by enhancing peristalsis (the wave-like muscle motion that moves food through). Yellow dock also contains a low dose of stimulant laxative anthraquinone glycosides alongside a modest amount of tannins that tighten and tone the gut mucosa and stanch diarrhea. Combined, these effects tonify and improve elimination, which is why you'll see it recommended for *both* diarrhea and constipation. The antimicrobial tannins also curb gut dysbiosis.

IRON FORTIFICATION

Another benefit of yellow dock root is its ability to increase iron levels and fight anemia. It not only contains a modest amount of the mineral but also encourages the liver to release iron from storage. This property is a boon for people who don't respond to iron supplementation alone, and combining it with iron-rich blackstrap molasses synergizes its effects. The leaf poultice helps stop nettle sting (though not quite as well as jewelweed, plantain, or comfrey).

THE RIGHT DOSE

Yellow dock's colon-regulating properties only go so far. Taking megadoses may cause explosive diarrhea followed by massive constipation. Like other plants in the buckwheat family (rhubarb, spinach, chard), yellow dock contains oxalic acid, which may be problematic in large doses for people with a tendency to develop kidney stones.

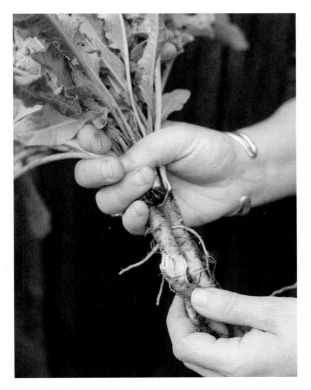

Harvesting, Preparing, and Using Yellow Dock

Dig up the taproots in spring or fall. Poor soil produces stronger roots. Use fresh or dried.

Parts Used: roots

Tea: 1 teaspoon dried root/cup, decoction, 1-3 cups daily

Tincture: 1-3 ml, 1-3 times daily, solo or in formula
• Fresh 1:2 in 95 percent alcohol, dried 1:5 in 50-60 percent alcohol, or double-extraction. Add 10% glycerine to stabilize tannins.

Syrup, Vinegar, Oxymel, Glycerite: 1 heaping teaspoon as needed, preferably with high-iron molasses

Capsules/Powder: 500–2,000 mg crude herb daily

Recipes: Multimineral Vinegar, page 86; Mineral-Rich "Coffee" Syrup, page 87; Bitter Brew Coffee Substitute, page 158

The best yellow dock grows in rocky, compact, poor soil. The yellower the root, the stronger the herb is.

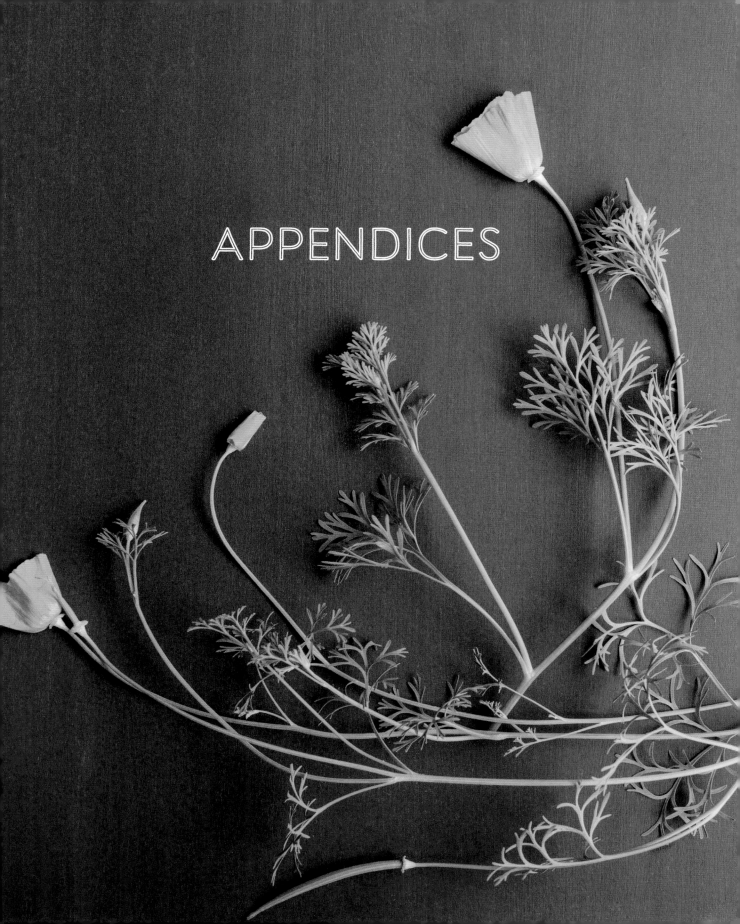

APPENDICES

COMMONLY USED HERBS BY CONDITION

Some herbs are especially known for the capacity to address certain conditions or promote wellness in certain areas.
The herbs here are listed in order of potency and preference for each condition.

Nutritious
Nettle
Oatstraw
Calendula
Violet
Rose Hips
Dandelion
Red Clover
Horsetail
Raspberry
Chicory
Burdock

Flavorful
Korean Mint
Anise Hyssop
Lemongrass
Lemon Verbena
Fennel
Mint
Stevia
Holy Basil
Roses
Rosemary
Lemon Balm
Bee Balm
Chamomile
Lavender

Base Flavor
Nettle
Oatstraw
Marshmallow
Lady's Mantle
Raspberry
Lemon Balm

Cholesterol
Artichoke
Garlic
Holy Basil
Lemon Balm
Hawthorn

Color/Flowers
Roses
Calendula
Bee Balm

Korean Mint
Purple Basil
Violets
Marshmallow
Anise Hyssop
Bronze Fennel

Stress & Energy
Holy Basil
Gotu Kola
Ashwagandha
Milky Oat Seed
Roses
Peppermint
Lemon Balm
Bacopa

Brain Boosters
Gotu Kola
Bacopa
Rosemary
Lemon Balm
Mint
Sage
Holy Basil
Ashwagandha

Antidepressant
St. John's Wort
Mimosa
Roses
Holy Basil
Lemon Balm
Mint
Motherwort
Ashwagandha
Betony
Lemon Verbena
Lemongrass
Peppermint

Anxiety/Relaxation
Motherwort
Holy Basil
Skullcap
Lemon Balm
Ashwagandha
Milky Oat Seed

Blue Vervain
Betony
Passionflower
Linden
Lavender
Rose

Sleep
Valerian
Skullcap
California Poppy
Passionflower
Chamomile
Lemon Balm
Lavender
Ashwagandha
Linden
Blue Vervain
Betony

Digestive Bitter
Artichoke
Catnip
Chamomile
Lemon Balm
Dandelion
Burdock
Yellow Dock
Chicory
Goldenseal
Barberry
Oregon Grape
Elecampane
Rosemary
Yarrow

Digestive Carminative
Fennel
Korean Mint
Anise Hyssop
Mint
Chamomile
Dill
Elecampane
Lemon Balm
Catnip
Holy Basil

Rosemary
Lavender
Culinary Seeds

Soothing
Marshmallow
Plantain
Meadowsweet
Fennel
Violet

Gut Healing
Plantain
Calendula
Meadowsweet
Gotu Kola
Chamomile
Lemon Balm
Horsetail

Gut Antimicrobial
Berberines
Oregano
Bee Balm
Garlic
Elecampane
Yellow Dock
Holy Basil
Roses
Chamomile
Calendula
Thyme

**Gut Astringent/
Diarrhea**
Roses
Raspberry
Plantain
Yellow Dock
Lady's Mantle

Constipation
Yellow Dock
Artichoke
Dandelion
Burdock
Marshmallow
Violet

Liver Detoxification
Dandelion
Burdock
Artichoke
Yellow Dock
Chicory

**Lymph
Detoxification**
Violet
Red Clover
Calendula
Echinacea

**Kidney
Detoxification/
Diuretic**
Nettle
Dandelion
Horsetail
Parsley
Burdock
Chicory
Birch Leaves

**Immune Simulant/
Infection Support**
Elder
Echinacea
Bee Balm
Oregano
Garlic
Thyme
Elecampane
Rose Hips
Berberines

Immune Modulator
Ashwagandha
Mushrooms

Cancer Prevention
Dandelion
Ashwagandha
Holy Basil
Thuja
Mushrooms

Antimicrobial
Bee Balm
Oregano
Garlic
Thyme
Elecampane
Rosemary
Sage
Lavender
Berberines
Yarrow
Calendula
Chamomile
Korean Mint
Anise Hyssop
Roses

Clear Lungs
Mullein
Elecampane
Wild Cherry
Horehound
Peppermint
Thyme

Soothe Lungs
Mullein
Marshmallow
Plantain
Honey
Wild Cherry
Violet
Korean Mint
Anise Hyssop
Fennel

Cough
Wild Cherry
Horehound
Honey
California Poppy
Fennel
Korean Mint
Anise Hyssop
Peppermint
Thyme
Marshmallow
Plantain
Mullein

Sore Throat
Echinacea
Berberines
Honey
Bee Balm
Oregano
Thyme
Marshmallow
Garlic

**Antihistamine/
Allergies**
Nettle
Goldenrod
Horehound
Ashwagandha
Elderflower

Congestion
Horehound
Bee Balm
Oregano
Thyme
Goldenrod
Peppermint
Berberines

Skin Care
Lavender
Rose
Calendula
Plantain
Gotu Kola
Comfrey
Lemon Balm
St. John's Wort

Wounds/Scars
Honey
Yarrow
Gotu Kola
Calendula
St. John's Wort
Berberines
Horsetail
Lavender
Comfrey

Bleeding
Yarrow
Cayenne

**Hemorrhoids/
Varicose Veins**
Yarrow
Calendula

**Rashes/Itchy Skin/
Bug Bites/Poison
Ivy**
Calendula
St. John's Wort
Plantain
Lavender
Peppermint

Insect Repellent
Yarrow
Lavender
Catnip
Rosemary

**Topical
Antimicrobial/
Antifungal/
Infections**
Berberines
Thuja
Bee Balm
Oregano
Thyme
Lavender
Garlic
Calendula
Horsetail

Herpes
St. John's Wort
Lemon Balm

Topical Pain Relief
St. John's Wort
Cayenne
Peppermint
Comfrey
Elder Leaf
Birch
Meadowsweet
Cramp Bark
Solomon's Seal

**Muscle Pain/
Relaxers/
Antispasmodics**
Peppermint
Rosemary
Birch
Meadowsweet

Black Cohosh
Betony
Blue Vervain
Valerian
Fennel
Cramp Bark
Skullcap
California Poppy

**Joints/Tendons/
Ligaments/Sprains**
Solomon's Seal
Mullein Root
Horsetail
Comfrey (topical)

Nerve Pain
St. John's Wort
Skullcap
California Poppy

Gladden Heart
Hawthorn
Linden
Rose
Motherwort
Lemon Balm
Holy Basil
Passionflower

**Circulation/Blood
Vessels**
Garlic
Cayenne
Rosemary
Yarrow
Gotu Kola

Heart Tonic
Hawthorn
Linden
Garlic
Motherwort
Cayenne

Hypertension
Dandelion
Burdock
Chicory
Nettle
Parsley
Hawthorn
Linden

Passionflower
Motherwort
Valerian
Cramp Bark

Hyperglycemia
Artichoke
Holy Basil
Barberry
Bitters
Garlic
Nettle
Lemon Balm

**Female
Reproductive
Hormonal**
Black Cohosh
Red Clover
Sage
Motherwort
Blue Vervain

**General
Reproductive
Tonics/Toners**
Raspberry
Lady's Mantle
Roses
Nettle

**Male Reproductive
Tonics/Toners**
Ashwagandha
Nettle Root
Horsetail
Mullein Root

Thyroid
Ashwagandha
Lemon Balm
Motherwort
Bacopa

Strong Bones
Nettle
Oatstraw
Horsetail
Red Clover
Dandelion
Black Cohosh

COMMONLY USED FLOWER ESSENCES BY CONDITION

Deep Healing & Vital Force
Comfrey
Echinacea
Garlic

Pain Support & Relief
Blue Vervain
Comfrey
Dandelion
Lavender
Lemon Balm

Community & Social Connections
Artichoke
Cramp Bark
Korean Mint
Anise Hyssop
Mimosa
Red Clover
Sage
Yarrow

Spiritual Connection & Consciousness
California Poppy
Elecampane
Holy Basil
Lavender
Meadowsweet
Mimosa
Passionflower

Earth Connection
Lady's Mantle
Meadowsweet
Sage

Communication & Relationships
Bee Balm
Calendula
Fennel
Goldenrod
Barberry
Oregon Grape
Hawthorn
Horehound
Marshmallow
Mimosa
Motherwort
Mullein
Nettle
St. John's Wort
Skullcap
Violet
Chokecherry
Yarrow

Forgiveness
Marshmallow
Raspberry
Solomon's Seal

Sensuality & Sexuality
Holy Basil
Lady's Mantle

Healing from Trauma
Comfrey
Lady's Mantle
Rose

Flexibility & Adaptability
Birch

Joy, Spark, Renewal, Restore
Bacopa
Bee Balm (red/ *didyma*)
Cayenne
Elder
Lemon Balm
Linden
Rose
Rosemary

Antianxiety & Relaxation
Betony
Lavender
Lemon Balm
Linden
Skullcap
Valerian

Confidence, Protection, Courage
Garlic
Goldenrod
Horehound
Meadowsweet
St. John's Wort
Violet
Yarrow

Soothing Belly & Solar Plexus
Chamomile
Dill

Lift Depression & Darkness
Black Cohosh

Grounding & Centering
Betony

Tension Release
Blue Vervain
Dandelion
Linden

Cleansing & Renewal
Burdock
Elder
Garlic
Goldenseal
Linden
Spearmint

Life's Purpose
Gotu Kola
Milky Oat Seed
Blackberry

Live in the Present
Rose
Thyme

Heart Care & Self-Love
Hawthorn
Rose

Mental Clarity & Cognition
Dill
Fennel
Gotu Kola
Horehound
Peppermint
Rosemary
Sage
Chokecherry

Creativity
Passionflower
Wild Black Cherry

HERBS FOR SPECIFIC CLIMATES

Hot & Damp
Bacopa
Gotu Kola
Holy Basil
Passionflower

Hot & Dry
Ashwagandha
California Poppy
Horehound
Lavender
Mullein
Rosemary
Sage
Thyme

Damp
Bacopa
Bee Balm
Blue Vervain
Elder
Gotu Kola
Horsetail
Linden
Marshmallow
Meadowsweet
Mints
Nettle
Skullcap
Thuja

Shade
Black Cohosh
Goldenseal
Lady's Mantle
Lemon Balm
Parsley
Solomon's Seal
Violet
Wild Cherry

MEASUREMENTS AND METRIC CONVERSIONS

An "ounce" can refer to weight or volume, and for some items they will not be the same. Herbs can vary widely in how their weight and volume compare.

1 ounce volume = 30 ml

1 ounce weight = 28 grams

1 gram = 1,000 mg

1 liter = 1,000 ml = about 1 quart (32 ounces)

1 ml = ⅕ teaspoon = approximately 1 squirt = approximately 30 drops

3 teaspoons = 1 tablespoon

2 tablespoons = ⅛ cup

4 tablespoons = ¼ cup

1 cup = 8 ounces = 240 ml (about ¼ liter)

2 cups = 16 ounces = 1 pint = 480 ml (almost ½ liter)

4 cups = 32 ounces = 1 quart = 960 ml (almost 1 liter)

8 cups = 62 ounces = ½ gallon

16 cups = 124 ounces = 1 gallon

TINCTURE MEASUREMENTS AND CONVERSIONS

1:2 fresh extract
Standard Measurements: 1 ounce herb (weight) in 2 ounces of alcohol (volume)
Metric Measurements: 1 gram herb (weight) in 2 milliliters of alcohol
To fill an 8-ounce mason jar, use 2⅔ ounces herb covered in approximately 5⅓ ounces alcohol.
Each 1 ml of a finished 1:2 tincture contains 500 mg of herb

1:5 dry extract
Standard Measurements: 1 ounce herb (weight) in 5 ounces of alcohol (volume)
Metric Measurements: 1 gram herb (weight) in 5 milliliters of alcohol
To fill an 8-ounce mason jar, use 1⅓ ounces herb covered in approximately 6⅔ ounces alcohol.
Each 1 ml of a finished 1:5 tincture contains 200 mg of herb
For comparison, 1 crude herb capsule contains approximately 500 mg of herbs, so each squirt (milliliter) of tincture equals approximately one pill.

CHOOSE YOUR TINCTURE VESSEL

JAR SIZE	WEIGHT OF HERB	YIELD
4 oz.	1½ oz. fresh or ⅔ oz. dry	1–3 oz.
8 oz.	2⅔ oz. fresh or 1⅓ oz. dry	5–7 oz.
12 oz.	4 oz. fresh or 2 oz. dry	8–11 oz.
16 oz.	5⅓ oz. fresh or 2⅔ oz. dry	10–15 oz.
32 oz.	10⅔ oz. fresh or 5⅓ oz. dry	20–30 oz.

TINCTURES VERSUS BOOZE

TINCTURE DOSE (60% ABV, some fresh tinctures will have a tad more, dried, a tad less)	EQUIVALENT BEER OR HARD CIDER (5% ABV)	EQUIVALENT WINE (12% ABV)	HARD LIQUOR (40% ABV)
1 ml	12 ml (~½ oz.)	5 ml (1 tsp)	1.5 ml (~⅓ tsp)
1 tsp (5 ml)	60 ml (2 oz.)	25 ml (~1 oz.)	7.5 ml (¼ oz.)
1 oz. bottle (30 ml, 6 tsp)	360 ml (12 oz.)	150 ml (5 oz.)	45 ml (1½ oz.)

MAKING SENSE OF PROOF AND ALCOHOL PERCENTAGE

PROOF	% ALCOHOL	EXAMPLES	BEST FOR
190	95%	Ethanol (grain, grape, sugarcane)	Fresh plants, resins (preferred), diluting with water for other % alcohol
151	75%	Grain alcohol, vodka	Fresh plants, resins
100	50%	Vodka	Dried plants, acceptable for fresh plants
80	40%	Vodka, brandy	Topical liniments, acceptable for dried and fresh plants

DECOCTION TINCTURE CHEAT SHEET TO THE PROOFS

For the sake of simplicity, here's a cheat sheet to get 25 percent alcohol in your finished product. Note that you can use fresh plant material instead of dried, but you'll want to bump up your alcohol percentage a tad to compensate.

PROOF	% ALCOHOL IN SPIRIT	USE THIS MUCH WATER	USE THIS MUCH SPIRIT
151-proof vodka or grain alcohol	75% alcohol by volume	66.67% (⅔)	33.33% (⅓)
190-proof ethanol (made from grain, grapes, sugarcane, or corn)	95% alcohol by volume (treat it like 100%)	75%	25%
100-proof vodka	50% alcohol by volume	50%	50%
80-proof vodka or brandy	40% alcohol by volume	~35%	~65%

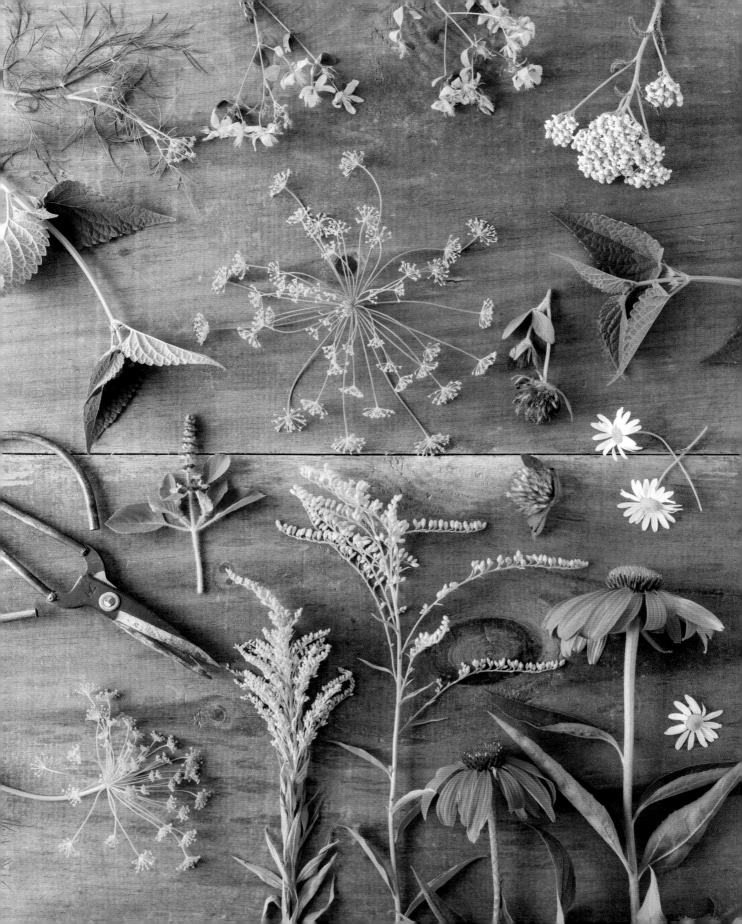

RESOURCES

General Information

American Herbalists Guild
americanherbalistsguild.com

American Botanical Council
herbalgram.org

Herb Society of America
herbsociety.org

Herbal Products

Gaia Herbs
gaiaherbs.com

Herb Pharm
herb-pharm.com

Mountain Rose Herbs
mountainroseherbs.com

Oregon's Wild Harvest
oregonswildharvest.com

Wise Woman Herbals
wisewomanherbals.com

Zack Woods Herb Farm
zackwoodsherbs.com

Seeds

Baker Creek Heirloom Seeds
rareseeds.com

Fedco Seeds
fedcoseeds.com

High Mowing Organic Seeds
highmowingseeds.com

Strictly Medicinal Seeds
strictlymedicinalseeds.com

Seedlings

Companion Plants
companionplants.com

Crimson Sage Nursery
crimson-sage.com

Growers Exchange
thegrowers-exchange.com

Mountain Gardens
mountaingardensherbs.com

Richters
richters.com

Grow Zones
To find your USDA Hardiness Zone, go to the USDA website and enter your zipcode: planthardiness.ars.usda.gov

FURTHER READING

For more resources and book recommendations, visit www.wintergreenbotanicals.com.

Flower Essences

The Essential Writings of Dr. Edward Bach: The Twelve Healers and Heal Thyself by Dr. Edward Bach

Flower Essence Repertory: A Comprehensive Guide to North American and English Flower Essences for Emotional and Spiritual Well-Being by Patricia Kaminski and Richard Katz

Flower Power: Flower Remedies for Healing Body and Soul through Herbalism, Homeopathy, Aromatherapy, and Flower Essences by Anne McIntyre

Lichenwood Herbals: lichenwood.com

Herb-Drug Reactions

American Herbal Products Association's Botanical Safety Handbook, 2nd edition, edited by Zoë Gardner and Michael McGuffin

Mosby's 2019 Nursing Drug Reference, 32nd edition, by Linda Skidmore-Roth, RN, MSN

Herbal Plant Propagation

Homegrown Herbs: A Complete Guide to Growing, Using, and Enjoying More Than 100 Herbs by Tammi Hartung

The Medicinal Herb Grower: A Guide for Cultivating Plants That Heal by Richo Cech

Medicinal Herbs

Alchemy of Herbs: Transform Everyday Ingredients into Foods and Remedies That Heal by Rosalee de la Forêt

Body into Balance: An Herbal Guide to Holistic Self-Care by Maria Noël Groves

Encyclopedia of Herbal Medicine by Andrew Chevalier

Herbal ABCs: The Foundation of Herbal Medicine by Sharol Tilgner

Herbal Medicine: From the Heart of the Earth by Sharon Tilgner

Medical Herbalism: The Science and Practice of Herbal Medicine by David Hoffmann

Rosemary Gladstar's Medicinal Herbs: A Beginner's Guide by Rosemary Gladstar

Plant Families

Botany in a Day: The Patterns Method of Plant Identification by Thomas J. Elpel

INDEX

Page numbers in *italic* indicate images; page numbers in **bold** indicate main entries.

G

garbling, 30, *30*
garden aromatics blend tea, 94
gardens. *See also specific gardens*
    in containers, 22–25
    harvesting and, 25–27
    planting, care, and maintenance of, 13–19
    preservation and, 27–31
    propagation and, 21
    started from plants or seeds, 19–21
garlic (*Allium sativum*), **268**
    for circulation, *234*, 235, 236, 237
    for immune and respiratory health, *166*, 167
    time until harvest, 20
genus names, **5**
geranium, for insect repellents and bite care, 204
Get the Blood Moving Garden
    overview of, 224, 233
    plants in, *234*, 235
    recipes, 236–237
Gladden the Heart Garden
    overview of, 224, 227
    plants in, *228*, 229
    recipes, 230–231
Gladstar, Rosemary, 3, 66, 236, 287
gluten, 290
glycerine, topical remedies and, 60
glycerine transfer, 51
glycerites, **50**, *50–51*
    aromatherapies and, 57
    for digestion, 140
    for gladdening the heart, 231
    for relaxation and restoration, 125
    stress relief and, 107
    syrups and, 52
    for uplifting, 119
goldenrod (*Solidago* spp.), **269**
    for immune and respiratory health, *180*, 181, 182
goldenseal (*Hydrastis canadensis*), **270–271**
    for immune and respiratory health, *180*, 181
Good Mood Tincture, 119
gotu kola (*Centella asiatica*), *18*, **272**
    for brain boost, *110*, 111, 112

for circulation, *234*, 235, 237
    for daily skin care, *190*, 191, 193
    for skin first aid, 198
    stress relief and, *104*, 105, 107
Gotu Kola-Calendula Cream, 193
grape root, Oregon (*Mahonia* spp.), 271
grindelia, for insect repellents and bite care, 205
growing conditions, herb selection and, 7
Gut-Healing Broth, 153
Gut-Healing Tummy Teas, 152

H

hand plows, 18
Happy Tea, 118
hardening off, 16
hardiness zones, **18**
harmonizer herbs, **69**
harvesting, **25–26**
hawthorn (*Crataegus* spp.), **273**
    for brain boost, 112
    for circulation, *234*, 235, 237
    for gladdening the heart, *228*, 229, 230, 231
    for heart issues, *224*
    time until harvest, 20
Hawthorn Tincture, 230
heading cuts, *25*, 26
heart and love
    Get the Blood Moving Garden, 232–237
    Gladden the Heart Garden, 226–231
    hawthorn and, 273
    herb types for, 224–225
    overview of, 223
    Woman's Garden, 238–243
Heart Tonic Tincture Blend, 237
heavy metals, infusions, teas and, 78
herb butters, 31
herb infusions, 35
Herbal Insect Repellent, 204
Herbal Nutri-Broth with Mushrooms, *81*
herb-pack compresses, 61
herbs, definitions of, 3
Holy basil blend tea, 94
holy basil (*Ocimum sanctum*), **274**
    for aches and pains, 220

beverages containing, 124
    for brain boost, 112
    flavor and, 94
    for gladdening the heart, 231
    hydrosols and, 58
    for relaxation and restoration, *122, 123*, 125
    stress relief and, *104*, 105, 107
    uplifting preparations and, *116*, 117, 118, 119
Holy basil tea, 107
Holy rose water, 107
honey, **48–49**
    for brain boost, 112
    extractions and, 48, *48–49*
    for immune system, 170
    oxymels and, 47
    raw wild cherry, 177
    for respiratory health, 177
    syrups and, 52
honey-alcohol syrups, 49
horehound (*Marrubium vulgare*), **275**
    for immune and respiratory health, *180*, 181, 182
    for respiratory health, *174*, 175, 177
Horehound Cough Syrup, 177
hormone balancers, **225**
horsetail (*Equisetum arvense*), **276**
    for aches and pains, *218*, 219, 220
    Nutritive Forager Garden and, *84*, 85
    for pain relief, 208
Hoxsey formula, 295
Hydrastis canadensis. See Goldenseal
hydrosols, **58**
    aromatherapies and, 57, *59*
    for daily skin care, 192
    topical remedies and, 60
Hypericum perforatum. See St. John's wort

I

ice cubes
    floral, 96, *96*
    freezing in, 31
    teas and, 36
iced tea, 36
Ick Stick Thuja Salve, 199

CULTIVATE BETTER HEALTH, NATURALLY,
with *More Books from Storey*

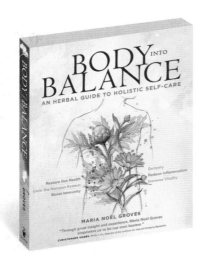

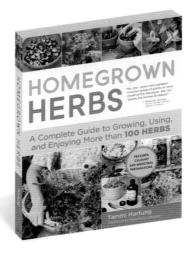

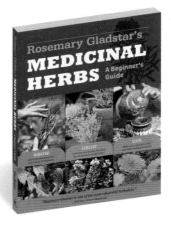

by Maria Noël Groves
Achieve your optimal health by learning to use herbs most effectively. Step-by-step photographs and in-depth instructions help you read the clues of your body's imbalances while also teaching you how to minimize your use of pharmaceuticals.

by Tammi Hartung
With complete information on growing and using more than 100 herbs for beauty, flavor, and health, this valuable primer offers gardeners of any level thorough guidance on seed selection, planting and maintenance, harvest, and more.

by Rosemary Gladstar
Stock your home medicine chest with safe, all-natural, low-cost herbal preparations, and enjoy better health! Profiles of 33 common and versatile healing plants show you exactly how to grow, harvest, prepare, and use them.

Join the conversation. Share your experience with this book, learn more about Storey Publishing's authors, and read original essays and book excerpts at storey.com. Look for our books wherever quality books are sold or call 800-441-5700.